Volume 1
SAGE Annual Reviews of Community Mental Health

PREVENTION IN MENTAL HEALTH

Research, Policy, and Practice

edited by
Richard H. Price
Richard F. Ketterer
Barbara C. Bader
John Monahan

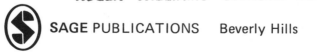

SAGE PUBLICATIONS   Beverly Hills   London

RA
790
P773

10-7-80

For information address:

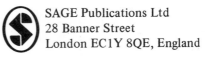

SAGE Publications, Inc.
275 South Beverly Drive
Beverly Hills, California 90212

SAGE Publications Ltd
28 Banner Street
London EC1Y 8QE, England

Printed in the United States of America

Library of Congress Cataloging in Publication Data
Main entry under title:

Prevention in mental health.

    (Sage annual reviews of community mental health ;
v. 1)
    Bibliography: p.
    1. Community mental health services.   2. Mental
illness—Prevention.   I. Price, Richard H.   II. Series.
[DNLM: 1. Community mental health services.
2. Community psychiatry. W1 SA125TC v. 1. / WM31.5
P9445]
RA790.P773   362.2'04256   80-14676
ISBN 0-8039-1468-7
ISBN 0-8039-1469-5 (pbk.)

FIRST PRINTING

CONTENTS

PREFACE

The community mental health movement in the United States first received national recognition and support with the inception of the Community Mental Health Centers Act of 1963. In the ensuing years, a number of major developments in the field of community mental health have occurred. There are now hundreds of federally funded community mental health centers in the United States in addition to thousands of community-based mental health facilities in clinics and hospitals throughout the country.

The growth of the community mental health movement also is reflected in the recent report to the President from the President's Commission on Mental Health (1978). This report clearly documents the degree to which the mental health movement has moved and will continue to move in the direction of community-based services for children, the elderly, recently released mental patients, minority groups, and other members of underserved populations in the community.

In addition, community mental health is exhibiting a rapidly growing concern and interest in what Peter Berger has called the "mediating structures" of society. These community structures include neighborhoods, families, kinship systems, churches, self-help groups, and voluntary associations, all of which play vital roles in the mental health of citizens and serve as structures that mediate between the individual and the larger bureaucratic health systems in the United States. New knowledge about these mediating structures and their role in the mental health of individuals will be vital to the continued growth and increased effectiveness of the community mental health field.

Community mental health has, with the rest of society, lived through a series of rapid economic and social changes over the past two decades.

New concerns with patient rights and the impact of the economy and new policy thrusts such as the concern with deinstitutionalization as well as the link between the health and the mental health fields are recent and vital preoccupations.

All of this means that the content, knowledge, and technology of community mental health is far more complex and is expanding much more rapidly than President Kennedy could have imagined when he first inaugurated the Mental Health Center Act in 1963. Thus, legal, economic, political, sociological, and organizational perspectives now are as important to the field of community mental health as is the more traditional concern with the psychological well-being of individuals. Indeed, we now realize that these larger social and economic forces and the psychological well-being of individuals are intertwined.

The *Sage Annual Review Series in Community Mental Health* is designed to respond to these new complexities and challenges by providing policy makers, researchers, and practitioners with timely reviews of the literature in the field of community mental health. Each volume will be devoted to a single major topic or problem and will provide an overview of theoretical developments, empirical findings, and new methods emerging in that problem area.

We have made the deliberate decision to solicit contributions from a broad range of researchers, policy makers, and practitioners who are developing innovative methods and approaches in the field. We believe that each of these very different perspectives must be represented if the complexities of the field are to be adequately portrayed. Thus, the *Sage Annual Review Series* is intended to expand the knowledge base in the field of community mental health and to bridge the gaps among theory, practice, and policy formulation. We expect the *Series* to provide a forum for controversy, a sourcebook of innovative practices, and a distillation of new research developments in the field. This first volume is devoted to new developments in the field of prevention in mental health. Future volumes will survey still other topics and issues that emerge as major developments in community mental health.

—Richard H. Price
John Monahan

1

Prevention in Community Mental Health
The State of the Art

Richard H. Price
University of Michigan
Barbara C. Bader
Richard F. Ketterer
*Center for Human Services Research,
Ann Arbor, Michigan*

If we mark the beginning of the community mental health movement in the United States with the enactment of the Community Mental Health Centers Act of 1963, then the field is only 17 years old. At that time, President John F. Kennedy called for a "bold new approach" to mental health. He argued that in the field of mental health,

> prevention is far more desirable for all concerned. It is far more economical and it is far more likely to be successful. Prevention will require both selected specific programs directed especially at known causes, and the strengthening of our fundamental community, social welfare, and vocational programs which can do much to eliminate or correct the harsh environmental conditions which often are associated with mental retardation and mental illness [Kennedy, 1963].

Now, only 17 years later, interest in the goal of prevention in the community mental health field is beginning to gain momentum. A substantial number of articles and volumes devoted to the topic of primary prevention in mental health have appeared in the last five years (for example, Albee & Joffe, 1977; Klein & Goldston, 1977; Bloom, 1979). Numerous conferences sponsored by the federal and state government, the National Council of Community Mental Health Centers, and other groups have raised the prospect of the development of viable prevention programs in the field of mental health. In addition, the President's Commission on Mental Health (*Task Panel Report on Prevention,* 1978) strongly emphasized prevention and made explicit recommendations for new initiatives and federal activity in this area. Partly as a consequence of this vigorous advocacy, the National Institute of Mental Health has developed a new Center for Prevention.

In short, it is fair to say that the goal of prevention is now more broadly accepted than ever in the field of community mental health. However, the routes to that goal are far from clearly mapped. In fact, the field of prevention is presently struggling with a number of critical issues; some are conceptual, others political, some are organizational, and still others are operational. Let us turn to several of the most important issues currently facing the field of prevention.

Conceptual Issues

Perhaps the most important issue facing the field of prevention is conceptual. Most readers are familiar with the traditional public health distinctions between tertiary, secondary, and primary prevention. Briefly, tertiary prevention programs are designed to reduce the severity and disability associated with a particular disorder. In fact, "tertiary prevention" is not prevention at all; it is more correctly termed rehabilitation. Secondary prevention, on the other hand, involves efforts to reduce the prevalence of a disorder by reducing its duration. Thus, secondary prevention programs are directed at persons who show early signs of disorder, and the goal is to shorten the duration of the disorder by early and prompt treatment. Finally, primary prevention efforts are those directed at reducing the incidence (rate of occurrence of new cases) in the community. Primary prevention efforts are directed at people who are essentially normal but believed to be "at risk" for the development of a particular disorder. In the past, these distinctions have served researchers and practitioners very well indeed, particularly when addressing specific diseases with known predisposing factors such as a lack of proteins or vitamins or the invasion of a particular bacillus.

Where specific diseases or other causal factors were easily identifiable, this model of prevention has been quite useful. However, in the field of mental health, precise definitions and specific disease entities with known etiologies are the exception rather than the rule. Partly in response to these conceptual difficulties, two important new developments have occurred in the field. As Bloom (1979) has noted, the first development has been a shift of interest from predisposing factors to precipitating factors as causal agents in the development of psychological disorders. That is, instead of searching for a specific underlying precondition associated with a particular pattern of maladaptive behavior, researchers have begun to focus their interests much more directly on stressful life events which appear to be capable of triggering patterns of maladaptive behavior in a proportion of the population that experiences those events. Thus, researchers have begun to shift their attention from "high risk populations" to "high risk situations" and events (Dohrenwend & Dohrenwend, 1974; Price, 1974; 1980). As Bloom puts it,

> four vulnerable people can face a stressful life event—perhaps a collapse of their marriage, or the loss of their job. One person may become severely depressed; the second may be involved in an automobile accident; the third may head down the road to alcoholism; the fourth may develop a psychotic thought disorder, or coronary artery disease [1979: 183].

Thus, according to this conceptualization, a variety of stress-producing precipitating events may be associated with the development of a number of disorders or negative outcomes, with stress being the common denominator.

A second important development in the field of mental health prevention has been a shift in interest from the prevention of specific disorders such as schizophrenia or endogenous depression to a substantial interest in health promotion. Bloom describes health promotion as "a variety of non-specific practices; for example, the provision of crisis intervention services or social supports during times of stress, may have a positive effect on health in general and may, in fact, prevent a variety of forms of disorder behavior" (Bloom, 1979: 181).

While the shift from an emphasis on predisposing conditions of psychological disorders to precipitating or "triggering" events is both conceptually promising and pragmatically sensible, the shift from the goal of prevention to one of health promotion raises still other issues. For example, one does not escape definitional ambiguity by pursuing health promotion, since "health" is no easier to define than is "disease." In fact, the definitions are interdependent. Second, it is often implied that health promotion or competence-building activities will automatically have preventive effects. This does not follow logically and, indeed, is an empirical question in each case. That is, whether or not a particular health promotion activity actually prevents any disorder from occurring must be demonstrated empirically, and claims of prevention should be greeted with the proper skepticism and empirical scrutiny.

Practice Methods

Because prevention is a relatively new field, knowledge about the nature and range of prevention services and methods has been limited. Despite the lack of an extensive body of practice knowledge, prevention professionals for years have been employing methods drawn from other fields, such as clinical and community psychology, community organization, and education, tailoring these methods to achieve prevention goals. For example, prevention practitioners have used behavioral techniques developed by clinical psychologists in order to achieve preventive goals in school systems. Similarly, prevention professionals have employed intervention strategies from community organization in order to modify social systems and make them more responsive to human needs.

Although some progress has been made in transferring methods from other fields, this process has not been systematic. What is needed is research and development efforts aimed at identifying practice-relevant knowledge, retrieving and organizing such knowledge, and disseminating it to prevention professionals.

Implementing such research requires that closer links be established between prevention researchers and practitioners. Efforts in this direction are currently evolving. For example, Ketterer and Bader (1977) collaborated with consultation and education staff in four community mental health centers (CMHCs) in carrying out research designed to improve C&E practice. These and similar efforts are needed before an adequate knowledge base for prevention can be developed.

Prevention Policy and Its Implementation

Although prevention services have been offered in community mental health centers since their inception, issues at the policy level have hampered effective implementation of these services. First, the broad goal of preventing mental disorders and promoting mental health has never been adequately specified in terms of policy and program guidelines. Second, until recently, there has been no federal agency or system which has provided leadership and support for prevention policy and programs, and federal funding for prevention programs has been limited.

Paralleling the realities at the federal level, state departments of mental health have been slow in developing systems to fund and support prevention programs. As late as 1975, only two state departments had created prevention units, while in 1979 a total of only seven had been established. As a result of the lack of support at both federal and state levels, local prevention programs have often floundered. For example, consultation and education programs, historically the preventive arm of community mental health centers, have remained underdeveloped (Ketterer and Bader, 1977). Funding for prevention programs has been uncertain and programming erratic. Moreover, in the absence of adequate state and federal guidelines, resources for preventive programs at the local level have often been eroded by demands for clinical services.

Despite these deficiencies, recent policy developments show promise. The President's Commission on Mental Health highlighted the need for national policy on prevention and health promotion. An Office on Prevention has been established within the National Institute of Mental Health to promote the development of research and policy on prevention. States have begun to develop plans for prevention programming in response to federal intentions to decentralize control of prevention resources to the states. Finally, prevention professionals have begun working with state and federal policymakers to develop better guidelines for prevention programs and to advocate for additional resources.

Research and Evaluation

A final issue in the field of prevention concerns the evaluation and assessment of prevention programs. Such efforts have important implications for both researchers and practitioners. From a research standpoint, evaluation provides an opportunity to study key variables associated with individual health and well-being as well as factors placing people at risk for mental and behavioral disorders. Practitioners, on the other hand, can use evaluation results as a means of improving preventive programs. From a policy standpoint, evaluation provides a critical means of accountability and provides important data for program planning and decision-making.

Despite the potential benefits of evaluation research, relatively little progress has been made in applying existing research methods to the evaluation of prevention programs. As Price (1978) and Heller, Price, and Sher have suggested in the present volume, considerably more effort will be required in the specification of program targets, program elements, and program goals before adequate evaluation evidence is available.

Overview of the Volume

As we noted earlier, one of the most important gaps to be closed in the field of primary prevention is between researchers on the one hand and practitioners on the other. Although the ultimate success of their prevention efforts requires interdependence and collaboration, all too often little or no dialogue exists between the two groups. In the present volume, the editors have made an explicit decision to include contributions from researchers who are substantive experts in particular fields of concern to prevention and contributions from practitioners at federal, state, and local levels who are much closer to the day-to-day realities of implementing primary prevention programs. This dialogue between practitioners and theorists is one that badly needs to be nurtured in the field of prevention and in still other fields in community mental health. *Sage Annual Reviews of Community Mental Health* have the fostering of this dialogue as an explicit goal.

Problem Focus for Prevention

The first four chapters in this volume are problem focused. Economic change, domestic violence, child abuse and neglect, and divorce are four of the most visible problems of our time. It is a truism that the potential for preventive intervention in a problem area depends upon how the problem is formulated. Each of the chapters described below offers insights for intervention based on thoughtful problem theoretical and empirical formulations.

Catalano and Dooley discuss current perspectives on primary prevention and raise two important issues. First, they discuss the distinction between activities which prevent the occurrence of risk factors and those which attempt to improve coping responses following exposure to stressors, calling these approaches "proactive primary prevention" and "reactive primary prevention," respectively. Second, they discuss issues related to the level of intervention, from micro-level prevention efforts to macro-level interventions. They note that little more than lip service is paid to interventions which reduce stressors in the larger environment, and they point to the recommendations of the President's Commission on Mental Health, which primarily supports microlevel reactive strategies.

Catalano and Dooley argue that macro-level proactive primary prevention strategies should be more carefully considered, although such efforts are often resisted or viewed with resignation. Sources of resistance to such strategies are identified, including clinically oriented disciplinary biases and lack of skills in the measurement and manipulation of macroeconomic variables. These biases result in lack of consideration of the contribution of ecological variables to behavioral disorders and lead to unthinking acceptance of economic and social conditions as "givens" with which individuals must cope.

A major part of Catalano and Dooley's discussion is devoted to a review of one ecological variable—economic change—and its relationship to behavior disorders. The authors provide evidence that "the status of an economy affects the psychological well-being of the population it supports," and they note that proactive primary prevention strategies can include efforts to manipulate the economy. Behavior disorders are viewed as an accountable cost, and behavioral cost accounting is seen as an important part of public management of economic change.

The potential for influencing corporate decision-making through behavioral cost accounting is also discussed. The increasing emphasis on "social audits" in the review of corporate performance is noted (with social audits viewed as opportunities for both proactive and reactive primary prevention efforts). It is suggested that such audits may force industries to consider behavioral costs in their decision-making.

Drawing on social psychological, sociological, and clinical evidence, Carlson and Davis examine the causes, myths, theories, and consequences of domestic violence. With this background, they focus on violence against the wife in the family unit, and suggest a number of short-term programmatic initiatives as well as long-term efforts and reforms that may reduce the incidence of domestic violence. The authors also remind us how deeply embedded domestic violence is in society, and that we must examine the cultural assumptions underlying our style of human service delivery if we are to offer effective preventive services.

In Chapter 4, Garbarino discusses the origins of child maltreatment, drawing on both scientific and cultural definitions of child abuse. He identifies a variety of factors that can place a family in jeopardy and lead to child maltreatment, and discusses five principal causes of abuse: psychopathology, temperamental incompatibility, family dynamics, interpersonal deficiencies, and culturally based attitudes and expectations about child rearing and development.

Garbarino offers four propositions on the prevention of child maltreatment, stating that conventional, individually oriented prevention programs are "doomed to failure." He suggests that to prevent child maltreatment we must concentrate on its necessary conditions, concentrate on social rather than psychological forces, engage in those aspects of our culture and socioeconomic system that undermine parental competence. Finally, Garbarino argues that we must prevent the social impoverishment of families and identifies a number of general strategies for reaching these goals. Garbarino calls for an end to the misuse of parental and institutional power and advocates an approach which empowers children as well as elements in the community that support the value and respect of children.

Divorce is unquestionably one of the most dramatically increasing stressful life events in the experience of contemporary Americans. This life transition and its consequences for the child and the parents has attracted considerable attention because of its obvious potential for preventive programming. In their chapter on the children of divorce, Felner, Farber, and Primavera examine the recent literature on stressful life events and suggest that it provides a useful framework for conceptualizing the impact of marital disruption on children. In examining the existing literature, they note that both characteristics of the child and a variety of situational mediators are critical in understanding the impact of divorce on the child. They suggest that divorce is not a unitary stressful event with which a child must cope. Instead, divorce sets in motion a number of changes in family patterns that may demand adaptation on the part of the child extending over a period of several years. They also caution that despite the substantial amount of interest in the impact of divorce on children, very little systematic data yet exist to aid in effective program development.

Settings for Prevention Efforts

The next four chapters are concerned with the settings and social environments that provide both the context and the opportunity for prevention programs. Schools, diversion programs, industrial settings, and social networks are each considered in detail.

In Chapter 6 Jason offers us a conceptual system for the development of behavioral preventive interventions in the schools and illustrates his framework with concrete examples of programs developed in a variety of school settings. Jason's model includes intervention strategies where the person is the primary target of intervention as well as in which some aspect of the social environment is the primary target. Although the framework is illustrated with behaviorally oriented approaches, other technologies could be placed in the framework just as easily. In addition to illustrating the wide range of prevention possibilities in school settings, Jason's framework helps to specify the multiple dimensions of preventive intervention programs more precisely.

Vandenbos and Miller describe the practice of diverting delinquent youths from the juvenile justice system as a strategy for further preventing more serious problems in this population. Because adolescents selected for diversion programs have generally exhibited delinquent behavior, these programs are classified as secondary prevention efforts. Despite a lack of unequivocal evidence regarding the causes of delinquency, a number of projects have been developed. The authors describe exemplary diversion projects, citing the results of evaluative data studies and offering prescriptive guidelines for developing and implementing diversion programs.

Foote and Erfurt focus on industrial settings and employee assistance programs as a promising context for preventive efforts. They note that community mental health has been relatively slow to recognize the potential of industry as a setting in which preventive efforts can be mounted and evaluated. Their focus is largely on early intervention efforts, and their rationale for retaining this emphasis is carefully reasoned. One of the interesting features of Foote and Erfurt's chapter is the way in which they have specified the potential linkages between industrial settings and human service organizations. They show how employee assistance programs, in particular, can serve as an important linking mechanism between the community mental health center on the one hand and the industrial setting on the other.

Few practitioners or researchers have directly addressed the question of patterns of client use of prevention programs. What are the factors that lead to underutilization of programs, and how can we understand them better? Gottlieb and Hall address the problem of prevention service underutilization and show how social network concepts can be brought to bear on the problem. Using a case example of one agency's attempt to design and deliver prevention programming to low income families, Gottlieb and Hall show how the social network of the potential recipients of prevention programs can (1) directly affect access to information about the program, (2) affect the type of information about the program received by members of a social network, or (3) even provide alternative preventive or supportive services. Community mental health centers will need a clearer understanding of the social context of the potential recipients if they are to assure that their program efforts will, in fact, actually be used by high-risk populations. Gottleib and Hall make an excellent beginning in formulating and understanding this critical problem.

Perspectives on Policy and Practice

The remaining chapters focus on the pragmatics of prevention. Large-scale efforts mounted in the name of prevention require large-scale mobilization of resources. Federal policy can create an initial monetary impetus, but critical resources also consist of organizational arrangements, manpower and skills, and technical research and evaluation expertise. Chapters 10-15 provide a perspective on recent policy developments at the federal level as well as examples of innovative practice at the state and local levels.

Federal policy on prevention will substantially shape and direct the content and mode of delivery of prevention programs at the local level. Thomas Plaut, Director of the Office of Prevention at the National Institute of Mental Health, is in a unique position to comment from the federal perspective and does so in Chapter 10. He recounts the development of the newly formed Office of Prevention and identifies several key policy issues, including the adequacy of the current knowledge base, appropriate targets for prevention activities, factors to consider in choosing prevention objectives, the currently diffuse boundaries of mental health prevention, and problems of program evaluation. Finally, Plaut articulates key principles involving the current federal mental health prevention program designed to move the federal effort foreward.

Swift reviews the increasing support for primary prevention programs throughout the health care system, traces the development of federal prevention policy, documents the commitment to prevention at the federal level and in community mental health centers, and projects emerging issues for prevention in the field. Federal prevention policy, as reflected in the Mental Health Systems Act and the establishment of the Office of Prevention within NIMH, is discussed in the context of the recommendations of the President's Commission on Mental Health. The current federal commitment to primary prevention in mental health cites the addition of primary prevention as the fourth mission of the Alcohol, Drug Abuse and Mental Health Administration. A review of CMHC staffing and budget commitments shows that NIMH has spent an estimated $128 million on CMHC primary prevention efforts since 1965. The current reduction in C&E (consultation and education) programs across the country is seen as a result of both a decrease in available federal dollars and an increase in the practice of labeling C&E services as clinical services to meet third-party reimbursement requirements.

Swift looks ahead to identify prevention issues for the 1980s in the community mental health field. She expects that they will include a reconceptualization of prevention, possible separation of prevention and treatment service delivery, decentralization of power from federal to state governments, prevention programs aimed at systems change, and a growing constituency for prevention and cost effectiveness. Evaluation and cost effectiveness are seen as survival issues for primary prevention in the eighties, and examples are given of projected savings between prevention and treatment programs.

Tableman describes the development of one of the first prevention units created within a state department of mental health. Since states are expected to play an increasingly important role in the development of prevention programs, policymakers and professionals interested in the development of statewide prevention units may find Chapter 12 especially valuable.

Tableman outlines the history, structure, and major goals of the state prevention unit in Michigan. Created in 1975 as the result of new legislation mandating prevention services, the prevention unit has evolved during the intervening years into an innovative, though relatively small, demonstration program. The chapter highlights key developmental issues, such as the need to gain internal and external support for prevention services as well as the need to specify the goals, target groups, and outcomes expected to result from specific demonstration projects. In regard to the latter, the chapter underscores the crucial, yet problematic, role of evaluation in the development of a viable prevention unit.

Too often it is assumed that once policy issues are clearly defined, local issues will take care of themselves. Nothing could be further from the truth. Speaking from the perspective of a center director, Saul Cooper discusses key political, definitional, organizational, and technical constraints in implementing prevention programs in community mental health centers. Cooper highlights the current lack of coordination that exists between prevention programs sponsored by various state and federal funding sources. Similarly, he discusses the inadequacy of funds for prevention services and political and technical barriers to evaluating the outcome of prevention programs. Given these constraints, Cooper suggests a number of pragmatic strategies for local program development and warns that future efforts in prevention must be approached with enthusiasm, but caution.

Ketterer, Bader, and Levy discuss strategies and skills for promoting mental health. Five types of mental health promotion strategies are described—strategies aimed at increasing competencies of normal and at-risk groups and at modifying social policies and social systems to make them more responsive to human needs: consultation to natural support systems, consultation to caregivers, organizational consultation, community network and coalition building, and mental health education. Necessary skills of mental health promotion specialists are then identified and discussed, including skills in consultation, education, community organization, and action research. Finally, implications for policy, research, and training in the field of mental health promotion are explored.

Regardless of the target of intervention, the technology deployed, or the context of the program, evaluators and researchers will be asked to evaluate the impact of preventive programs both to assure accountability and to develop new knowledge. Prevention-oriented programs in community mental health offer a variety of unique challenges to the evaluator and researcher, as Heller, Price and Sher note in Chapter 15. They examine the political impediments, unique conceptual issues, and methodological problems facing the evaluator of prevention programs. They then offer a set of guidelines for evaluation that focus on three separate conceptual areas: (1) the target of the intervention, (2) the program itself, and (3) the program goals and objectives. They observe: "It is our strong conviction that prevention proponents will lose the political battle for funding without good data capable of documenting the effectiveness and social utility of prevention programs."

We believe the present volume illustrates that, in the 17 years since the beginning of the community mental health movement, progress toward the goal of prevention has been substantial. Progress in the 1980s will require even more effective collaboration between researchers and practitioners and even more rigor in turning prevention goals into mental health realities.

References

Albee, G.W. & Joffe, J.M. (Eds.). *Primary Prevention of Psychopathology. Volume I. The Issues.* Hanover, NH: University Press of New England, 1977.

Bloom, B.L. Prevention of mental disorders: Recent advances in theory and practice. *Community Mental Health Journal,* 1979, *15,* 179-191.

Dohrenwend, B.S., & Dohrenwend, B.P. (Eds.). *Stressful Life Events: Their Nature and Effects.* New York: John Wiley, 1974.

Klein, D.C., & Goldston, S.E. (Eds.). *Primary Prevention: An Idea Whose Time Has Come.* Washington, DC: U.S. Government Printing Office, 1977.

Kennedy, J.F. *Message from the President of the United States Relative to Mental Illness and Mental Retardation.* 88th Congress, First Session, U.S. House of Representatives Document No. 58. Washington, DC: U.S. Government Printing Office, 1963.

Ketterer, R.F., & Bader, B.C. *Issues in the Development of Consultation and Education Services.* Final report submitted to the Michigan Department of Mental Health, December, 1977.

Price, R.H. Etiology, the social environment, and the prevention of psychological dysfunction. In P. Insel and R.H. Moos (Eds.), *Health and the Social Environment.* Lexington, MA: D.C. Heath, 1974.

Price, R.H. Evaluation research in primary prevention: Lifting ourselves by our bootstraps. Presented at the Primary Prevention Conference sponsored by the Community Mental Health Institute, National Council of Community Mental Health Centers, Denver, Colorado, June 11, 1978.

Price, R.H. The social ecology of treatment gain. In A.P. Goldstein & F.H. Kanfer (Eds.), *Maximizing Treatment Gains: Transfer Enhancement in Psychotherapy.* New York: Academic Press, 1979.

Price, R.H. Risky situations. In D. Magnusson (Ed.), *The Situation: An Interactional Perspective.* Hillsdale, NJ: Lawrence Erlbaum, 1980.

Task Panel Report on Prevention. Submitted to the President's Commission on Mental Health, 1978, Volume 4.

2

Economic Change in Primary Prevention

Ralph Catalano*
David Dooley

*Public Policy Research Organization
and Program in Social Ecology,
University of California, Irvine*

Discussions of primary prevention of behavioral disorder rarely pay more than lip service to interventions which reduce stressors from larger environments (for example, the urban community or regional economy). The origins of this orientation away from macro-level prevention may be both substantive (perceived feasibility or efficiency of such interventions) and paradigmatic (habits of psychological thinking which favor individual-level, reeducative change). After distinguishing several approaches to prevention, we will consider the case of one macroenvironment which has measurable consequences for behavioral disorder—the economy. After overviewing the evidence for the economy-disorder linkage, we will discuss a variety of possible interventions for primary prevention.

To no one's surprise, the President's Commission on Mental Health (1978) stated as a goal for the next decade that we should "undertake a concerted national effort to prevent mental disabilities" (I, 10). After recognizing the three traditional levels of prevention, the commission chose a noncommital definition of prevention which "embraces a broad range of activities which help individuals avoid becoming 'patients' " (I, 51). Such an all-encompassing approach to prevention may reflect the split between the Prevention Task Panel and the Research Task Panel (Herbert, 1979). The Prevention Task Panel favored action for primary prevention (eliminating causes of disorder by reducing risk factors), while the Research Task Panel urged caution and much more research before promis-

*Order of authors determined by toss of coin. This research was supported by National Institute of Mental Health Grant MH 28934-1 OA1.

ing "the country more than we are able to deliver" (President's Commission on Mental Health, 1978: IV, 1820).

The three traditional levels of prevention of Caplan (1964) are discussed in more detail elsewhere (Cowen, 1973; Heller & Monahan, 1977; Rappaport, 1977). Secondary prevention is invoked after the earliest detection of symptoms to prevent the disorder from becoming more serious or chronic (e.g., crisis intervention, Dohrenwend, 1978). Tertiary prevention involves the rehabilitation of chronically symptomatic individuals and the use of maintaining and correcting therapies to minimize the resulting disability. All three levels are portrayed in Figure 2.1.

The debate on the current practicality of primary prevention has left relatively unattended two other issues which bear on the specific types of primary prevention to be pursued. The first issue entails the distinction between preventing the occurrence of the risk factor and improving the coping response triggered by stressors. To borrow from public health terminology, this distinction is the one between eliminating or avoiding the noxious or causal agent (for example, eliminating breeding grounds of malaria-carrying mosquitos) and strengthening individuals' resistance to the agent (in this example, vaccinations for polio and small pox). The first strategy assumes that the causal agent itself is controllable or preventable, while the second strategy assumes that the agent, if unavoidable, is resistible.

For convenience we will call the first approach "proactive primary prevention" and the second "reactive primary prevention." Reactive primary prevention can occur before or after the stressor but is aimed at preparing the individual to react effectively to the stressor. For example, mental health education to cope with divorce could be required before the issuing of marriage licenses. Most commonly, however, such training is provided after separation or divorce. In contrast, proactive primary prevention attempts to avoid the stressor altogether. As illustrated in Figure 2.1, both these approaches occur before secondary and tertiary prevention. The President's Commission (1978), insofar as it favored primary prevention, seemed particularly in favor of reactive primary prevention where adults are concerned. For example, the Prevention Task Panel called for programs aimed at reducing the stressful consequences "associated with major later-life crises such as ... bereavement [and] ... marital disruption" (1978: IV, 1854).

The second issue raised by primary prevention involves the level of intervention, particularly in regard to proactive primary prevention. Adaptation demands, or stressors, may come from a variety of sources on a continuum ranging from the micro to the macro (see, for example, the hierarchy of levels of Bronfenbrenner, 1977). For simplicity, Figure 2.1

FIGURE 2.1 Typology of Preventive Interventions

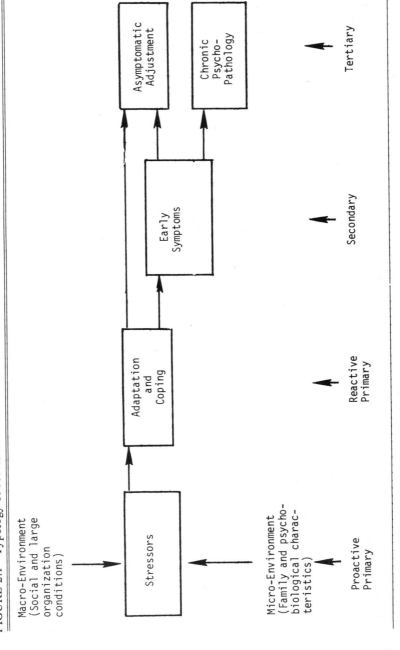

condenses this range of levels into two broad categories. At the micro level, proactive prevention might take the form of mental health education for expectant parents to prevent the occurrence of damaging parenting practices. At the macro level, proactive prevention might involve community-wide transportation planning to prevent excessive automobile lead exhausts and airport noise from occurring near school playgrounds.

Relatively micro-level sources or risk factors seem to appeal most to the commission members. For example, the Research Task Panel concluded that one of the most effective investments in prevention today is in "research on the brain and biological mechanisms that are relevant to mental disorders" (1978: I, 51). Greatest attention is to be devoted to child care including prenatal, parental, and foster and out-of-home care.

In contrast to the optimistic view of primary prevention at the biological and family levels, the attitude toward macro-level proactive primary prevention seems one of resignation. The Prevention Task Panel points to sources of societal stress "as factors capable of producing profound emotional distress in individuals" (IV, 1855). But the Task Panel "recognizes that the President's Commission on Mental Health has no magical power to eliminate" such sources (IV, 1855). Moreover, such conditions (as unemployment, discrimination, boring work, and the like) are possibly not "part of mental health's purview," and "such considerations may involve sufficiently controversial social values that it would be politically wise to avoid them" (IV, 1838). In sum, micro-level proactive and reactive primary preventive approaches are currently targeted for research and development, while macro-level proactive preventive approaches are, regrettably, beyond the province of mental health workers.

This chapter's thrust is that, contrary to the prevailing view of the commission, macro-level proactive primary prevention should be more carefully considered before being rejected. The sources of the resignation or resistance regarding macro-level prevention are probably many and varied. Some may stem from habits of thinking which are shaped by the mental health disciplines and their most favored paradigms. The psychological perspective habitually takes the individual as the unit of analysis and has little experience with or methodological equipment for aggregate-level analysis (Bronfenbrenner, 1977; Katona, 1979). Economic and social conditions are thus taken as givens with which individual patients must cope. Lacking skills in the measurement or manipulation of such macro variables, psychologically minded mental health workers naturally seek interventions which are within their competence. Hence, we have proactive preventive strategies which range from the psychobiological to the family level and reactive strategies, which capitalize on training in coping and the cultivation of social support (naturally occurring, quasi-therapeutic interventions). This posture is assumed without even the pretense of comparing empirically the relative contribution of stressors measured at different levels of analysis or the relative feasibility of manipulating variables at different levels. Presumably given even less consideration is the possibility that the interaction of variables from different analytic levels might account for a significant share of disorder.

As a practical matter, such disciplinary biases may be appropriate in terms of optimizing the use of current mental health talent. Nevertheless, it must be emphasized that such biases are unlikely to give a fair evaluation of the contribution of ecological variables to behavioral disorder. To leave such variables out of the equation because of unfamiliarity with appropriate methodologies or because of political risk may cause us to miss an important ingredient in the prevention of disorder. The questions of the President's Commission in regard to prevention should not be arbitrarily circumscribed by the wearing of unidisciplinary blinders. They are: "What factors contribute to the risk and what is the relative importance of each of these factors?" "Can we effectively reduce or eliminate the most significant of these risk factors?" (1978: I, 51).

In the remainder of this chapter we will review one ecological variable as a possible cause of disorder—economic change. We demonstrate that there is a literature addressing this linkage and discuss a variety of strategies for primary prevention. Space does not permit similar treatment for other ecological variables (such as prejudice, poverty, and environmental stressors), but this example points the way for the systematic inclusion of such variables in future analysis of primary prevention.

Economic Causation of Disorder

As alluded to above, the President's Commission has noted that most of the environmental factors implicated in the etiology of behavioral disorders are beyond the control of the mental health community. While this may be so, it does not follow that such phenomena cannot be societally regulated to reduce the incidence of disorder. Those trained in the behavioral sciences often believe that change in such environmental factors as noise, job demands, housing quality, and economic opportunities is random. There is, however, considerable precedent for modeling such change as a manifestation of shifts in the ecology of institutions which produces and distributes goods and services (Catalano, 1979a). This ecology is usually operationalized as the "economy" and its effect on the incidence of behavioral disorder has come under increasing scrutiny in recent years.

The economic change-behavioral disorder literature has been reviewed in detail elsewhere (Dooley & Catalano, 1980). This literature includes several classic case studies and ethnographic analyses of the effect of adverse economic conditions on individuals and families (Bakke, 1940; Cavan & Rauck, 1938; Jahoda, Lazarsfeld & Zeisel, 1971; Komarovsky, 1940). More recent empirical work has found that measures of economic stability are inversely related to institutionalizations for behavioral problems at the state (Brenner, 1969, 1973; Marshal & Funch, 1979), metropolitan area (Catalano & Dooley, in press; Barling & Handel, 1980) and catchment area (Sclar & Hoffman, Note 1) levels. While these time-series analyses have been criticized on several grounds (Dooley & Catalano, 1979; Eyer, 1977; Kasl, 1979), the relationship appears real, if little understood.

Attempts to explain the relationship between service utilization and economic instability have been separated into two groups (Catalano & Dooley, 1977). The first assumes that the utilization of inpatient services varies longitudinally with economic change because the latter provokes behavioral disorder. The second group assumes that the incidence of disorder remains fairly constant over time and that economic change influences inpatient case openings by changing either or both the tolerance for disorder or the availability of specialty or nonprofessionally based outpatient treatment. The provocation position has been supported by both aggregate- and individual-level findings. The aggregate research, conducted in Kansas City, reported that monthly (October 1971-January 1973) sample means of life events, depression, and psychological symptoms are longitudinally related to measures of economic change (Catalano & Dooley, 1977; Dooley & Catalano, 1979). While depression and symptoms were inversely related (most strongly among low-income persons) to directional measures of economic climate, the sample mean for stressful life events tended to vary more strongly with measures of change per se.

Several prospective analyses of individually experienced economic life events also support the provocation hypothesis (Cohn, 1978; Parnes & King, 1977; Theorell et al., 1975; Cobb & Kasl, Note 2). Perhaps the best of the individual-based analyses has been Cobb and Kasl's (Note 2) prospective monitoring of male workers in two closing industrial plants. Both physiological and psychological symptoms varied with the phases of anticipation of plant closing, unemployment, probationary employment, and stable employment. The complex findings suggest that the adverse effect of anticipated and actual unemployment is greatest among those with low social support who live in urban communities.

A recent evaluation of income maintenance programs in Denver and Seattle lends support to the provocation hypothesis. Thoits and Hannan

(1979) report that guaranteed annual incomes did not decrease self-report of symptoms in any population groups, but actually increased symptoms among married males and females and among unmarried black females. The authors attributed the effect to stressful life events associated with economic improvement.

The uncovering hypothesis, on the other hand, has been supported by the finding (Catalano & Dooley, in press) that while mean sample scores of untreated disorder, as measured by the Langner-22, vary with the economy, neither untreated disorder nor stressful life events is related to subsequent variation in aggregate inpatient case openings. Marshall and Funch (1979) report, moreover, that the availability of facilities explains a portion of the variation in the institutionalization data analyzed by Brenner (1973).

The literature summarized above suggests that while the economic climate may influence inpatient case openings by "uncovering" existing disorders, the incidence of untreated disorder and/or subclinical symptoms (depressed mood) may be increased by economic instability. The findings, however, do no converge on subgroup reactions, and there is considerable controversy over methods employed by both the aggregate-level (Kasl, 1979) and individual-level (Dooley & Catalano, 1980) analyses. Despite these problems, the sum of the findings indicates that the status of an economy affects the psychological well-being of the population it supports.

Public Management of Economic Change

In light of the above literature, efforts to manipulate the economy become germane to a discussion of proactive primary prevention. The public sector exercises considerable control over private entrepreneurial behavior. This control is justified by long-standing political theory which asserts that the government, assuming democratic processes, has the duty to protect the general health, welfare, and safety at the expense of individual liberty. Keynesian economic theory, moreover, has made public intervention conceptually congruent with capitalist principles on the grounds that market inefficiencies can be reduced by enlightened taxing and spending policies. These political and economic concepts are operationalized as regulations and programs which range from Federal Reserve Board policy to local zoning codes. These interventions are supposedly initiated only when a comparison of likely impacts suggests that the ratio of public costs to benefits is smaller for interceding than for nonintervention (Mishan, 1976).

These cost/benefit analyses, either intuitive or formal, assume three steps. The first is the forecasting of the outcomes of alternative courses of action. Projecting impacts is essentially a technical problem which assumes an ecological model of the system being manipulated.

The second step is separating the projected impacts into costs and benefits. This implies establishing a point of reference. One person's cost is often another's benefit, and no formal decision system can function without establishing a reference.

Weighting the categories of outcomes is the third cost/benefit step. Weighting refers to the process of establishing values for types of outcomes which are not inherently comparable (Hill, 1968). The comparison of one suicide to the loss of one dollar of tax revenue, for example, requires some weighting scheme before the forecasting of either has meaning to a decisionmaker.

The second and third steps of cost/benefit analysis inherently involve conflict among those who are likely to benefit from or pay for the alternatives being considered. Another term for this conflict is politics, and, unlike the first step, which assumes technical expertise, steps two and three clearly involve what the President's Commission refers to as "controversial social values."

Before describing the role of behavioral cost accounting in decision-making, an important point regarding cost/benefit analysis needs to be made. While explicit use of sophisticated decision systems is not widespread, the reader should be careful not to dismiss the concept of behavioral costs as having limited value in primary prevention. The fact is that while formal systems are rare, the implicit use of the cost/benefit paradigm is nearly universal among managers and decisionmakers. The weightings used in these implicit systems may be so obscure as to make decisions appear arbitrary, but this does not mean that decision behavior cannot be changed by insisting on the conceptualization of behavioral disorder as an accountable cost.

The concept of behavioral cost accounting and its place in decision-making has been discussed elsewhere (Dooley & Catalano, 1977; Catalano & Dooley, in press). The thrust of that discussion and of the preceding paragraphs is that primary prevention could theoretically be enhanced if the mental health outcomes of economic policy alternatives were anticipated and included in implicit or explicit cost/benefit analyses. This argument assumes that proactive primary prevention could be served by the selection of policy alternatives which minimize the incidence of disorder, or that reactive primary prevention can be initiated when adverse impacts are at least anticipated. The former of these assumptions will be considered first.

The inclusion of behavioral costs among the accounted outcomes of policy alternatives certainly appears technically possible. The research issues are tractable, and decisionmakers, at least at the federal level, are willing to consider mental health outcomes. The Joint Economic Committee, for example, commissioned an analysis of behavioral and health outcomes for its debate of the Humphrey-Hawkins Full Employment Bill (Brenner, 1976). The main impediment to wider use of such information is probably the preliminary nature of the research itself. The facts that remarkably few empirically oriented researchers are in the field and that their findings do not always converge raise the issue of whether the knowledge base is solid enough to guide policy.

Even if the direction and degree of impact of economic change are established statistically for various subgroups, the policy significance of the relationship may remain an issue. Time-series analyses measure the correlation between longitudinal variance in economic change and disorder. As Luft (1978: 198) has observed, we must not confuse the variation with the larger, invariant baseline of mental health problems.

While the forecasting of mental health outcomes demands most of the attention of the research community, more difficult and frustrating problems probably wait at steps two and three of the cost/benefit decision process. As noted earlier, separating costs and benefits and establishing weights are inherently political acts. If all persons were equally affected by economic change, the political problem would reduce to establishing a consensus on weightings. The fact is, however, that the impact varies across geographic regions and across demographic and socioeconomic subgroups.

There are no federal attempts to influence the economy which affect all regions in the same way. There is no "national" economy, but rather a collection of regional economies which are constantly evolving. Because of differences in the economic bases of these regions, no two will benefit or suffer equally from market forces or government policies (Sternlieb & Hughes, 1977). Politicians know this and their reaction to policy alternatives is often guided by regional rather than national concerns. A federal policy to increase defense spending, for example, will benefit the "Sunbelt" more than the Northeast, and the behavioral impacts will therefore vary across regions.

Perhaps more complicated than the geographic variations are the demographic and socioeconomic differences. The research indicates, for example, that the poor are most seriously affected by downturns (Dooley & Catalano, 1977) but that women and the elderly are adversely impacted by expansion (Brenner, 1973; Catalano & Dooley, in press). The picture is even further complicated by the literature which suggests that expansion is related to increased incidence of physiological problems in the same population behaviorally affected by downturns (Catalano, 1979b; Eyer, 1977)!

Although economic *interventions* may be politically impractical at the national level, there is reason for pursuing behavioral cost accounting at the national level. As alluded to above, federal decisionmakers have requested behavioral impact forecasts, and these estimates have become part of the debate surrounding the employment-versus-inflation controversy (*APA Monitor,* 1978). Claims are already being made that include estimates, for example, of the number of suicides that could have been avoided had full employment policies been in place over the past decade (Brenner, 1977). Interest groups have inevitably begun to use such claims in their efforts to influence employment policy (New York *Times,* October 31, 1976). It is inevitable that the mental health community, especially those involved in primary prevention, will be called upon to contribute to this debate (New York *Times,* April 19, 1976). That contribution will be neither responsible nor informed if the President's Commission's view that the issue is not "part of mental health's purview" is taken seriously.

The authors believe that the most effective proactive primary prevention would be at the regional level. The use of public power to manipulate economic conditions at the regional and local levels has not traditionally been used to achieve social ends. This power is most frequently operationalized as land use regulation. To the degree that such regulation has had goals larger than orderly physical development, it has been used to maximize economic growth or diversity (Pfouts, 1960). Recent years, however, have seen an exponential increase in legislative reforms which require that the social impact of new development be considered in the decision process (Catalano et al., 1975). It has already been argued, for example, that community psychologists should be involved in land use regulation to reduce adverse behavioral impacts of new development (Catalano & Monahan, 1975). This movement, referred to as "social impact assessment," has spawned a multidisciplinary research tradition (see, for example, Christenson, 1976; Finsterbusch & Wolf, 1977).

The inclusion of behavioral costs in social impact assessments has been precipitated by recent events in several communities adversely affected by plant closures (Beck-Rex, 1978). These assessments offer meaningful opportunities for proactive primary prevention for technical as well as political reasons. The technical reasons reflect the fact that the task of forecasting the impacts of economic changes is more tractable on the regional than national level (Catalano & Dooley, 1977, in press). Economic techniques of long standing allow regional economic forecasts (Isard,

1976; Isserman, 1977), and the smaller unit of analysis reduces the problem of "ecological" fallacy (Firebaugh, 1978; Kasl, 1979).

The political complexities of establishing a point of reference and of weighting classes of impacts are also reduced at the regional or local level. The impact of policies is more homogeneous than at the national level, increasing the chances of political consensus. The political behavior of local areas has, moreover, been the subject of considerable analyses, many of which offer empirically based advice on strategies for effective intervention (for example, Coplin & O'Leary, 1972). The prospects of successful use of economic regulation as a tool for proactive primary prevention are, in summary, greater at the local than national level.

Another advantage of local approaches to the primary prevention problem is that the forecasting exercise offers valuable information for reactive prevention even if the proactive stance is politically precluded. Knowing that a community is likely to experience an increase in environmental risk factors offers an opportunity heretofore seldom used to prepare populations to cope with adaptation demands. The potential of these opportunities is discussed in more detail in a subsequent section of this chapter.

Influencing Corporate Decisions

The above discussion reflects the traditional approach to managing adverse economic impacts in that the regulatory power of the public sector has been emphasized. The potential for influencing corporate decision-making through behavioral cost accounting should not, however, be overlooked. As will be discussed below, employer-sponsored "stress innoculation" programs offer an ideal setting for reactive primary prevention among those workers likely to be affected by a company's economic fortunes. The expansion of worker's compensation to cover more than accidents or illnesses caused by toxins may, moreover, encourage corporations to increase their involvement in "stress management" projects.

Corporate decision-making may also prove a useful point for intervening for proactive prevention. There has been an increasing emphasis on "social audits" in the accounting of corporate performance (Estes, 1976). These audits are attempts to identify the costs and benefits realized by communities as a result of a corporation's management policies. Such costs and benefits should, it is argued (Dilley & Weygandt, 1973), be included in corporate reports to stockholders so that the social responsibility of an industry can be monitored.

The National Association of Accountants (NAA) has prepared guidelines for social audits (NAA Committee on Accounting for Corporate

Social Performance, 1974). These guidelines are prefaced with the following statement:

> Social performance of corporations is of increasing concern to management, investors and the general public, but this performance is not measured and reported in a systematic manner. . . . Areas of social performance need to be identified in order to assist management: 1) in establishing goals, objectives and priorities; 2) in planning the use of monetary, physical and human resources; and 3) in measuring progress [1974: 40].

The guidelines recommend that social performance be disaggregated into (1) community involvement, (2) human resources, (3) physical resources and environmental contribution, and (4) product or service contribution. Of particular importance to the current discussion are two examples of social benefits listed by NAA in the human resources area: 1) "Employment Continuity—scheduling production so as to minimize layoffs and recalls, maintaining facilities in efficient operation condition so that they will not have to be abandoned because of deterioration, and exploring all feasible alternatives to closing a facility"; and (2) "Drugs and Alcohol—providing education and counseling for employees to prevent or alleviate problems in these *and similar areas*" (1974: 41; italics added).

If the above corporate behaviors are conceived of as benefits to be accounted in social audits, the logical inference is that employment discontinuity and the failure to provide counseling for behavioral problems are accountable social costs. The social audit, therefore, offers an arena for arguing for both proactive (for example, job continuity) and reactive (for example, counseling) primary prevention.

There are precedents for social audits (Eastern Gas & Fuel Associates, 1974; First National Bank of Minneapolis, 1974; Scovil, 1972), and their use as aids in proactive prevention should be investigated. The threat of legal action similar to that inherent in the assertion of corporate liability for exposing communities to toxins may increase the willingness of industry to consider behavioral costs in their decision-making.

Community and worker purchase of production facilities is another form of nonpublic sector primary prevention which has emerged in response to those situations in which corporate decisions threaten community stability. Corporate decisions to close a plant or curtail employment do not necessarily reflect the economic viability of the particular facility (Whyte, 1977). Conglomerates make such decisions based on the status of overall holdings and may close or neglect potentially profitable facilities to improve cash flow or decrease tax liabilities (Nadel, 1976). Communities based on these facilities suffer economic stressors which could be avoided if corporate management were more sensitive to local conditions. One means of achieving increased sensitivity is worker and/or community participation in corporate ownership. The concept of worker ownership is not new (Bellas, 1972; Bernstein, 1977) and has led to several worker purchases of corporations in the United States (Berman, 1967; Whyte, 1977). Community ownership is a newer concept (Whyte, Note 3) but has already been suggested in the case of Youngstown, Ohio (Beck-Rex, 1978). Moreover, legislation in the form of the Community Stabilization Act (HR 12094) has been proposed (1978) which would provide federal loans to communities to assume ownership of economically viable facilities threatened with closure.

Implications for Reactive Primary Prevention

As the above section on proactive primary prevention suggests, the dissemination of information about economic change may assist individuals in avoiding or ameliorating certain kinds of stressful life events by providing early warning and permitting time for anticipatory coping. In this section we will briefly note some of the possibilities for individual-level interventions predicated on the assumption that economic changes are unavoidable. Interventions which assist individuals in reacting effectively to stressful life changes may be either event-specific or general. The scope and focus of this chapter do not allow an extensive treatment of general stress inoculation methods (see Jarenko, 1979, and Novaco, in press, for a review of these methods). As a brief illustration of this class of intervention, we will describe elements of a training and counseling program tailored for individuals about to lose or having just lost their jobs. Other less catastrophic economic changes which also warrant similar types of inoculative training include retirement, promotion to more intense responsibilities, underemployment (reduction of hours or responsibilities), and job strains (difficulties with boss, colleagues, or quality of work life).

A job-loss stress inoculation program would consist of three major components: education, cognitive restructuring, and behavioral skill acquisition. The educational component would provide information about stress responses in general and reactions to job loss in particular. Cognitive restructuring would focus on the attributional and emotional response to job loss. The behavioral component would deal with techniques for adapting to the job loss and for actively coping by changing the situation.

Education

A job-loss-specific education component would include preparation for two dimensions of the job loss experience. The first is the variety of changes entailed in job loss: (a) loss of income and reduction in material resources; (b) change in social role and possible loss of social support at a time when it may be most needed; (c) loss of self-esteem, mood changes, and possibly even physiological symptoms; and (d) the potential for additional stressful life events consequent on or in adaptation to job loss. These changes are interrelated and probably operate reciprocally. The second dimension is the sequence of stages from anticipation (from announcement of job loss) through termination (immediate and short-term responses to job loss) to reemployment or chronic long-term unemployment. Different symptom patterns have been recorded for these different phases of the unemployment experience (Cobb & Kasl, Note 2). Different types of loss or change may be differentially salient at different steps in this process. For example, for some the job loss experience may be initially positive—a break from an unloved job and an opportunity for refreshment and review. Later, the dwindling of savings and the embarrassment of an undesirable social role may lead to depression. Awareness of the types of losses and phases may provide the individual with time for psychological preparation and possibly even a heightened sense of control, both elements thought to be positive factors in handling stress (Glass & Singer, 1972; Schulz, 1976; Sherrod, 1974).

This educational component would also include two other kinds of information. The first category includes accurate, current data on the prevailing labor market conditions. As will be seen later, such information may be useful not only as general context, but in assisting the individual in making emotionally positive attributions of his or her experience. The second category of information includes referral data for utilizing available resources such as job retraining, unemployment compensation, and counseling. Such public services, paid for in part by the individual through taxes or voluntary contributions, have been found to be underutilized through ignorance (Gutek, Note 4).

Cognitive Restructuring

The central feature of cognitive restructuring is helping the individual identify negative self-statements or attributions and replacing them with more positive ones. The main target of this intervention is the loss of self-esteem. Negative statements related to job loss might include self-blame for the termination and "catastrophizing" worry about the duration or consequences of the unemployment. Correct attributions of the termination may require information regarding the prevailing economic climate and insights into the corporate and public policies which affect unemployment levels. Some evidence exists that prevailing unemployment levels are already being taken into account to destigmatize job loss. Cohn (1978) found that psychological distress in those having lost jobs was higher when the prevailing unemployment rate was lower. However, another study found a similar result, not for the relatively well-publicized unemployment rate, but for a technical measure of economic expansion/contraction which could not be available to large numbers of people (Dooley et al., Note 5). Whatever the actual state of the economy surrounding the unemployed individual, the bulk of cognitive restructuring is likely to consist of cognitive behavioral techniques aimed at correcting irrationally punitive self-judgments.

Behavioral Training

The most general physical approach to stress inoculation is the teaching of relaxation in the face of the stressful stimuli. The client is taught to monitor his or her mental and physical reactions and to control them through deep breathing, systematic muscular relaxation, and cognitive strategies such as distraction or mental imagery.

While this general relaxation approach may be useful in reducing the cost of unavoidable stressful stimuli, particularly those underlying physiological stress disorders, more active behavioral coping could be aimed at changing the situation. Such active coping would be focused on the objective impacts of unemployment including loss of income, loss of social support or social role, and other life events. The most obvious example of such active coping interventions is the training of new job skills and assertion and self-presentation interpersonal skills which can facilitate interviewing for and obtaining a new job.

A less obvious but perhaps equally important benefit of interpersonal skills training and counseling pertains to social support. Social support appears to buffer the impact of job loss (Gore, 1978). Termination may dislocate existing social role relationships with spouse and family, with friends and neighbors, and especially with friends and colleagues from the work place. Individuals may need to learn how to repopulate and rely on their social networks. The acquisition of such interpersonal approach and assertion skills should also yield tangible gains in terms of seeking and obtaining unemployment compensation and social service benefits (including professional social support).

Finally, it may be anticipated that job loss will produce additional life changes as the individual reorganizes his or her schedule, personal finances, and social arrangements. Later, the individual must find another job with the possibility of a residential move; change in job tasks, responsibilities, and hours; and introduction to new colleagues and a modified social-occupational role. Anticipation of such changes (from the education component) may ameliorate some of their impact. Moreover, the individual can exercise control over the volitional life changes with an eye to minimizing both current life change and the likelihood of future changes. Thus, the whole episode of job loss and adaptation can be treated as a learning experience about the individual's responsiveness to and management of occupational change.

Staging Stress Inoculation Programs

The offering of such individual-level reactive programs for job loss raises issues of sponsorship and timing. Employers, unions, community mental health centers, schools, and government social service agencies dealing with health and employment are all candidates for sponsoring such inoculation programs. Different sponsors may better serve at different stages in the job loss experience. Prior to termination, schools may be the most feasible sites for stress inoculation programs. For morale reasons, employers and unions may prefer not to emphasize the threat of job loss before actual termination. Walsh and Taber (Note 6) have described a plant-based project utilizing fellow employees as counselors who facilitated the adjustment of workers in the anticipation phase. Such corporate- or union-sponsored projects could be guided by teams of community mental health center staff on short notice if the job-loss coping programs have been prepackaged and rehearsed. Following actual job loss, mental health centers could sponsor self-help group coping programs. Similarly, government employment offices could offer parallel programs or refer their more vulnerable clients to such programs. All such agencies and programs could also facilitate secondary prevention by serving as referral sources for individuals beginning to show psychological symptoms.

Summary

It behooves the mental health community to concern itself with proactive primary prevention. While clinical education has not emphasized the role of environmental factors in the etiology or treatment of disorder, the behavioral implications of managing those factors are of increasing societal concern. If the mental health community is unwilling or unable to provide insights into the choice of alternative management policies at least at the regional level, major opportunities for both proactive and reactive primary prevention will be lost.

Proactive primary prevention will be politically difficult at the national level because few federal policies, particularly economic policies, have uniform impact across regions. The mental health community should, however, be prepared to contribute in an informed way to the inevitable debate which will arise over the human impact of federal economic policies.

The regional level offers great potential for proactive primary prevention. The modeling of change at the regional level is technically possible and should allow prediction of periods of increased adaptation demands. This knowledge could be used proactively to alter the proposed or anticipated change or to deploy reactive prevention programs.

The mental health community should also insist that the private sector recognize its responsibility in proactive prevention of health and behavioral problems. The philosophical and mechanical prerequisites for social audits exist and should be utilized. Worker and community participation in corporate ownership should not be overlooked as effective means of proactive prevention.

Reactive primary prevention may be made more immediately operational than the proactive strategies listed above. Reactive programs would, however, be most effective when based on the behavioral cost accounting model assumed by the proactive strategies. Modeling communities to predict periods of increased adaptation demands would allow optimum deployment of preventive resources such as stress inoculation.

Reference Notes

1. Sclar, E.D., & Hoffman, V.J. *Planning Mental Health Service for a Declining Economy.* Final report to the National Health Services Research. Waltham, MA: Brandeis University, January, 1978.

2. Cobb, S., & Kasl, S.V. *Termination: The Consequences of Job Loss.* Report No. 76-1261. Cincinnati, Ohio: National Institute for Occupational Safety and Health, Behavioral and Motivated Factors Research, June, 1977.

3. Whyte, W.F. The voluntary job preservation and community stabilization act: Government support for worker participation and ownership in the United States. Presented to the Ninth World Congress of Sociology, August, 1978.

4. Gutek, B.A. Government's role in the amelioration of the impact of unemployment: In *Ameliorating the Impact of Unemployment: Established Programs Versus Individual Needs.* Symposium presented at the American Psychological Association Convention, Washington, D.C., 1976.

5. Dooley, D., Catalano, R., & Barthrop, A. The relation of economic conditions and individual life change to depression: Towards a cross-level analysis of behavioral disorder. In B. Lubin (chair), *Ecological Models: Contributions to Current Social and Mental Health Issues.* Symposium presented at the meeting of the American Psychological Association, New York, September, 1979.

6. Walsh, J.T., & Taber, T.D. Assessing the effectiveness of nonprofessional counseling during a plant closing. In *Ameliorating the Impact of Unemployment: Established Programs Versus Individual Needs.* Symposium presented at the American Psychological Association Convention, Washington, D.C., 1976.

References

APA Monitor Political points. July 1978, *9,* 9.

Bakke, E.W. *Citizens Without Work: A Study of the Effects of Unemployment upon the Workers' Social Relations and Practices.* New Haven, CT: Yale University Press, 1940.

Barling, P., & Handel, P. Incidence of utilization of public mental health facilities as a function of short term economic decline. *American Journal of Community Psychology,* 1980, *8,* 31-40.

Beck-Rex, M. Youngstown: Can this steel city forge a comeback? *Planning,* 1978, *44,* 12-15.

Bellas, C.J. *Industrial Democracy and the Worker Owned Firm.* New York: Praeger, 1972.

Berman, K. *Worker-Owned Plywood Companies: An Economic Analysis.* Pullman: Washington State University Press, 1967.

Bernstein, P. *Democratization at the Workplace.* Ohio: Kent State University Press, 1977.

Brenner, M.H. Patterns of psychiatric hospitalization among different socioeconomic groups in response to economic stress. *Journal of Nervous and Mental Disease,* 1969, *148,* 31-38.

Brenner, M.H. *Mental Illness and the Economy.* Cambridge, MA: Harvard University Press, 1973.

Brenner, M.H. *Estimating the Social Costs of Economic Policy: Implications for Mental and Physical Health, and Criminal Aggression.* Report to the Congressional Research Service of the Library of Congress and Joint Economic Committee of Congress. Washington, DC: U.S. Government Printing Office, 1976.

Brenner, M.H. Personal stability and economic security. *Social Policy,* 1977, *8,* 2-5.

Bronfenbrenner, V. Toward an experimental ecology of human development. *American Psychologist,* 1977, *32,* 513-531.

Caplan, G. *Principles of Preventive Psychiatry.* New York: Basic Books, 1964.

Catalano, R. *Health, Behavior and the Community.* New York: Pergamon, 1979. (a)

Catalano, R. Health costs of economic expansion: The case of manufacturing accident injuries. *American Journal of Public Health,* 1979, *69,* 789-794. (b)

Catalano, R., & Dooley, D. Economic predictors of depressed mood and stressful life events in a metropolitan community. *Journal of Health and Social Behavior,* 1977, *18,* 292-307.

Catalano, R., & Dooley, D. Does economic change provoke or uncover behavioral disorder: A preliminary test. In L. Ferman and J. Gordus (Eds.), *Mental Health and the Economy.* Kalamazoo, MI: Upjohn Foundation, in press.

Catalano, R., & Monahan, J. The community psychologist as social planner: Designing optimal environments. *American Journal of Community Psychology,* 1975, *3,* 327-334.

Catalano, R., Simmons, S., & Stokols, D. Adding social science knowledge to environmental decision-making. *American Bar Association Natural Resource Lawyer,* 1975, *8,* 24-41.

Cavan, R.S., & Rauck, K.H. *The Family and Depression: A Study of One Hundred Chicago Families*. Chicago: University of Chicago Press, 1938.

Christenson, K. *Social Impacts of Land Development*. Washington, DC: The Urban Institute, 1976.

Cohn, R.M. The effect of employment status change on self attitudes. *Social Psychology*, 1978, *41*, 81-93.

Coplin, W.D., & O'Leary, M.K. *Everyman's Prince: A Guide to Understanding Your Political Problems*. North Scituate, MA: Duxburg Press, 1972.

Cowen, E.L. Social and community intervention. *Annual Review of Psychology*, 1973, *24*, 423-472.

Dilley, S.C., & Weygandt, J.J. Measuring social responsibility: An empirical test. *The Journal of Accountancy*, September 1973, *136*, 62-70.

Dohrenwend, B.S. Social stress and community psychology. *American Journal of Community Psychology*, 1978, *6*, 1-14.

Dooley, D., & Catalano, R. Money and mental disorder: Toward behavioral cost accounting for primary prevention. *American Journal of Community Psychology*, 1977, *5*, 217-227.

Dooley, D., & Catalano, R. Economic, life, and disorder changes: Time-series analyses. *American Journal of Community Psychology*, 1979, *7*, 381-396.

Dooley, D., & Catalano, R. Economic change as a cause of behavioral disorder. *Psychological Bulletin*, 1980, *87*, 450-468.

Eastern Gas & Fuel Associates. *Annual Report*. Boston: Author, 1974.

Estes, R. *Corporate Social Accounting*. New York: John Wiley, 1976.

Eyer, J. Does unemployment cause the death rate peak in each business cycle? *International Journal of Health Services*, 1977, *7*, 625-661.

Finsterbusch, K., & Wolf, C.P. *Methodology of Social Impact Assessment*. New York: McGraw-Hill, 1977.

Firebaugh, G. A rule for inferring individual-level relationships from aggregate data. *American Sociological Review*, 1978, *43*, 557-572.

First National Bank of Minneapolis. *Annual Report*. Minneapolis: Author, 1974.

Glass, D.C., & Singer, J.E. *Urban Stress*. New York: Academic Press, 1972.

Gore, S. The effect of social support in moderating the health consequences of unemployment. *Journal of Health and Social Behavior*, 1978, *19*, 157-165.

Heller, K. & Monahan, J. *Psychology and Community Change*. Homewood, IL: Dorsey Press, 1977.

Herbert, W. The politics of prevention. *American Psychological Association Monitor*, 1979, *10*, 7-9.

Hill, M. A goals-achievement matrix for evaluating alternative plans. *Journal of the American Institute of Planners*, 1968, *34*, 19-29.

Isard, W. *Introduction to Regional Science*. Englewood Cliffs, NJ: Prentice-Hall, 1976.

Isserman, A. The location quotient approach to estimating regional economic impacts. *Journal of the American Institute of Planners*, 177, *43*, 33-41.

Jahoda, M., Lazarsfeld, P.F., & Zeisel, H. *Marienthal: The Sociology of an Unemployed Community*. Chicago: AVC, 1971.

Jarenko, M.E. A component analysis of stress innoculation: Review and prospectus. *Cognitive Therapy and Research*, 1979, *3*, 35-48.

Kasl, S.V. Mortality and the business cycle: Some questions about research strategies when utilizing macro-social and ecological data. *American Journal of Public Health*, 1979, *69*, 784-788.

Katona, G. Toward a macropsychology. *American Psychologist*, 1979, *34*, 118-126.

Komarovsky, M. *The Unemployed Man and His Family: The Effect of Unemployment upon the Status of the Man in 59 Families.* New York: Dryden Press, 1940.

Luft, H.S. *Poverty and Health: Economic Causes and Consequences of Health Problems.* Cambridge, MA: Ballinger, 1978.

Marshall, J.P., & Funch, D.P. Mental illness and the economy: A critique and partial replication. *Journal of Health and Social Behavior,* 1979, *20,* 282-289.

Mishan, E.J. *Cost Benefit Analysis.* New York: Praeger, 1976.

Nadel, M. *Corporations and Public Accountability.* Lexington, MA: D.C. Heath, 1976.

National Association of Accountants Committee on Accounting for Corporate Social Performance. Accounting for corporate social performance. *Management Accounting,* February 1974, *55* (part 2), 39-41.

New York *Times* The recession takes its toll: Family discord, mental illness. April 19, 1976, p. 32.

New York *Times* U.S. study links rise in jobless to deaths, murders, and suicides. October 31, 1976, p. 1.

Novaco, R.W. The cognitive regulation of anger and stress. In P. Kendall & S. Hollan (Eds.), *Cognitive-Behavioral Interventions: Theory, Research, and Procedures.* New York: Academic Press, in press.

Parnes, H.S. & King, R. Middle-aged job losers. *Industrial Gerontology,* 1977, *4,* 77-95.

Pfouts, R.W. (Ed.) *The Techniques of Urban Economic Analysts.* Trenton, NJ: Chandler-Davis, 1960.

President's Commission on Mental Health. *Report to the President from the President's Commission on Mental Health,* Vols. *1, 4.* Washington, DC: U.S. Government Printing Office, 1978.

Rappaport, J. *Community Psychology: Values, Research, and Action.* New York: Holt, Rinehart & Winston, 1977.

Schulz, R. Effects of control and predictability on the physical and psychological well being of the institutionalized aged. *Journal of Personality and Social Psychology,* 1976, *33,* 563-573.

Scovil Corporation. *Annual Report.* Waterbury, CT: Author, 1972.

Sherrod, D.R. Crowding, perceived control, and behavioral aftereffects. *Journal of Applied Social Psychology,* 1974, *4,* 171-186.

Sternlieb, G. & Hughes, J.W. New regional and metropolitan realities of America. *Journal of the American Institute of Planners,* 1977, *43,* 226-241.

Theorell, T., Lind, E., & Floderus, B. The relationship of distrubing life-changes and emotions to the early development of myocardial infarctions and other serious illnesses. *International Journal of Epidemiology,* 1975, *4,* 281-293.

Thoits, P. and Hannan, M. Income and psychological distress: The impact of an income maintenance experiment. *Journal of Health and Social Behavior,* 1979, *20,* 120-138.

Whyte, W.F. The emergence of employee owned firms in the United States. *Executive,* 1977, *3,* 22-24.

3

Prevention of Domestic Violence

Bonnie E. Carlson
Liane V. Davis

School of Social Welfare,
State University of New York at Albany

Introduction

The family has traditionally been viewed as a buffer between the individual and society, providing a safe haven in which the individual can grow while protected from both internally generated psychological conflicts and external societal stresses and strains (see, for example, Goode, 1966; Vincent, 1966). Some theorists, taking issue with this view, have considered conflict to be an inherent part of family structure; however, they have been in the minority (Safilios-Rothschild, 1970; Sprey, 1969). In recent years, however, a growing body of empirical research has forced the recognition that the American family is one of our most violent social groups, surpassed only by the police and the armed forces (Straus, in press). Simultaneously, "wife beating" has become increasingly visible as a social problem as a result of concerted efforts by local women's groups to develop supportive networks which encourage abused women to bring the issue out of the privacy of their homes.[1]

We define violence as any "act carried out with the intention of, or perceived as having the intention of, physically hurting another person" (Gelles and Straus, 1979: 554). By choosing this definition, we are accepting the view that it is the *intent,* not the *outcome,* which defines an act as violent. Included in this definition are those acts which many people consider to be the "normal" way to discipline children; that is, physical

Special thanks to Deb Burkhalter, Claudia Purcell, and Anita Williams, who assisted in preparation of the literature review.

punishment. Our position rests on the belief that people, within the privacy of their family, should be subject to the same norms and laws which govern their behavior outside the boundaries of the family. Therefore, any act which would be considered assault when carried out against an unrelated person is also a violent act when carried out against a family member. The range of acts thus extends from a slap of the hand to the use of a gun.

Family violence may be categorized in a number of ways. One can consider the potential consequences of the act, making a distinction between those acts which entail a high risk of physical injury (such behaviors as kicking, biting, beating up, threatening with a weapon, stabbing, and shooting) and those whose potential consequences are less severe (slapping, shoving). A second means of categorization is in terms of the act's intended purpose. Some violence has as its goal the induction of change in the victim's behavior (instrumental violence), while for other acts of violence the primary goal is the infliction of pain and injury (expressive violence). A third type of categorization, which cross-cuts but is not orthogonal to the second, makes a distinction between legitimate (or normal) and illegitimate (or abnormal) violence. The National Commission on the Causes and Prevention of Violence, in the first comprehensive national assessment of attitudes toward violence, found that one out of four men and one out of six women approved of a husband slapping a wife *under certain circumstances* (Stark & McEvoy, 1970). Such normative approval legitimates some domestic violence. The identity or role of the victim is the fourth variable by which family violence can be categorized. When the victim is a child, it is child abuse; when it is husband or wife, it is spousal abuse or domestic violence. This chapter will focus on the latter, violence which occurs between husband and wife.

Inferences drawn from a recent survey of a representative sample of 2143 American couples lead to the conclusion that 26 to 30 percent of all husbands and wives in the United States would admit to using physical force against one another. Serious physical violence would be expected to occur in three million American households, with 1.8 million wives and 2 million husbands being physically abused each year.[2] There are a number of reasons to think that these statistics grossly underestimate the actual incidence of domestic violence (Straus, 1977). When violence has become integrated into the life of the family, minor incidents are likely to be disregarded. At the other end of the spectrum, severe violence is likely to be underreported out of fear, guilt, and shame. This underreporting may be sex-based with greater underreporting by male than female victims. This would be consistent with society's condemnation of aggressive women and passive men. More specific to the sample is the fact that only intact couples were surveyed. Since physical abuse is a primary complaint of women seeking divorce,[3] omission of this increasingly large segment of the population would result in a significant underestimate of the extent of domestic violence.

These data demonstrate that men and women are almost equally likely to be the victims, as well as the perpetrators, of domestic violence. We agree with Straus, Gelles, and Steinmetz (1978), however, in believing that "it would be a great mistake if that fact distracted us from giving first attention to wives as *victims*" (p. 6). There are a number of reasons for giving top priority to wife abuse. The data reflect acts whose intent is the infliction of pain or injury; they do not take into account the *actual* injury sustained. Men's average superiority over women in physical strength makes it likely that they are capable of both inflicting greater harm to women and minimizing the impact of the attacks on them by women. Neither do the data address the issue of which spouse is the most likely instigator. It has been noted that while men and women are equally likely to murder their spouses, women are seven times more likely to do so in self-defense (Pleck et al., 1977). We do know that more husbands than wives beat up their spouses and do so with greater frequency (Straus, 1977a); that a large number of these attacks occur when the wife is pregnant, thus posing a danger to the fetus as well as to the mother (Gelles, 1976); and, perhaps more importantly, that women are less likely to have, or perceive they have, alternatives to remaining in an abusive marriage. For these reasons, this chapter is devoted primarily to those instances of domestic violence in which the woman is the victim.

Causes of Domestic Violence

Prior to discussing the causes of domestic violence, it is necessary to consider the discrepancy between our common assumptions about family life (namely, that it is characterized primarily by love, peace, and harmony) and the reality that violence is "a major feature of American life" (Gelles and Straus, 1979: 552). Why should the family be the locus of so much violent behavior when compared with other social groups?

There are a number of characteristics of the family as a social unit which may predispose it to violence. People spend a great deal of time interacting in the context of the family. The range of activities and events occurring there is quite broad, and family members differ in terms of sex, age, ability, and access to resources. All of these factors contribute to a high potential for disagreement and conflict. Membership in the family is more involuntary than membership in most other social groups and carries with it the implicit right to influence the behavior of other members, even to the point of using physical force in the case of children. The inherently unstable and ever-changing nature of family structure also results in chronic, high levels of change and stress. In addition, beliefs about the sanctity of family privacy tend to discourage many from taking problems outside of the family when they cannot be adequately resolved using internal family resources, thus causing unresolved problems to fester and often erupt into violence. Finally, the family is the primary training ground for violence, the setting in which most people are not only first exposed to violence but also come to associate violence with love and learn that those who love you most are often those who physically hurt you most.[4] It seems clear that we need to revise our assumptions about the nature of family interaction and assume not that harmony and equilibrium are what best characterize family interaction, but rather that conflict is *normative,* as has been observed by Sprey (1969) and others.

Myths about the Causes of
Family Violence

There are a number of commonly held beliefs about causes of or factors contributing to domestic violence which have not received empirical support and which are potentially dangerous and misleading in terms of prevention and treatment of the problem. For example, it is widely believed—particularly among victims—that excessive consumption of alcohol causes men to physically abuse their wives. Numerous papers have, in fact, suggested an association between abuse of alcohol and physical violence (Carlson, 1977; Hanks and Rosenbaum, 1977), but the exact nature of the relationship has not been specified. Generally, it is asserted that alcohol acts as a disinhibitor; inhibitions are reduced which would normally serve to suppress violent behavior. Since this disinhibiting effect has only been observed in men and does not appear to operate to the same degree in relation to violence against children as it does in relation to violence against women (Coleman and Straus, 1979), it appears important to consider other explanations. Perhaps "being drunk may provide individuals with a convenient excuse [which serves to] neutralize the deviance of violence toward family members" (Gelles and Straus, 1979: 561).

Closely related to the idea that alcohol consumption leads to family violence is the notion that temporary loss of control is responsible for incidents of violence against family members. If the man who beats his wife has "lost control," why, then, as Straus has asked repeatedly, doesn't he go on to stab her, shoot her, or run over her with his car? Obviously, some degree of control has been maintained. It seems clear that certain norms continue to influence this man's behavior and permit him to hit his wife, while proscribing more serious forms of violence (Gelles and Straus, 1979).

Another common misconception is related to the catharsis hypothesis which asserts that keeping anger and frustration pent up inside (that is, not expressing it) will result in more serious, explosive aggressiveness or violence. Proponents of this view maintain that (1) viewing violence leads to vicarious gratification of the instinctual need to express aggression, and (2) engaging in less serious forms of aggressiveness (such as verbal aggression) will serve to discourage the expression of violence in the future. A widely used book offering advice to married couples counsels that intimates *must* fight (albeit in the context of rules) and further that "affection grows deeper *when it is mixed with aggression*" (Bach and Wyden, 1974: 107; italics added). The authors further imply that a relationship is not intimate unless it involves fighting and go on to advocate fighting "in front of [one's] friends and children [as well as] before, during, and after intercourse" (Bach and Wyden, 1974: 99). Is there any evidence that verbal aggression or mild forms of aggression defuse more serious forms of aggression or violence? Little, if any, supporting evidence can be found; on the contrary, both vicarious participation in aggressive activities and participation in verbal aggression have been shown to *enhance* the likelihood of physical aggressiveness (Bandura, 1973; Gelles, 1974).

The final myth to be addressed pertains to the role of psychopathology or mental illness in the etiology of family violence, either against children or adults. It is widely believed that people who use violence against their children or marital partners must be "crazy." Undoubtedly, some individuals who use violence against family members are truly mentally ill. But there is no sound evidence supporting the idea that those who commit violent acts in the context of the family are any more likely to be mentally ill than those who do not, or that mentally ill persons are more likely to commit violence against a family member (Straus, 1979).

Theories on the Origin of
Family Violence

To date, no comprehensive theory of family violence per se has been formulated. However, several intraindividual, social-psychological, and sociocultural theoretical approaches attempting to explain aggression and or violence have been identified and are discussed at length by Gelles and Straus (in press). It is not possible to review them all here, and since no single theory is in and of itself adequate to account for family violence, an attempt will be made to briefly discuss those approaches at the social-psychological and sociocultural levels, which have received the most empirical support thus far. As it turns out, there is considerable overlap across the various approaches and remarkable complementarity.

At the social-psychological level, social learning theory appears to best explain family violence. Learning theorists maintain that violence, like other behavior, is learned. There are two mechanisms by which aggression and violence are acquired: through direct reinforcement and by means of observational learning or modeling, which does not require reinforcement. When applied to the family, this approach recognizes the fact that for most people the family serves as a training ground for violence—this is the context in which force and violence are simultaneously observed and rewarded. While this process may not be intentional on the part of family members, it is nonetheless extremely powerful. In fact, the association between violence observed and/or experienced as a child and used and/or experienced later as an adult has been widely documented (Ball, 1977; Flynn, 1977; Gelles, 1977; Ganley and Harris, 1978; Pfouts, 1978), although the precise relationship has not been identified. Certainly, the almost universal use of physical punishment on American children of all ages both models the use of force and violence and establishes its legitimacy as a means of achieving certain ends, thus contributing to the learning of violence as an appropriate response to problem-solving.

Another theoretical approach at the social-psychological level related to social learning theory asserts that an additional source of interpersonal violence lies in negative self-attitudes—that is, low self-esteem—arising from devaluing psychosocial experiences. Low self-esteem is said to predispose individuals to deviant behavior patterns in the attempt to obtain attention and ultimately more positive self-attitudes. Many anecdotal reports have documented the pervasiveness of poor self-concept among both victims and perpetrators of family violence (for example, Carlson, 1977). The major limitation of this framework is that it does not account for why some individuals with low self-esteem resort to aggressive behavior while others do not (Gelles and Straus, 1979).

At the sociocultural level, theories attempting to explain family violence have focused on the contributions of social structural factors, norms, and institutional arrangements to the causation of violence.

Cultural norms operate in several ways to both subtly and overtly encourage family members to engage in violence against one another. It has been observed that the marriage license is in many ways a "hitting license" (Straus, in press). Acknowledging the fact that while loving, affectionate, and supportive behaviors are expected between marital partners, hostile and aggressive behaviors which would not be normatively approved among unrelated adults are also tolerated. While it is no longer legally permissible to use physical violence against one's spouse, historically this prerogative has been granted to husbands under certain circumstances, and the right to use physical punishment is currently granted to parents in relation to their children in all states. Although the cultural norms regarding marital partners are not legally codified, they are still extremely powerful.

The intrafamily resource theory has been promulgated most strongly by Goode (1971) and Straus and identifies socioeconomic factors as being central to the causation of family violence. Briefly, the theory argues that in order for a member to maintain a superior position in the family he or she must have superior resources in the form of education, occupation, income, interpersonal skills, and so on. When the person desiring to be dominant, usually the husband, does not have superior resources as described above, he may resort to physical force or violence as the "ultimate resource" (Gelles and Straus, 1979). A variation on the family resource theory is the "status inconsistency" hypothesis which holds that when a wife's resources are superior to those of her husband, he may resort to violence in the attempt to equalize the resource imbalance. The existence of status inconsistency among couples in which violence has been identified as a problem has been noted by several of those working in this area (Allen and Straus, in press; Carlson, 1977; Flynn, 1977; Tidmarsh, 1976). This raises two additional issues: the role played by social-structural factors which ensure that both socioeconomic resources and stresses are not evenly distributed across all groups within the population; and the role played by sexism and inequality between the sexes. It seems clear that these factors contribute to and/or perpetuate domestic violence independently and in an interactive fashion.

For example, men in this culture are socialized to believe that they will be dominant or superior in relation to their wives. However, social structural factors ensure that men in the lower and working classes often do not have access to the resources to back up that superior status in the family. It may be the case that as women begin to make progress toward sexual equality with respect to valued resources, men who have been socialized to think of themselves as having superior ascribed status will feel increasingly threatened. This may have the unfortunate short-term consequence of increasing the rates of intrafamily violence between the sexes (Whitehurst, 1974). Another manifestation of sexism is the fact that as a result of being discriminated against educationally and occupationally, many women are locked into physically abusive marriages because they know they cannot economically support a family on their own. For them, the alternative to a violent marriage is poverty or public assistance (Straus, 1977a).

The role played by stress in the etiology of domestic violence has not been specified but is alluded to in virtually all of the studies available and appears to operate on more than one level. In its simplest form, stress can operate directly as a precipitating factor. However, it can also function in a cumulative manner. For example, Gelles (1979) reports the highest rates of spousal violence in blue-collar families, families with low income, where the partners have less than a high school education, where there are four to six children, where the husband is unemployed, and which live in large urban areas. In fact, several of the theories discussed point to circumstances which have a high stress potential. Unemployment of the spouse, for example, might simultaneously cause financial hardship, status inconcistency, and low self-esteem. These stress factors may in turn interact with past learning, cultural norms permitting family violence, and social isolation (a form of interpersonal resource limitation noted by Ball [1977], Hanks and Rosenbaum [1977], Pfouts [1978], and Tidmarsh [1976]), to ultimately result in violence.

To conclude the discussion of causal factors, it is apparent that (1) there are many complex factors which contribute to the causation of domestic violence, and although we are not yet certain about the exact manner in which they operate, the data strongly suggest an interactive model, and (2) the most salient causes are deeply embedded in our culture (norms), family structure and organization, and socioeconomic structure.

Consequences

Long Term

In the long run the costs of domestic violence are inestimable. Dollar values cannot be placed on the pain and even death of family members, nor on the social and psychological consequences of family disorganization to all its members. The effects of domestic violence transcend the generations. When children grow up believing that violence is the normal way to resolve conflicts, they carry that belief into their own families of procreation, thus transmitting violence throughout the society. Society is affected in yet another way. It has been estimated that in some areas of the country over half of all police calls involve domestic violence. Since those who request and those who offer assistance often have conflicting perceptions of the police role in family disturbances, such interventions carry with them a high risk of injury and death to both the police and the family members (Bard and Zacker, 1971).

Immediate

Because women are affected disproportionately and adversely by the consequences of domestic violence, we now direct our attention briefly to what we know about their actions after experiencing serious physical abuse. How the female victims respond in the short run is affected by the severity and frequency of the violence they currently experience, their socioeconomic status and personal resources, their family constellation, and their childhood experiences with domestic violence. The best predictor of whether they will seek help of any sort is the severity of the violence (Gelles, 1976). The more severe it is, the more likely they will be to seek help. Other variables which increase the likelihood that the victims will seek help are the presence of adolescents in the home (perhaps because the victims fear that their adolescent children will fight back and themselves become victims) and the victims' accessibility to personal resources which enhance their alternatives to the marriage.

The source to which women turn when seeking assistance is also affected by a number of factors. Women of lower socioeconomic status and those who are most frequently and severely beaten are likely to call the police. Women who are less frequently abused often turn to the legal system and seek separation and/or divorce. Far fewer turn to the traditional social agencies, and these are apt to be women who, as children, experienced minimal family violence (Pfouts, 1978). It is suggested that this may be the only group for which family violence is perceived to be abnormal or problem behavior where counseling is appropriate.

Regardless of the institution to which the women turn, they are likely to find a similar response: minimization of the problem and a primary concern with maintaining the integrity of the family at the expense of providing adequate protection to the victim. Such informal police procedures and rules as the "cooling off" period[5] and the "stitch rule"[6] serve to minimize the severity of the victim's complaint and the need for immediate attention and may even serve to aggravate the problem.

Should the women turn to the court system for assistance, they may find, as is true in many states, that the court's response is to provide treatment for the offender, the victim, or the family rather than the sought-after protection. In many states familial and nonfamilial violence come under the jurisdiction of entirely different court systems. In New York for example, until 1977, domestic violence fell solely under the jurisdiction of the family court system, and nonfamilial violence was within the jurisdiction of the criminal court system. Recent changes now *allow* the victim to decide which court system should have jurisdiction. The victim, however, is advised of two facts relative to the choice to bring action in criminal court: a decision to bring such charges may result in incarceration of the offender (thus resulting in removing what is often her sole source of financial support) and the victim has only 72 hours to either drop charges or change the jurisdiction. After that time the state will proceed in criminal court regardless of the wishes of the victim. Thus, it is not surprising that few victims have chosen to press charges in criminal court.

When women turn to traditional social agencies they are likely to encounter caseworkers who, trained in psychoanalytic psychology, implicitly or explicitly blame the victim. Even when clinicians attempt to dispel the old myths of female masochism from their practice wisdom, it is often an impossible task. This difficulty is graphically illustrated in a recent article which appeared in *Social Casework* in which the author ably argued that widespread tolerance of the Freudian theory of female personality development played a crucial role in the failure of casework to effectively assist victims of domestic violence. However, as if to illustrate the difficulty of eshewing decades of Freudian indoctrination, the same author wrote:

> If the relationship between client and worker is strong enough and the client is motivated, a frank discussion of Freudian psychology in relation to the masochistic position may cause the client to examine her own motives more clearly [Nichols, 1976: 31].

The consequences of seeking, yet not receiving, help may actually aggravate the problem. Straus (1977a) has argued that a battering husband's hand may be strengthened when an abused wife is sent home by the police, the courts, or the social service agency, since the husband perceives, often correctly, that his wife has exhausted her alternatives.

Prevention

It seems apparent that for prevention to be effective we must have accurate information on the incidence of domestic violence and link preventive strategies to its causes. Since most of the causes of domestic violence are fundamentally ingrained in the nature of the American family and society, we believe that nothing short of radical social change ultimately will be successful in eliminating violence between marital partners. However, in terms of what can be accomplished immediately and what is feasible, it can also be argued that any type of intervention of an ameliorative nature will ultimately serve to prevent future family violence. These more immediate interventive measures will be discussed first; a discussion of preventive measures at the micro and macro levels will follow.

Intervention as Prevention

The Victims

The victims of domestic violence, often seeking help in a state of crisis, are in need of immediate and concrete assistance. Many need a protected environment in which to live, financial assistance, legal aid, and emotional support. And they need all of these services on an emergency basis. Traditional social welfare agencies are not equipped to meet these needs. Often the eligibility requirements act as a "catch-22," preventing those who are most in need from receiving the services. Legal aid and public assistance, for example, are often provided on the basis of family income. The woman needs the service for herself, and often her children, yet cannot qualify because her husband's income, which is unavailable to her, is included in calculating eligibility.

It is the authors' belief that there are deeply ingrained values embodied in traditional social service agencies which can prevent the victims of domestic violence from receiving appropriate services. In their discussion of barriers to service delivery, Pincus and Minahan (1973) note that agencies avoid providing services which may embroil them in controversy and therefore threaten funding. Certainly, providing services to victims of domestic violence can be highly controversial, since it involves intervening in the private lives of families. And so, as is the case when needed services are not provided by traditional agencies, alternative services have developed, often sponsored by community feminist organizations. When such services are available, the influx of clients suggests that they fill a service vacuum (see for example Carlson, 1977). While we agree with

Straus (1977a) that the most important single step which any community can take is to establish domestic violence shelters where women may make rational decisions in a safe and supportive atmosphere, we would underline the necessity for traditional social welfare agencies to look at the reasons for their failure to provide such services and prepare to fulfill these needs.

Other services may be needed to enable a woman to consider the option of leaving an abusive relationship. Pfouts' (1978) social exchange theory analysis of a sample of abused wives provides a useful basis upon which to formulate intervention strategies appropriate to different groups of domestic violence victims.[7] According to Thibaut and Kelley (1959), two factors are important in understanding why a person remains in a relationship. The comparison level, which is a person's perception of the ratio between his or her contributions to and benefits from the relationship, determines satisfaction with the relationship. Thus, the more the benefits outweigh the costs, the more satisfied a person will be, while the more the costs outweigh the benefits, the more dissatisfied a person will be. However, dissatisfaction is not a sufficient reason to terminate a relationship. The second factor is the comparison level for alternatives, or the person's evaluation of how the relative benefits of the present relationship compare with the relative benefits available in the next best alternative. Thus, even if a wife is dissatisfied with a marriage, she may remain if the next best alternative does not appear any more satisfying.

Using this framework, Pfouts has identified four groups of women who respond differently to domestic violence and for whom intervention strategies must be designed. The classic victims are those who are dissatisfied within the relationship, yet see no better alternative. They become totally dependent on the abuser and are unlikely to voluntarily leave. Treatment of these women is extremely difficult and, to be successful at all, must be directed toward enhancing the women's self-esteem and assisting them to mobilize other material resources (such as public assistance and jobs) so that alternatives become both available and attractive. The second group consists of those women who, despite the violence, obtain some satisfaction from the relationship while finding no satisfactory alternatives outside. They are likely to respond to abuse by fighting back, sometimes against their husbands, more often against their children. Pfouts believes that this is the most difficult group to treat, since intervention must be directed toward resocializing them into nonviolent ways of behaving. One frequently mentioned strategy to be used both with victims and abusers is assertiveness training to teach people how to express themselves in nonviolent ways (see for example Ganley and Harris, 1978; Nichols, 1976; Straus,

1977a). Those women who are dissatisfied within their marriages and see better alternatives outside form the third group. These are the women who need the least help, as they either disengage at an early stage or force the abusive spouse to change his behavior. The fourth group consists of those women who have devoted many years to a marriage which they finally decide provides them with little satisfaction. Since they have demonstrated a pattern of giving their husbands one last chance, they are the most in need of immediate emotional and financial support if they are to carry out their decision to leave.

The social exchange analysis makes it apparent that one major goal of intervention with abused women is to change their perceptions of the benefits both within and outside of the marriage to enable them to make an active decision about whether to remain in the abusive relationship; to remain only if the husband agrees to, and actually does, change his behavior; or whether to leave the relationship entirely. Thus, any strategy which either increases the salience of the costs of remaining in an abusive relationship or enhances the available alternatives may serve to make being a victim less tolerable and motivate the woman to actively consider her alternatives. It has been noted, for example, that many victims of domestic violence have low self-esteem (Carlson, 1977; Nichols, 1976). Interventions which are designed to enhance a woman's self-esteem have multiple effects. A woman who has a heightened sense of self-esteem will find an abusive relationship less tolerable because she will place more value on what she brings to a relationship and will simultaneously expect to receive more from it. At the same time, more alternatives will become available to her both in the form of other relationships and in the form of educational or employment opportunities. An alternative strategy to accomplish the same goal is to provide her with the skills to obtain her own financial resources which will in turn affect how she feels about herself. Working serves additional functions for a woman who has been the victim of domestic violence. Contact with other people will decrease the sense of isolation which has been identified among women who are victims (Carlson, 1977; Tidmarsh, 1976), as well as making their victim status appear deviant and less tolerable (Gelles, 1976). All of these factors combine to make obtaining employment an important goal in the treatment of domestic violence.

Leaving a violent relationship is not the only solution. Unless the victim has this option, however, she is powerless to effect any change. Once a woman is protected from further assaults, it is vital that the notion that she has deserved the abuse be dispelled. We believe that this can best be accomplished through consciousness-raising and therapeutic support groups. It may also be appropriate to help the victim understand if she contributed in any way to her victimization (Ball, 1977). We are not implying that women are responsible for the abuse bestowed upon them. We are suggesting, however, that some women may unwittingly feed into an abusive marriage by engaging in behaviors which trigger their husbands' violent response or by enhancing their husbands' power. For example, a woman may not realize that continual threats to leave which never result in her actually leaving may serve to increase a husband's power and his perceived right to use violence (Straus, 1977a). The final objective of all interventions is to make violence totally unacceptable to the victims.

The Batterers

Less attention has been given to the intervention strategies for abusive husbands than for either abused wives or for the abusing couple. One reason for the lack of attention to the batterer per se has been the implicit assumption that domestic violence is a function of the marital relationship, with batterer and victim enmeshed in a mutually gratifying relationship. While it may be useful to reeducate the couple into nonviolent means of conflict resolution (see Blechman et al., 1976 for some innovative approaches), to focus on the couple as the unit of treatment is to imply shared responsibility for the abuse. We agree with Ganley and Harris (1978), whose major assumption behind the design of their program to treat batterers is that violence is not a function of the relationship, but is the way the male batterer expresses and resolves stress and conflict. Therefore, treatment of the male batterer must be focused primarily on training the male, through whatever methods may be effective, to stop being assaultive and to resolve conflicts in nonviolent ways. This may be accomplished through assertiveness training (Ganley and Harris, 1978), behavior modification (Saunders, 1977), or problem-solving training (Blechman et al., 1976). Both substance abuse and stress contribute to domestic violence. It is important, therefore, to treat the alcohol and drug abuse as well as to ensure employment opportunities for men. However, the basic message which must be conveyed in the treatment of battering husbands is that the use of physical force is never acceptable.

Service Providers

Since service providers may unwittingly contribute to the problem of domestic violence, intervention strategies must also focus on their reeducation and training in order to facilitate appropriate and effective ways of helping both the victim and the abuser. Extensive effort must be directed toward police training, especially in those communities where they are the most likely source of assistance (see Bard and Zacker, 1971, for details of an excellent police training program).

The community as a whole may contribute to the treatment of domestic violence by establishing an environment in which abuse is not tolerated and one in which services are both available and visible. Community efforts must focus on compilation of local statistics and counteracting the pervasive "it can't happen here" attitude which often greets those seeking to bring out in the open what many wish to hide.

Prevention at the Micro Level

Prevention at the micro level refers to measures which can be taken among individuals and families to reduce the likelihood that marital partners will resort to violence against one another. One obvious target is the way in which we socialize our children. Sex-role socialization is, in effect, where the double standard begins. We train little boys to be strong, independent, and aggressive, while little girls are taught to be passive, dependent, and submissive. Further, boys are taught, subtly or overtly, that they will be dominant, while girls learn to expect to play secondary, supportive, and nurturing roles. And yet, there is a growing body of literature which suggests that independent, assertive people who can adapt to the demands of the situation rather than rigidly adhering to sex-stereotyped behaviors constitute the most well-adjusted group of adults (Kaplan and Bean, 1976). When people can choose their adult roles on the basis of interest and ability rather than on the basis of socially prescribed sex roles, we may expect a reduction in several powerful sources of interpersonal conflict—for example, expectations regarding dominance and submission, low self-esteem, and poor match between interests and prescribed role.

Another measure which can be taken at the family level derives from the recognition of the inevitability of problems and conflict in family life. It also acknowledges the fact that problem-solving and conflict resolution are skills which can be taught. Various models of problem-solving and nonviolent conflict resolution should become a regular part of our school curricula, starting in the very early grades. We must also have community resources available to reeducate adult family members about nonviolent conflict resolution skills. At the same time, we should be teaching assertiveness to both children and adults, emphasizing the distinction between standing up for yourself and making your needs known in a nondestructive and nonhurtful manner (assertiveness), and using force and violence to impose your will on another person in a hurtful manner (aggressiveness). Children can be taught to distinguish between these two different approaches at a surprisingly early age. Although we tend to equate assertiveness training with women, there is reason to believe that many men, especially those who resort to force to make their needs known, can benefit from a program that gives them alternative means to achieve their goals. Ganley and Harris (1978) found that many of the male batterers they saw in their program had difficulty verbally expressing their thoughts, feelings, and needs; this problem was treated through provision of assertiveness training. This is doubly important since verbal skills are an important component of family communication which can serve as a valuable resource for conflict resolution. When healthy family communication defuses potential disagreement and conflict, the likelihood of things getting out of control and resulting in serious violence can be reduced.

Prevention at the Macro Level

Because so many of the causes of family violence are deeply rooted in the nature of American society, there are numerous changes that can and must occur at this level. If we are really serious about wanting to eliminate violence between family members, one of the most basic changes is to take whatever steps are necessary to reduce the amount of violence in society as a whole. This might entail, for example, stringent gun control measures, as well as a reduction in the amount of violence shown on television, not only to children but to adults as well. In fact, all media, including the film industry, magazines, and newspapers, should be induced to limit their depiction of violence, particularly against women. This issue is currently being brought to public attention in relation to pornographers, who use the protection of the First Amendment rights to free speech to legitimate depiction of violence against women.

The second line of attack at the macro level is to change the norms which make the marriage license a hitting license. The first step is to make people explicitly aware of the norm. Then we must convince people that behavior which is not tolerated outside of the context of the family—that is viewed as assault—will not be tolerated within the family. As long as we legitimize the use of force by parents against children, the norm of family violence will remain, and the family will continue to serve as the major "training ground for violence" (Straus, 1977a). Therefore, we must follow the lead taken this year by Sweden and ban the physical punishment of children. While acknowledging the difficulty of enforcing the new law, officials from the Swedish Ministry of Justice say it is the first step toward changing people's attitudes about physical punishment. The law will be supplemented by a large-scale public relations campaign about children's rights and alternative means of child discipline (Vinocur, 1979). It is recognized that this is a very radical step and one which would probably not be as well received in the United States as it was in Sweden, but it may be that the only way to change a norm or attitude as deeply ingrained as the one pertaining to family violence is to legislate such a change. There is evidence in the social-psychological literature which strongly suggests that not only do attitudinal changes lead to behavioral changes, but also that changes in behavior can and do lead to changes in attitudes. Support for this can be seen in the area of race relations, where court action was necessary to ensure changes in behavior (that is, school desegregation), which would probably still not have come about if we had waited for people's biased attitudes about blacks and other minorities to change first (see the chapter on prejudice in Aronson, 1972).

Another major arena in which change is essential pertains to the role of women in American society and the family. First, these changes should address the numerous remaining instances of sex discrimination in the educational and occupational spheres which serve to limit women's options and material resources, ultimately locking them into abusive relationships. There is ample evidence that when women can leave and support themselves and their children, they will do so. Passage of the Equal Rights Amendment would be one efficient way of ensuring progress along these lines. Discrimination against women in the strongly male-oriented legal system must also be eliminated. Communities must let law enforcement officials know that the antiwoman attitudes embodied in informal policies such as "stitch rules" and "cooling off" periods, which serve as powerful barriers preventing women from taking advantage of what limited legal protection they do have, will not be tolerated. Likewise, judges with preconceived notions about the inherent superiority of intact families over single-parent families must be educated and not permitted to penalize women who opt to leave their violent spouses.

The other needed changes must address the issue of women's positions in the family. Traditionally, being a woman has been virtually synonymous with playing the nurturant, supportive role—being wife and mother and subordinating her interests and needs to those of her husband and children. Any historical conditions which may have legitimated male superiority over women in the past, such as differentials in physical size and strength, can no longer be seen as justifying the perpetuation of male dominance. However, men have continued to be thought of as heads of the household, even when their wives are employed and fulfill all of the household and child care responsibilities. For women, the wife-mother role has been considered not only mandatory but also primary in their lives, whereas for men the husband-father role has been seen as more secondary and voluntary. We need to carefully reexamine the notion of "head of household" and either assume it applies equally to both spouses irrespective of the family roles they assume or, better still, eliminate it entirely from our beliefs about family life. Straus (1977: 209) has strongly recommended that

> no woman should enter marriage without it being firmly and *explicitly* understood that the husband is not the head of the family. Unless stated otherwise, the implicit marriage contract includes the "standard" clause about male leadership.

Family role responsibilities (for example, economic support, household management, and child care) should not be assigned primarily on the basis of sex, as this perpetuates the low value placed on activities internal to the home which are typically carried out by women. Rather, the spouse who assumes responsibility for a particular family role should be determined on the basis of ability and interest; when disagreements arise they should be negotiated.

Not only should family role responsibilities be distributed on a more equal basis, but family decision-making should also be shared between spouses. This tends to be the case when both spouses share responsibility for the breadwinning role and is reflected in the national survey data, where Gelles (1979) found that egalitarian decision-making was inversely related to the incidence of domestic violence.

As delineated in the section above on causes, several of the factors contributing to domestic violence are stress-related and have their origins in social structural factors which ensure that certain groups in the population experience disproportionate rates of poverty and unemployment. While the frustration-aggression hypothesis has received limited empirical support, it is clear that economic deprivation is a frustrating experience which often results in violent behavior. This may be especially true for men who are expected to fulfill the breadwinner role in their families and yet are unable to do so because of the constant unemployment our economy continues to sustain. While some feel that the impact of full employment on our economy would not be entirely favorable, this may be a goal we can no longer afford to ignore as a result of the exorbitant social costs of continued high unemployment. At least one author (O'Brien, 1969) has asserted that a priority should be placed on job training and employment opportunities for *men* rather than women, because of the societal expectations regarding male fulfillment of the breadwinning role and in order to equalize "status inconsistency." While this may be justifiable in the short run, in the long run it will perpetuate assumptions about males' "rightful" position as heads of households. Therefore, it is recommended that men and women be given equal opportunities to obtain the prerequisites necessary to become employed.

If we fail to choose the option of full employment, or cannot achieve it, then we must remove the stigma attached to being a recipient of public assistance. Let us move toward a guaranteed annual income which neither demeans its recipients nor ensures that their lives remain highly stressful because they are not "productive contributors" to society. In fact, in a broad sense, any measure which tends to reduce poverty or redistribute societal resources toward the "have nots" will tend to eliminate some of the direct or indirect causes of domestic violence. Increasing the availability of low-cost day care is an example of such a measure.

The last major preventive measure to be proposed is the formation of a permanent commission at the federal level to monitor the effects of all governmental policies on families. While we give lip service to the importance of the American family, rarely if ever have we taken it seriously enough to be willing to systematically analyze the consequences for family life of actions taken in the public sector. A specific focus of such a commission should be examination of existing and future policies with regard to their implications for domestic violence. Another purpose of such a commission might be to promote public education about the causes and consequences of family violence, as well as alternatives. One aspect of such a public education campaign should be to encourage the formation of domestic violence task forces in every community to study the problem, educate citizens about it, and take action against it. This approach has been used successfully in most of those communities which have been in the forefront in providing services to victims of domestic violence.

Although domestic violence is an extremely serious and complex social problem in terms of both its causes and consequences, there are steps that individuals and communities can and must take in order to alleviate it. We have identified several of those approaches here. Violence is learned behavior, and the preponderance of evidence suggests that unless we actively take responsibility to assist people in *un*learning this maladaptive behavior pattern and eliminate the conditions giving rise to it, it will continue to take its toll on our families.

Notes

1. Whether there has been an increase in the rate of "wifebeating" or an increase in the rate of reporting of "wifebeating" appears to be an unanswerable, although important, question. There is little doubt that the changing social norms toward equality between the sexes have made being a victim less acceptable for abused women. At the same time, these social norms may be further undermining the ascribed power of otherwise powerless men, thus increasing their need to turn to what Straus, (1977b) refers to as the "ultimate resource" to reassert their power.

2. We have chosen to rely on the Straus, Gelles, and Steinmetz (1978) data for these statistics, as we believe that theirs is the first study which provides a data base which has been obtained using adequate methodological control.

3. Levinger (1966) found that 36 percent of the women seeking divorce in one large metropolitan area reported physical abuse as a complaint.

4. This discussion is a highly condensed summary of several aspects of the family which must be considered in the attempt to explain intrafamilial violence, and is based on a more extensive discussion by Gelles and Straus. See their chapter in Burr et al. (1979) for a more detailed elaboration of these issues.

5. The police, believing that charges brought by women in the heat of the argument or under the stress of the beating are less likely to result in court action than are charges brought after due consideration, tend to discourage attempts to take immediate action. They accomplish this through informal rules which prevent women from filing complaints against their husbands for anywhere from three to 14 days after the incident has occurred (until she has "cooled off").

6. The "stitch rule," informally applied in many localities, is that charges of abuse may not be brought unless the injury is sufficient to require medical action.

7. While this analysis draws heavily on Pfouts (1978), it goes beyond that study in explaining the theory and incorporating additional intervention implications.

References

Allen, C., & Straus, M.A. Resources, power, and husband-wife violence. In M.A. Straus & G.T. Hotaling (Eds.), *The Social Causes of Husband-Wife Violence.* Minneapolis: University of Minnesota Press, in press.

Aronson, E. *The Social Animal.* San Francisco: W.W. Freeman, 1972.

Bach, G.R., & Wyden, P. Why intimates must fight. In S.K. Steinmetz & M.A. Straus (Eds.), *Violence in the Family.* New York: Harper & Row, 1974.

Ball, M. Issues of violence in family casework. *Social Casework,* 1977, *58,* 3-12.

Bandura, A. *Aggression: A Social Learning Analysis.* Englewood Cliffs, NJ: Prentice-Hall, 1973.

Bard, M., & Zacker, J. The prevention of family violence: Dilemmas of community intervention. *Journal of Marriage and the Family*, 1971, *33*, 677-682.

Blechman, E.A., Olson, D.H.L., Schornagel, C.Y., Halsdorf, M. & Turner, A.J. The family contract game: Technique and case study. *Journal of Consulting and Clinical Psychology*, 1976, *44*, 449-455.

Burr, W.R., Hill, R., Nye, F.I., & Reiss, I.L. (Eds.). *Contemporary Theories about the Family*. New York: Free Press, 1979.

Carlson, B.E. Battered women and their assailants. *Social Work*, 1977, *22*, 455-460.

Coleman, D.H., & Straus, M.A. Alcohol abuse and family violence. Presented at the meeting of the American Sociological Association, February, 1979.

Flynn, J.P. Recent findings related to wife abuse. *Social Casework*, 1977, *58*, 13-20.

Ganley, A.L., & Harris, L. Domestic violence: Issues in designing and implementing programs for male batterers. Presented at the meeting of the American Psychological Association, Toronto, 1978.

Gelles, R.J. *The Violent Home: A Study of Physical Aggression Between Husbands and Wives*. Beverly Hills, CA: Sage, 1974.

Gelles, R.J. Violence and pregnancy: A note on the extent of the problem and needed services. *Family Coordinator*, 1975, *24*, 81-86.

Gelles, R.J. Abused wives: Why do they stay? *Journal of Marriage and the Family*, 1976, *38*, 659-668.

Gelles, R.J. No place to go: The social dynamics of marital violence. In M. Roy (Ed.), *Battered Women: A Psychosociological Study of Domestic Violence*. New York: Van Nostrand Reinhold, 1977.

Gelles, R.J. The myth of battered husbands—and new facts about family violence. *MS.*, 1979, *8*, 65-73.

Gelles, R.J., & Straus, M.A. Determinants of violence in the family: Toward a theoretical integration. In W.R. Burr, R. Hill, F.I. Nye, and I.L. Reiss (Eds.), *Contemporary Theories about the Family*. New York: Free Press, 1979.

Goode, W.J. Force and violence in the family. *Journal of Marriage and the Family*, 1971, *33*, 624-636.

Goode, W.J. Marital satisfaction and instability. In R. Bendix and S.M. Lipset (Eds.), *Class, Status and Power*. New York: Collier-Macmillan, 1966.

Hanks, S.E., & Rosenbaum, C.P. Battered women: A study of women who live with violent alcohol-abusing men. *American Journal of Orthopsychiatry*, 1977, *47*, 291-307.

Kaplan, A.G., & Bean, J.P. *Beyond Sex-Role Stereotypes: Readings Toward a Psychology of Androgyny*. Toronto: Little, Brown, 1976.

Levinger, G. Source of marital satisfaction among applicants for divorce. *American Journal of Orthopsychiatry*, 1966, *36*, 804-806.

Nichols, B.B. The abused wife problem. *Social Casework*, 1976, *57*, 27-32.

O'Brien, J.E. Violence in divorce-prone families. *Journal of Marriage and the Family*, 1969, *31*, 692-698.

Pfouts, J.H. Violent Families: Coping responses of abused wives. *Child Welfare*, 1978, *57*, 101-111.

Pincus, A., & Minahan, A. *Social Work Practice: Model and Method*. Itasca, IL: F.E. Peacock, 1973.

Pleck, E., Pleck, J., Grossman, M., & Bart, P. The battered data syndrome: A comment on Steinmetz's article. *Victimology: An International Journal*, 1977, *2*, 680-683.

Safilios-Rothschild, C. The study of family power structure: A review 1960-1969. *Journal of Marriage and the Family,* 1970, *32,* 539-551.

Saunders, D.G. Marital violence: Dimensions of the problem and modes of intervention. *Journal of Marriage and Family Counseling,* 1977, *3,* 43-52.

Sprey, J. The family as a system in conflict. *Journal of Marriage and the Family,* 1969, *31,* 699-705.

Stark, R., & McEvoy, J. III. Middle-class violence. *Psychology Today,* 1970, *4,* 52-65.

Straus, M.A. Sexual inequality, cultural norms, and wife beating. In E. Viano (Ed.), *Victims and Society.* Washington, DC: Visage Press, 1976.

Straus, M.A. A sociological perspective on the prevention and treatment of wife beating. In M. Roy (Ed.), *Battered Women.* New York: Van Nostrand Reinhold, 1977. (a)

Straus, M.A. Wife beating: How common and why? *Victomology: An International Journal,* 1977, *2,* 443-458. (b)

Straus, M.A. A sociological perspective on the causes of family violence. In M.R. Green (Ed.), *Violence and the American Family,* in press.

Straus, M.A., Gelles, R.J., & Steinmetz, S.K. Physical violence in a nationally representative sample of American families. Presented at the meeting of the 9th World Congress of Sociology, Uppsala, Sweden, August, 1978.

Thibaut, J.W., & Kelley, J.H. *The Social Psychology of Groups.* New York: John Wiley, 1959.

Tidmarsh, M. Violence in marriage. *Social Work Today,* 1976, *7,* 36-38.

Vincent, C.E. Familia spongia: The adaptive function. *Journal of Marriage and the Family,* 1966, *28,* 699-706.

Vinocur, J. Swedes shun Norse adage, ban spanking. New York *Times,* April 4, 1979.

Whitehurst, R.N. Violence in husband-wife interaction. In S.K. Steinmetz & M.A. Straus (Eds.), *Violence in the Family.* New York: Harper & Row, 1974.

4

Preventing Child Maltreatment

James Garbarino

Center for the Study of Youth Development,
The Pennsylvania State University

Introduction

In his treatise on the ecology of human development, Urie Bronfenbrenner (1979) recalls what he fondly refers to as "Dearborn's Maxim" in honor of his first mentor in graduate school, Walter Fenno Dearborn: "If you want to understand something, try to change it." Dearborn's Maxim speaks loudly to the topic of preventing child maltreatment. In fact, only by trying to change it *will* we understand it. The voluminous and evergrowing corpus of research, theory, clinical experience, and speculation concerning the origins and consequences of child abuse and neglect is testimony to this. Several good reviews of this field are available (Belsky, 1980; Friedman, 1976; Garbarino, 1977; Parke & Collmer, 1975; Polansky, 1976), and such a review is not intended here. Rather, my goal in this discussion is to ask how we can improve our understanding of child maltreatment by trying to prevent it. I think, given the very primitive state of the art when it comes to preventing child abuse and neglect, that the best bet is to consider some propositions about prevention and use them to organize what we know about maltreatment as a community mental health issue. I do this in the hope of enticing the reader into giving the prevention program implicit in these propositions a try, and with the full recognition that this topsy-turvy, cart-before-the-horse approach is not without dangers.

To summarize the conclusions with which I will begin, consider the following four propositions.

- *To prevent child maltreatment concentrate on its necessary conditions:* By removing or otherwise thwarting the necessary conditions for child abuse and neglect, the problem is effectively "disarmed." This implies the need to establish a community climate inimicable to the growth and maintenance of abusive and neglectful patterns of family life.

- *Concentrate on social rather than psychological forces:* The ethical and practical limitations of preventive efforts focused at individual psychologies are enormous. They effectively negate programs aimed at reforming individual personality through direct, one-to-one intervention. The strategy of preference seeks to generate countervailing social forces that can override the deficiencies of individual parents and children.

- *Preventing child maltreatment is inextricably linked to community development:* The front lines in preventing child abuse and neglect lie in efforts to humanize and reform those aspects of our culture and the broader socioeconomic system that undermine parental competence. In the absence of such social and cultural reform, such as is implicit in efforts to alter our ideology concerning the use of force as punishment and the concept of children as disposable property of their parents, conventional intervention programs are "doomed to failure."

- *To successfully prevent child maltreatment we must prevent the social impoverishment of families:* Social impoverishment refers to the isolation of families from potent, pro-social support systems, be that isolation imposed from the outside or initiated from the inside. Socially impoverished families are cut off from the *essential* nurturance and feedback that serve to support adults in the role of parent and to protect children.

In the course of this chapter I will seek to clarify and document the rationale for these four propositions. In so doing, I will draw upon the review articles cited above, new reports and projects currently in progress, and my own work in this area. The first step is to briefly review what I think we know about the origins of child maltreatment.

The Origins of Child Maltreatment

Child abuse and neglect are perhaps best thought of as indicators of families in trouble. As such, they reflect a mixed bag of causes and associations. There are many, far too many, factors that can place a family in jeopardy and lead to child maltreatment. This multiplicity of causes (actually, "sufficient conditions" in the sense of the term proposed by

Bronfenbrenner and Mahoney in 1975) complicates the task of understanding origins of maltreatment. Further complicating this task is the fact that there is no single unified definition of child maltreatment that is adequate for all uses and purposes. As Parke and Collmer (1975) note in their excellent review of the topic, "a variety of definitions of child abuse have been offered and none is free of ambiguities." With a plethora of independent variables and a somewhat uncertain dependent variable, the task of understanding the origins of maltreatment would be difficult enough. When the inordinate sampling difficulties associated with the problem are added, the result is a confusing welter of seemingly unrelated, inconsistent, and dubious findings (Friedman, 1976). I think that while no definition of child maltreatment can be adequate for all purposes, for the conceptual use to which it is being put in this review, the following definition will suffice: "Child maltreatment consists of acts of omission or comission by parents or guardians that are judged by a mixture of community values and professional expertise to be seriously inappropriate and damaging to the child." This definition is an attempt to combine science and culture as a source of standards with which to evaluate parent-child relations. A complete explication of the rationale for this decision is beyond this study's scope (for such a discussion see Garbarino, 1978), but the definition does underlie many of my thoughts about what is to be changed in a program of prevention.

As Pfohl (1977) has made clear, the process of dealing with child abuse and neglect is as much one of "discovering" it as it is of "recognizing" it. Just as the actual behaviors constituting abuse and neglect are indicators of impaired family functioning, so the community's ability to evaluate those behaviors and act to prevent developmental damage to children is an indicator of its ideology. A "pro-child" community sets and enforces high standards of child care by providing a social and economic climate for families in which the "natural" care-giving relationship between parents and children is stimulated, nurtured, and reinforced. Thus, a community's inability to prevent child maltreatment is an *ipso facto* indictment of its ideology and social structure. This view of prevention is consonant with Albee's recent formulation: "I suggest that in primary prevention we attempt to *prevent* the arbitrary use of power in ways that damage others or reduce their opportunities" (Albee, 1979: 26). In this sense, child maltreatment is always a misuse of parental power. As we shall see, however, it is often linked to a misuse of institutional power as well.

With this in mind, I see five principal "causes" of child maltreatment: psychopathology, temperamental incompatibility, perverse family dynamics, interpersonal deficiencies, and culturally based inappropriate attitudes and expectations about child rearing and child development.

Psychopathology plays a role in some cases of child maltreatment. Although classifiable psychiatric disorders appear to be present in only a small proportion of the cases (the most commonly cited figure being 10 percent), borderline and marginal personality disorders are common among certain classes of abuse and neglect cases. "Sick parents" are a small, albeit important, part of the overall problem. When parents are not able to function normally because of mental illness, alcoholism, or drug abuse, their children are at risk. Caring for a child is a challenging proposition in any circumstance, but for a parent with impaired ability to cope with life it may be overwhelming. Even among abusive and neglectful parents, however, most are within the normal range. Neglecting parents seem particularly prone to what one investigator has called "the apathy futility syndrome" (Polansky, 1976), while abusers may be subject to some sort of "aggressive-impulsive syndrome" (Spinetta and Rigler, 1972).

Temperamental incompatibility seems to play a role in some cases. To match a parent with a hypersensitivity to infant crying with a colicky baby is to ask for trouble. Such a parent-child dyad may well be at much greater risk for abuse than a couple not so temperamentally mismatched. Likewise, to pair a lethargic and passive infant with a parent prone to neglect is much more likely to result in inadequate care than would be the case if the child were temperamentally inclined to activity and attention-seeking. The scope and precise interrelationship of these temperamental characteristics is a largely unexplored area.

Perverse family dynamics seem to play an important role in many cases of abuse and neglect. Families involved in mistreatment appear to become enmeshed in patterns of interaction that reinforce whatever destructive elements are present in the family. Burgess and Conger (1978) found that families involved in mistreatment had half the level of overall interaction, twice the propensity to respond to negative behavior, and half the likelihood of responding to positive behavior than were similar families not involved in mistreatment. Giblin and his associates (1978) found that when parents neglect their children, the children show affective deficits as a result. The scanty available research dealing with the abuse of adolescents (Garbarino, 1980c; Garbarino and Carson, 1979; Garbarino and Gilliam, 1980; Lourie, 1977) suggests that families with marginal coping skills built into their everyday patterns of interaction are most likely to fail at adolescence when the challenges to the social system of the family raised by the child's developmental changes are greatest. In sum, it seems that inadequate interactional patterns within families establish a climate of vulnerability which may easily slide into abuse and neglect.

When adults are deficient in the basic social skills of human interaction they are at greater risk for becoming involved in mistreating their children. From a variety of sources comes the proposition that lack of empathy is one of the best predictors of parental risk for abuse and neglect. Gray (1978) found that inadequate empathy was characteristic of parents who succumb to social stress and abuse children. Bavolek and his colleagues (1977) reported that the factor most distinguishing adolescent victims of mistreatment was poor ability to empathize. Many of the characteristics attributed to abusive parents (such as role reversal, intolerance, and impulsiveness) can be subsumed within the broader problem of inadequate empathy. In their study of the life course of neglecting parents, Polansky and his colleagues (1979) found a persistent record of inability to relate in normal social relationships. Clearly, deficient basic social skills are at the heart of many mental health problems, including child maltreatment, and often deficient patterns within the family parallel deficiencies in relating outside the family.

The abuse and neglect problem can neither be understood nor dealt with as simply a problem of individuals, however. Culturally based inappropriate attitudes and expectations about child rearing and child development play an essential role. They provide fertile soil in which individual problems can grow to become abusive and neglectful family relationships. They stimulate abuse and neglect by presenting a false picture of the world to parents. Naturally, individuals differ in the extent to which they partake of this "cultural poison." Indeed, historical progress in the treatment of children derives in large part from the efforts of those who transcend the poisonous aspects of their cultures to see their way clear to articulate and advance the legitimate needs of children for nurturance and a sense of support. In his cross- and trans-cultural study, Rohner (1975) finds that rejection is a universal threat to psychosocial development and mental health. Although cultures differ in the extent to which children are rejected and in the modalities in which this rejection is expressed, rejection is a psychologically malignant force. Rohner's findings, coupled with those of anthropologist Jill Korbin (1977), strongly suggest that when society's values lend support to social structures that isolate the parent-child relationship from "outside" adults with an enduring interest in the welfare of the child, abuse and neglect is more likely. Thus, to the extent that a culture places full and undivided responsibility for children in the hands of individual and isolated parents, it sets up those families for abuse and neglect (Korbin, 1977). This cultural support for an unrealistic concept of child rearing is exacerbated in many cases by the ideology supporting the use of force in interpersonal relations. Nonviolence makes good developmental sense, and a culture that endorses domestic violence is in the wrong. In a cultural climate poisoned in this way, the individual deficiencies of parents conspire with social experiences to place children in jeopardy. This is the overriding theme implicit in the available knowledge on the origins of child maltreatment. It provides the starting point for efforts to prevent abuse and neglect. It is to these efforts, as embodied in the four principles outlined at the start of this discussion, I turn next.

To Prevent Child Maltreatment, Prevent Social Impoverishment

I am not alone in thinking that conventional, individually oriented prevention programs will prove ineffective, that they are "doomed to failure" (Zigler, 1979). The history of efforts to develop and employ "screening" instruments to identify and thus provide a basis for intervening with individual families speaks to this point (Newberger and Daniel, 1979). While clinicians assert their ability to reliably and validly identify parents who either are at high risk for mistreating their children or who actually have done so, the available evidence belies this claim, particularly if one hopes to extrapolate from small-scale studies to massive prevention programs. Richard Light (1973) provided what may well be a definitive critique of the very concept of using comprehensive developmental screening to identify (setting aside the question of preventing) child abuse. He notes that because of the low overall base rate of the phenomenon in question (approximately one percent to four percent of the population), even a remarkably reliable instrument will generate a preponderance of false-positives, cases inaccurately "diagnosed" as child abuse. Figure 4.1 presents this thesis in simplified form. In the example given, using a base rate of four percent (an upper limit estimate according to most experts) even a 90 percent-accurate instrument would generate nearly three times as many false-positives (that is, nonabusive families who were "diagnosed" as abusive) as it would true-positives (that is, abusive families who were so diagnosed). As Light correctly points out, the effects of such a screening program on the nonabusive families might totally eliminate its ethical and practical merits. Unless the response to such a screening process were highly supportive and nonjudgmental, one would run the risk of pushing families into abuse merely by falsely "accusing" them of it.

FIGURE 4.1   Screening for Child Abuse in 1000 Children*

Actual Status

	Abusive (N=40)	Nonabusive (N=960)
Identified as:		
Abusive	36	96
	(true positives)	(false positives)
Nonabusive	4	864
	(false negatives)	(true negatives)

*Assuming a 4% prevalence rate and a 90% accurate instrument.

If Light's analysis shows us the problems of diagnosing abuse even after it has occurred, then the efforts spearheaded by Ray Helfer (1978) to develop a simple questionnaire-like screening instrument to identify high-risk parents before they abuse their children testifies to the problems of prevention when individuals are screened. Among other things, Helfer's group found that it was impossible to assign scores to some 40 percent of their abusive test subjects because these individuals tended to respond inconsistently. Overall, when efforts were made to validate the screening instrument on a broadly based sample of American parents, so many parents were classified as high risk as to make the procedure unusable for anything but the most generalized and nondiscriminating intervention programs. Helfer himself has concluded that a broadly based preventive program aimed generally at parents with the intent of improving their child-rearing skills is the best bet, given the limitations of individual screening.

I would expand upon these criticisms in a more categorical way. The precipitating or sufficient conditions for child abuse are many, and no program aimed at eliminating them will succeed without a massive intrusion and comprehensive intervention into the lives of the many individuals who appear "at high risk" for child abuse. Even Gray's results (1978), which document the role of inadequate empathy in mediating the effects of social conditions among child abusers, do not really offer hope of primary prevention.

Because of the practical and moral problems implicit in preventing anything so specific and relatively rare as each particular form of child abuse, no program will be cost effective (if it is effective at all) if it seeks a piecemeal solution to the problem. I think a better approach is one that focuses on the necessary rather than the sufficient conditions for child maltreatment. I have outlined the empirical and theoretical rationale for this approach elsewhere (Garbarino, 1977). It boils down to this: How can we effectively disarm or defuse the sufficient conditions for child abuse and neglect? How can we remove the fertile medium within which these predisposing factors operate? While scientific specification of necessary conditions is an extremely difficult task, and one that is rarely accomplished, for heuristic and even public policy purposes, I think we can identify at least two such necessary conditions.

For child maltreatment to occur—or at least for it to be maintained and produce long-term developmental damage to children—the individual deficiencies of parents must be set within a social and cultural context that is characterized by social isolation and antichild values. Such a context simultaneously legitimatizes the destruction of children and provides the social structure in which that destruction can take place unimpeded by whatever pro-child forces that do exist. For example, children seem to be at greatest risk for destructive maltreatment when the values of non-familial adults in their environment emphasize family privacy, parental autonomy, the authoritative use of force in socialization, and the concept of the child as chattel. When coupled with an environment deficient in adults who have an enduring and informed relationship with the child as well as with the parents, these factors almost ensure that when parental functioning is impaired—be it through alcohol misuse, psychopathology, social stress, or any of a host of "personality" characteristics—children will be damaged. For this reason, there are "ecological niches" within our society in which child maltreatment in all its forms flourishes. The principal goal of a prevention program is to reduce and hopefully eliminate the conditions that underlie such destructive ecological niches.

It is in this sense that preventing child maltreatment is inextricably linked to community development. Rather than focusing our efforts on "training" parents we should direct our attention to "training" the processes of social change through which the cultural and structural necessary conditions for child maltreatment are created and maintained. In this sense, child advocacy is synonymous with child protection, and both are related to the development of a pro-child and nurturing community. The process involved is a social parallel to applied behavioral analysis. That is, just as applied behavioral analysis seeks to examine the contingencies in interaction that generate and sustain problematic patterns of behavior, so this preventive approach (applied *social* analysis) seeks to alter the contingencies in community development. We need to provide norms and structures incompatible with antichild and socially impoverished family life. All aspects of the community can play a role. The mass media have an obligation to provide a climate which reinforces nonviolent resolution of conflict and promotes high standards of child care. In such a context, individual decisions can be expected to bend in the direction of the overarching principles articulated in the media. Individual recommendations (such as to avoid spanking, to reinforce positive behavior by the child, to reach out to isolated individuals, and to offer and accept help freely) will gain credence if such a media context is established. This credence function has been demonstrated with respect to Parents Anonymous.

The mass media are not alone in such a conception of prevention, however. Each significant element of the institutional life of the community must be involved. Thus, for example, governmental decisions affecting neighborhood life must be made with an eye to their consequences for parent-child relations and the social connectiveness of families. My own research suggests quite strongly that economically comparable neighborhoods can present radically divergent contexts for parent-child relations, in some measure because of institutional decisions that conspire with individual predilections to produce a socially disorganized and unsupportive social context (Garbarino, 1976, 1980a; Garbarino and Crouter, 1978a, 1978b; Garbarino and Sherman, 1980).

This research sought to validate the concept of "social impoverishment" as a characteristic of high-risk family environments. It was designed to identify the environmental correlates of child maltreatment which provided an empirical basis for "screening" neighborhoods to identify high- and low-risk areas. Multiple regression analyses were used to illuminate two meanings of high risk (Garbarino and Crouter, 1978a). The first, of course, refers to areas with a high absolute rate of child maltreatment (based on cases per unit of population). In this sense, concentrations of socioeconomically distressed families are most likely to be high risk for child maltreatment. SES accounts for about 40 percent of the variation across neighborhoods (defined grossly as census tracts).

It is the second meaning that is of greatest interest here, however. High risk can also be taken to mean that an area has a higher rate of child maltreatment than would be predicted knowing its socioeconomic character. Thus, two areas with similar socioeconomic (and even demographic) profiles may have very different rates of child maltreatment. In this sense, one is "high-risk" while the other is "low-risk," although both may have higher rates of child maltreatment than other, more affluent areas. Already available data were assembled to provide a preliminary and gross test of the hypothesis that neighborhoods identified as high risk using this strategy were indeed "socially impoverished" (Garbarino et al., 1977). The next step in this research program was to examine a pair of neighborhoods, one high risk and the other low risk for child maltreatment, matched on socioeconomic characteristics to test the hypothesis that the two neighborhoods present contrasting environments for child rearing. Relative to the low-risk area, the high-risk neighborhood was hypothesized to represent a socially impoverished human ecology. It did (Garbarino and Sherman, 1980).

What emerged from the data was the conclusion that those who need the most tend to be clustered together in settings that must struggle most to meet those needs. The picture that emerged from the high-risk area was one of very "needy" families competing for scarce social resources. The very high level of need compounded the problem of scarce social resources, of course. In their studies of informal helping networks, Collins and Pancoast (1976) used the concept "free from drain" to describe people who can afford to give and share. These people can afford to give and share because the balance of needs and resources markedly favors the latter. The low-risk area seemed "free from drain" in many respects. We found that people "keep up" their houses and their families. Therefore, they can afford to become involved in neighborly exchange without fear of exploitation (and they do so, according to our data). Houses and families are much more "run down" in the high-risk neighborhood. In such a stressful environment, we believe that parents are inclined to seek an advantage by getting all they can from others while giving as little as they can get away with. There is ambivalence about neighborly exchanges and a recognition that, overall, the neighborhood exerts a negative effect on families (as illustrated by interviews with mothers in which they gave a low rating to the neighborhood as a place to raise children and reported on the lack of interaction among the children).

From our perspective, the high-risk neighborhood presents a disturbing picture. In many respects it resembles what Pavenstedt (1967) described in her study of "the drifters: children of disorganized lower-class families"; what Elmer (1977) observed in her longitudinal study of child maltreatment; and what Maccoby and her colleagues (1958) saw in their comparison of two neighborhoods, one high risk for juvenile delinquency, the other low risk. We found that families in the high-risk neighborhood are struggling. The observations of our expert informants made it clear that family life is threatened from within and without. Our conclusion would match that offered by the mothers. The high-risk neighborhood is *not* a good place to bring up children. A family's own problems seemed to be compounded rather than ameliorated by the neighborhood context, dominated as it is by other needy families. Whatever the characteristics of individuals, the neighborhood seemed to set in motion negative "progressive conformity" (as Moos, 1976, uses that term to describe social climate).

Under such circumstances strong support systems are most needed, but least likely to operate, of course. The high-risk area needs outside intervention to increase its capacity to fend for itself and to strengthen families as a way of reducing the demands they place on already tenuous informal helping networks. The irony, of course, is that it is usually just such needy families and neighborhoods that are hardest to serve and organize, as the experience of our expert informants makes clear.

We augmented our case study with data from two other sources. The first included socioeconomic and demographic information obtained from the U.S. Census Bureau and local governmental sources, plus the results of a survey conducted by the Center for Applied Urban Analysis at the University of Nebraska at Omaha. The second source of data was an interview study of family stresses and supports we conducted for other purposes. We found that a neighborhood's "risk score" (the difference between actual and predicted child maltreatment rates) was uncorrelated with the battery of socioeconomic and demographic factors that usually account for variance among families (National Academy of Sciences, 1976). The algebraic origins of the risk score would themselves tend to produce this finding, of course. But they are worth noting in any case because they focus attention on the fact that in discussing neighborhood risk we are *not* simply examining socioeconomic factors under an assumed name. The risk factor operates independently of conventional socioeconomic variables.

We found that the risk score was associated with important aspects of family stresses and supports as perceived and reported by mothers in the interview study. The neighborhood risk score was found to be significantly and negatively correlated with the overall rating of the neighborhood as a place to raise children made by parents living in that neighborhood ($r = -.61$, $p < .001$), *even after controlling for family income and structure.* The less "risky" the neighborhood, the more positively mothers in that neighborhood rated it as a context in which to rear children. This finding was based on a sample of 13 neighborhoods in which we had conducted a total of 87 family interviews. In human terms, it suggests that parents are sensitive to the way neighborhood factors establish a particular climate for families and parent-child relations, that there really is a *community* psychology at work. Once again, this relationship is independent of major conventional socioeconomic and demographic indices. A second finding from this analysis merits noting. The interview provides an indication of a family's use of preventive and recreational community services (for example, the Boy Scouts) as opposed to treatment and rehabilitative services (such as the Family Service Association). The neighborhood risk score is significantly correlated with the use of treatment versus preventive services ($r = .52$, $p < .05$). The more risky the neighborhood, the more families report involvements with treatment rather than preventive agencies. This finding provides further support for the hypothesis that the risk score is an index of neighborhood social quality. High-risk neighborhoods are socially impoverished neighborhoods.

In this hypothesis Kromkowski's (1976) analysis of neighborhood quality is called to mind.

> The organic life of a neighborhood, created by the persons who live in a particular geographic area, is always a fragile reality. A neighborhood's character is determined by a host of factors, but most significantly by the kinds of relationships that neighbors have with each other. A neighborhood is not a sovereign power—it can rarely write its own agenda. Although neighborhoods differ in a host of ways, a healthy neighborhood has some sort of cultural and institutional network which manifests itself in pride in the neighborhood, care of homes, security for children, and respect for each other [Kromkowski, 1976: 228].

To engage in such primary prevention, professional human services must be redirected, in part, out of the one-to-one intervention and rehabilitation mode into a community consultation role. The "clients" are social networks and neighborhoods. To do this, they must be able to identify "high-risk" *neighborhoods* (rather than focus exclusively on high-risk individuals). Such high-risk areas have more than their share of socially impoverished families and exacerbate rather than compensate for those families' own individual deficiencies. They stand in contrast to "low-risk" neighborhoods in which the social structure is strong enough to protect both children and parents and to provide support for nurturant and effective family functioning. Professionals need to stand as liaison between existing, informal, helping resources ("natural helping networks") and the broader community. My associates and I have tried to develop the rationale for doing so, as well as some specific suggestions for both conducting such a needs assessment and providing the requisite "consultation" services (see Garbarino et al., 1980).

A preventive orientation to child maltreatment requires further that we look at family formation as an opportunity to alter social roles and expectations as a way of preventing the primary villains in this matter, namely, social impoverished and antichild ideologies. One of the most promising of these opportunities lies in viewing childbirth as a social event. To see childbirth as a social event is to recognize that beyond the physiological and psychological processes involved, the roles and status afforded the participants have an effect upon the developmental outcomes. Specifically, a family-centered approach to childbirth in which parents are given active, high-status roles can produce more physiologically and psychologically healthy family beginnings, a more healthy child and mother, a more intimately and effectively active father, and, still further, a better connection between the health care systems and the individual families. Promoting family-centered childbirth can be one of the corner-stones of a community program to prevent maltreatment (Garbarino, 1980b). Normally hard-to-reach families may be unusually accessible at this critical juncture (Gray et al., 1977). They may be more willing and more able to form connections with professional support systems and, where they are provided, volunteer family aides (Olds, 1980). By enmesh-ing families in such a nurturant and protective set of relationships, when they are most vulnerable to them, the overarching goal of primary preven-tion may be advanced. The latent antichild ideology in our culture may be overcome and replaced with a more nurturant pro-child ideology. At the same time, the structural problems associated with social impoverishment may be dealt with in a constructive manner, all without the potentially destructive effects of any screening and "diagnosis-oriented" program such as has been the foundation of other proposals. The "personality" deficits associated with inadequate empathy may be replaced with greater interper-sonal competence through changed patterns of social roles.

A related but different approach is to focus on the potential of adolescent peer groups as agents for preventing child maltreatment. Much has been said about the need for parent education in our schools. How-ever, there are good reasons to question the effectiveness of conventional parent education as primary prevention (see Bronfenbrenner, 1978). By incorporating efforts aimed at humanizing and better linking adolescent peer networks to pro-child values through nurturant adults, our preventive goals may be advanced, however. First, maltreatment contemporaneous with adolescence may be uncovered and dealt with (see Garbarino and Jacobson, 1978). What is more, however, the social impoverishment characterizing youths in trouble may be overcome. Polansky and his colleagues (1979) report that neglecting parents have a history of social isolation and social inability, extending backward into adolescence. By tackling this problem through a systematic approach to integrating peer networks into pro-child values and family life education, these alienated youths may be reached before they become parents. Once they assume the parental role, the characteristic expression of their social impoverishment is child neglect and abuse. Once again, we see here the opportunity for a preventive approach that does not require labeling and discriminatory intervention, but rather seeks to build the collective resources of the community in such a way that they will "naturally" provide care for children and protect them from harm. This proposal receives support from recent successful efforts to curb child abuse among apes in captivity by fostering social integration and peer groups of young simian mothers (Nadler, 1979; Rock, 1978).

Arthur Emlen has spoken of the need to evaluate our communities and, in fact, the individual lives of children in terms of the plentitude of "protective behaviors" in their immediate environments. Prevention in this sense is a form of "empowering the child." This brings us back to Albee's conception of prevention: "I suggest that in primary prevention we attempt to *prevent* the arbitrary use of power in ways that damage others or reduce their opportunities." I agree. To prevent child abuse we must empower children by socially enriching their environments. In so doing, we will enhance their mental health and their overall developmental well-being. We must also empower pro-child elements in the community, for these individuals and groups provide the necessary nurturance and feedback that constitute support systems for individual parents (see Caplan, 1974). There is a "social sanitation" job that needs doing. As the child is father to the man, so the community is parent to the child.

References

Albee, G. Politics, power, prevention and social change. Presented at the Vermont Conference on the Primary Prevention of Psychopathology, June, 1979.

Bavolek, S., Kline, D., McLaughlin, Jr., & Publicover, P. *The Development of the Adolescent Parenting Inventory (API): Identification of High Risk Adolescents Prior to Parenthood.* Logan: Utah State University, Department of Special Education, 1977.

Belsky, J. Child abuse in ecological perspective. *American Psychologist,* 1980, *35,* 320-335.

Bronfenbrenner, U. Who needs parent education? *Teachers College Record,* 1978, *79,* 767-787.

Bronfenbrenner, U. *The Ecology of Human Development.* Cambridge, MA: Harvard University Press, 1979.

Bronfenbrenner, U., & Mahoney, M. The structure and verification of hypotheses. In U. Bronfenbrenner & M. Mahoney (Eds.), *Influences on Human Development.* Hinsdale, IL: Dryden Press, 1975.

Burgess, R., & Conger, R. Family interaction patterns in abusive neglectful and normal families. *Child Development,* 1978, *49,* 163-173.

Caplan, G. *Support Systems and Community Mental Health.* New York: Behavioral Publications, 1974.

Collins, A., & Pancoast, D. *Natural Helping Networks.* Washington, DC: National Association of Social Workers, 1976.

Daniel, J., Newberger, E., Reed, R., & Kotelchick. Child abuse screening: Implications of the limited predictive power of abuse discriminants from a controlled family study of pediatric social illness. *Child Abuse and Neglect,* 1978, *2,* 247-260.

Elmer, E. A follow-up study of traumatized children. *Pediatrics*, 1977, *59*, 273-279.

Friedman, R. Child abuse: A review of the psychosocial research. In Herner et al. (Eds.), *Four Perspectives on the Status of Child Abuse and Neglect Research.* Washington, DC: National Center on Child Abuse and Neglect, 1976.

Garbarino, J. A preliminary study of some ecological correlates of child abuse: The impact of socioeconomic stress on mothers. *Child Development*, 1976, *47*, 178-185.

Garbarino, J. The human ecology of child maltreatment: A conceptual model for research. *Journal of Marriage and Family*, 1977, *39*, 721-736.

Garbarino, J. The elusive "crime" of emotional abuse. *Child Abuse and Neglect*, 1978, *2*, 89-100.

Garbarino, J. An ecological perspective on child maltreatment. In L. Pelton (Ed.) *The Social Context of Child Abuse and Neglect.* New York: Human Sciences Press, 1980. (a)

Garbarino, J. Changing hospital policies and practices concerning childbirth: A developmental perspective on child maltreatment. *American Journal of Orthopsychiatry*, 1980, *50*. (b)

Garbarino, J. Meeting the needs of mistreated youth. *Social Work*, 1980, *25*, 122-127. (c)

Garbarino, J., & Carson, B. Mistreated youth vs. abused children. Center for the Study of Youth Development. Boys Town, NE, 1979. (unpublished)

Garbarino, J., & Crouter, A. Defining the community context of parent-child relations: The correlates of child maltreatment. *Child Development*, 1978, *49*, 604-616. (a)

Garbarino, J., & Crouter, A. A note on the problem of construct validity in assessing the usefulness of child maltreatment report data. *American Journal of Public Health*, 1978, *68*, 598-599. (b)

Garbarino, J., & Gilliam, G. *Understanding Abusive Families.* Lexington, MA: D.C. Heath, 1980.

Garbarino, J., & Jacobson, N. Youth-Helping-Youth as a resource in meeting the problem of child maltreatment. *Child Welfare*, 1978, *57*, 505-512.

Garbarino, J., & Sherman, D. High-risk families and high-risk neighborhoods: Studying the ecology of child maltreatment. *Child Development*, 1980, *51*, 188-198.

Garbarino, J., Crouter, A., & Sherman, D. Screening neighborhoods for intervention: A research model for child protective services. *Journal of Social Service Research*, 1978, *1*, 135-145.

Garbarino, J., Stocking, H., & Associates. *Protecting Children from Abuse and Neglect.* San Francisco: Jossey-Bass, 1980.

Giblin, P., Starr, R., & Agronow, S. A comparison of abused and control children: Influence on parent and child attitudinal and behavioral variables on children's responsivity. 1978. (unpublished)

Gray, C. *Empathy and Stress: Their Role in Child Abuse.* Doctoral dissertation, University of Maryland, 1978.

Gray, J., Cutler, C., Dean, J., & Kempe, C.H. Prediction and prevention of child abuse and neglect. *Child Abuse and Neglect*, 1977, *1*, 45-58.

Helfer, R. *Report on the Research Using the Michigan Screening Profile of Parenting (MSPP).* Washington, DC: National Center on Child Abuse and Neglect, 1978.

Korbin, J. Anthropological contributions to the study of child abuse. *Child Abuse and Neglect*, 1977, *1*, 7-24.

Kromkowski, J. *Neighborhood Deterioration and Juvenile Crime.* U.S. Department of Commerce, National Technical Information Service, PB-260 473. Indiana: The South Bend Urban Observatory, August, 1976.

Light, R. Abused and neglected children in America: A study of alternative policies. *Harvard Educational Review,* 1973, *43,* 556-598.

Lourie, I. The phenomenon of the abused adolescent: A clinical study. *Victimology,* 1977, *2,* 268-276.

Maccoby, E., Johnson, J., & Church, R. Community integration and the social control of juvenile delinquency. *Journal of Social Issues,* 1958, *14,* 38-51.

Moos, R. Evaluation and changing community settings. *American Journal of Community Psychology,* 1976, *4,* 313-326.

Nadler, R. Child abuse in gorilla mothers. *Caring,* 1979, *5,* 1-3.

National Academy of Sciences. *Toward a National Policy for Child and Families.* Washington, DC: U.S. Government Printing Office, 1976.

Newberger, E., & Daniel, J. Knowledge and epidemiology of child abuse: A critical review of concepts. In R. Bourne & E. Newberger (Eds.), *Critical Perspectives on Child Abuse.* Lexington, MA: D.C. Heath, 1979.

Olds, D. Improving formal services to mothers and children. In J. Garbarino, S.H. Stocking et al. (Eds.), *Protecting Children from Abuse and Neglect.* San Francisco: Jossey-Bass, 1980.

Parke, R., & Collmer, C.W. Child abuse: An interdisciplinary analysis. In E.M. Hetherington (Ed.), *Review of Child Development Research, Vol. 5.* Chicago: University of Chicago Press, 1975.

Pavenstedt, E. *The Drifters: Children of Disorganized Lower-Class Families.* Boston: Little, Brown, 1967.

Pfohl, S. The "discovery" of child abuse. *Social Problems,* 1977, *24,* 310-323.

Polansky, N. Analysis of research on child neglect: The social work viewpoint: In Herner and Company (Eds.), *Four Perspectives on the Status of Child Abuse and Neglect Research.* Washington, DC: National Center on Child Abuse and Neglect, 1976.

Polansky, N., Chalmers, M., Buttenwieser, W., & Williams, D. The isolation of the neglectful family. *American Journal of Orthopsychiatry,* 1979, *49,* 149-152.

Rock, M. Gorilla mothers need some help from their friends. Smithsonian, 1978, *9* (4), 58-63.

Rohner, R. *They Love Me, They Love Me Not.* New Haven, CT: HRAF Press, 1975.

Spinetta, J.J., & Rigler, D. The child-abusing parent: A psychological review. *Psychological Bulletin,* 1972, *77,* 296-304.

Zigler, E. Controlling child abuse in America: An effort doomed to failure? In R. Bourne & E. Newberger (Eds.), *Critical Perspectives on Child Abuse.* Lexington, MA: D.C. Heath, 1979.

5

Children of Divorce, Stressful Life Events, and Transitions
A Framework for Preventive Efforts

Robert D. Felner
Stephanie S. Farber
Judith Primavera
Yale University

In recent years the need to develop effective strategies for the prevention of new cases of emotional disorder has become a matter of increasing concern. Dissatisfaction with the distribution and efficacy, of traditional, reconstructive approaches to mental health service delivery (Cowen et al., 1967), combined with the recognition that both manpower and financial resources are, indeed, limited (Albee, 1959), have contributed to an increased awareness that intervention efforts need to be refocused and new frameworks for conceptualizing and attacking such problems developed. Under the broad rubric of "primary prevention" a number of innovative approaches attempting to reduce the incidence of new disorders and enhance competency have been advanced. Cowen (1978) has argued that the focus of primary preventive efforts must be the understanding and modification of "impactful social systems" (p. 21) and the development and implementation of competency training, particularly for children (Cowen, in press). Heller (1979) and Gottlieb and Hall (1980) have stressed the importance of social support systems for preventive efforts. Still others (Bloom, 1979; Dohrenwend, 1978; Goldston, 1977b) have urged that preventive intervention programs be organized around the

The authors wish to thank Lisa G. Martin for her invaluable assistance in the preparation of this chapter.

mastery of stressful life events or life crises by individuals who experience them.

While these positions may, on the surface, appear to be distinct, and for the purpose of conceptual and empirical clarity may need to be presented separately, when applied to the development of primary prevention frameworks and programs they are, indeed, complementary. If, as Goldston (1978) has suggested, primary prevention efforts "must be characterized by *specific* actions directed at *specific* populations for *specific* purposes" (p. 27), then knowledge about social systems, support systems and individual competencies may serve to shape our actions while the understanding of stressful life events and their mastery may inform our goals and target populations. In this same vein, Dohrenwend (1978) has pointed to the need for a clear understanding of those personal, situational, and environmental variables which mediate an individual's response to a stressful life event.

In the first section of this chapter we will examine paradigms that have been employed for viewing the consequences of stressful life events and the processes by which individuals cope with them. Particular attention will be paid to those components which can serve to inform the organization of research and preventive intervention programs. Following that, we will discuss the impact of one such stressful event, parental divorce, on children who experience it. The framework developed for understanding stressful life events will guide an examination of the state of knowledge of those factors which may exacerbate or mitigate the impact of parental divorce on children. Current preventive efforts for children of divorce will be examined, and finally, we will elaborate on the strengths and limitations of a stressful life events approach to preventive programming and sugggest future directions for research.

Stressful Life Events

Two primary approaches have been employed in examining the impact of stressful life events on the individuals who experience them. One line of this research has focused on the relationship between the individual's experience of a number of recent life events and his or her current level of physical or emotional well-being. The second approach has examined the process by which individuals cope with particular, discrete life events. In the former approach, a number of scales have been developed for adults and children which attempt to assign stress weights to various life events (Coddington, 1972; Holmes & Rahe, 1967; Hough et al., 1976; Monaghan et al., 1979). A summary score of the total amount of stress the individual has recently experienced is, in turn, related to indices of psychological or physical disorder (Holmes & Masuda, 1974). While such work has been important for focusing attention on stressful life events as factors which may predispose an individual to emotional or physical disorders, Rabkin and Streuning (1976) pointed out that the correlations between stress and illness reported in the majority of these studies fall below .30 and have called for caution in their interpretation.

A major limitation of this approach is its failure to consider that individuals are not equally stressed by similar events. For example, for one individual a geographic relocation or job change may be highly stressful, while another may handle these events with relative ease, experiencing only moderate levels of stress. Recently, several authors have begun to recognize the need for such life event research to examine individual differences in the perception of and the response to similar events (Dohrenwend, 1978; Sarason et al., 1978). At least one stressful life events inventory has been developed which attempts to take into account not only the occurrence of a particular event but also its recency and the individual's perception of its desirability and impact (Sarason et al., 1978). In addition, other researchers have begun to try to identify situational and personal variables which may influence an individual's ability to cope with similar levels of stress. An examination of these variables may help to explain why two individuals with similar stress scores exhibit very different reactions, one displaying emotional or physical disorder and the other showing no such problem. For example, Kobasa (1979) examined differences in personality and event perception between two groups who had experienced similarly high levels of stress over a three-year interval as measured by the Holmes and Rahe (1967) Schedule of Recent Life Events but who displayed differing levels of physical illness. She concluded that individuals with higher degrees of feelings of personal control, social commitment, and perception of change as a challenge were better able to cope with the stress of such life events than those who scored lower on these dimensions.

An approach that explores the cumulative impact of stress which may result from multiple life events in an individual's history is assuredly helpful in both highlighting target populations toward whom preventive efforts may be addressed and in clarifying some of the processes which facilitate an individual's efforts to cope with stress. However, since this approach is primarily concerned with the identification of highly stressed individuals and the factors which influence their level of stress rather than with the management of stressful life events per se, it may not be the most fruitful tactic for those interested in developing primary prevention programming in this area.

A second approach for organizing preventive efforts around stressful life events focuses on identifying particular discrete life events which place those who experience them at high risk for emotional disorder and/or physical illness. This approach is based in part on the work described above which points to the role of stressful life factors in predisposing an individual to emotional and/or physical dysfunction. It also draws heavily from crisis theory which states that interventions keyed to central life points can reduce the incidence of emotional disturbance (Goldston, 1977a). Goldston (1977b), in defining primary prevention, argues that the ultimate goal of such programs is "to increase people's capacities for dealing with crises and for taking steps to improve their own lives" (p. 20). Life crises are thought to place demands on individuals which exceed their ability to handle them with normal coping resources (Caplan, 1964). Such life crises are believed to produce a heightened vulnerability to the development of enduring maladaptation as well as the potential for rapid psychological growth (Caplan, 1964; Goldston, 1978; Lindemann, 1956). In an attempt to help guide the organization of preventive efforts from this perspective, Bloom (1979) has outlined the following paradigm:

1. Identify a stressful life event that appears to have undesirable consequences in a significant proportion of the population. Develop procedures for reliably identifying persons who have undergone or who are undergoing that stressful experience.

2. By traditional epidemiological and laboratory methods, study the consequences of that event and develop hypotheses related to how one might go about reducing or eliminating the negative consequences of the event.

3. Mount and evaluate experimental preventive intervention programs based on these hypotheses [Bloom, 1979: 183].

Procedures for identifying potentially targetable stressful life events are relatively straightforward. One may focus on pinpointing predictable transition points or normative crises in individuals' lives which are potential periods of heightened stress. For example, kindergarten entry, promotion to high school, or retirement may all be viewed as normative life crises. The identification of events classified as normative life crises may "proceed by informal observation or by deductions from the analysis of changing role performance requirements in the developing individual" (Bloom, 1978: 83).

The examination of epidemiological data may also help in identifying stressful life events by highlighting high-frequency events which occur at unpredictable times in an individual's life. These events may precipitate "accidental" crises (Caplan, 1964) and concomitant physical or emotional dysfunction.

The second and third steps that Bloom (1979) suggests are not as easily dealt with as the first. While investigators may rather easily identify some of the gross consequences of an event by comparing groups of individuals who have experienced that event to similar groups who have not on a variety of criterion measures, all individuals do not respond to an event in the same fashion or to the same extent. Some individuals cope well with an event, displaying little evidence of trauma, while others experience serious emotional or physical difficulties as a consequence.

In order to understand the differential impact of life events and to design and develop effective preventive intervention programs, we must go beyond the simple question of what are the consequences of a particular event on a person's well-being. Rather, we should seek to understand which factors differentially facilitate an individual's ability to adapt to such an event and to achieve a healthy postcrisis adjustment. Lazarus and Launier (1978) underscore the importance of answering this latter question by stressing that any intervention designed to facilitate adaptation and social competence must be based on a knowledge of the specific difficulties confronted by the population, the contribution of these difficulties to distress and the range and efficacy of coping strategies that may be employed to alleviate them.

Several conceptual frameworks have been suggested for understanding the process by which individuals cope with life stress in general and with stressful life events in particular. In their attempt to clarify the process by which individuals cope with stress per se, Lazarus and his colleagues (Lazarus & Cohen, 1977; Lazarus & Launier, 1978) define the process involved as a transaction between the individual and a threatening environment. Within their model, the individual's cognitive appraisal of the event is viewed as central in determining the amount of stress the event generates for him or her. This approach is supported by the finding of Kobasa (1979) that individuals who perceived stressful events as challenges rather than as threats were better able to cope with them. The question remains, however, what leads to differential appraisals of an event by different individuals. To explain these differences, Lazarus and Launier (1978) postulate that the characteristics of the individual and the psychological and situational coping resources available to him or her interact with the stressors present to shape the individual's unique response.

Dohrenwend (1978) has presented a similar model addressed specifically to an individual's attempts to cope with a particular stressful life event. Stressful life events are described as events which involve change, and the amount of change, as well as the individual's perception of the desirability of that change, may influence the degree of stress experienced. The first stage of Dohrenwend's model focuses on the extent of the individual's responsibility for the occurrence of the event. That is, some events such as a natural disaster or the death of a loved one are primarily the result of environmental factors which are beyond the individual's control, while the occurrence of other events such as marital separation or divorce are typically more open to the influence of those involved.

The second stage of the model postulates the occurrence of an immediate stress reaction following the event. Dohrenwend (1978) posits that this stress reaction is inherently time-limited and that the outcome depends on the mediation of psychological and situational factors that define the context in which the transient stress reaction occurred. Situational mediators include characteristics of the external situation which impinge on the individual such as social and material supports as well as additional environmental stressors (Lazarus & Cohen, 1977). Individuals lacking in social support or experiencing additional stressors engendered by the life event itself are more likely to have difficulty adapting than those with adequate social support and minimal additional stress. Other factors that contribute to the adaptive process are the specific characteristics of the individual. Background and personality factors such as age, sex, cognitive and emotional development, the resolution of previous coping experiences, and the coping abilities and competencies of the individual may all contribute to shape the adaptation of the individual to the stressful life event (Dohrenwend, 1978; Turk, 1979).

Finally, Dohrenwend (1978) states that there may be three possible outcomes of the coping process: substantial growth and adaptive change where the individual develops new skills and capabilities; the individual may develop some form and degree of psychopathology; or the individual may display no discernible change in emotional or physical functioning.

In summary, while several avenues exist for the study of stressful life events, the one we shall concern ourselves with for the purpose of our discussion of the impact of parental divorce on children draws heavily from crisis theory and the recent emphasis by mental health professionals on identifying precipitating, rather than predisposing, factors for psychopathology. This position emphasizes the need to identify a high-frequency life event which has a potentially negative impact on a significant proportion of those who experience it, and to elaborate those factors which may influence the relative success of the individual's coping efforts as necessary precursors to the establishment of primary prevention programs.

Incidence and Impact of
Marital Disruption on Children

Employing the framework for organizing preventive intervention around stressful life events in this section and the one which follows, we will (1) examine the current incidence of divorce, (2) consider studies which have focused on the global impact of divorce on children and parents, and (3) discuss those factors which studies of marital dissolution indicate may be potential mediating variables. Particular attention will be paid to those variables which are either amenable to programmatic intervention or aid in the targeting of intervention efforts. For example, while variables such as custodial arrangements, parent-child interactions, or the availability of social support may inform the shape and nature of our intervention efforts, other variables such as age or sex may be helpful in targeting preventive efforts and resources. Wherever possible, the interaction of variables will be emphasized, as they may inform efforts to further tailor preventive efforts to the particular populations being served.

Incidence of Marital Disruption

For the period 1975-1977, it has been estimated that over one million divorces per year occurred involving an average of 1.08 children per divorce (Glick & Norton, 1977; National Center for Health Statistics, 1977). Norton and Glick (1979) note that in 1975, six out of ten divorces involved couples who had children.

Several variables have been shown to be related to the incidence of marital disruption and divorce. Age, level of education, and income have been found to be negatively correlated with the rate of divorce for first marriages (Glick & Norton, 1977; Norton & Glick, 1979). In addition, when considering ethnic/racial differences, Norton and Glick (1979) state: "Although blacks and whites display generally similar patterns of divorce by social and economic characteristics, the incidence of divorce is uniformly higher for blacks than for whites" (p. 15).

While divorce rates are high, so too are rates of remarriage, particularly for persons under age 30 (Bloom, 1978). Norton and Glick (1979) have estimated that approximately four out of every five persons who divorce will remarry. Since young couples are clearly the most likely to be the ones to have young children, we may anticipate that part of the post-divorce adjustment process for a significant number of children may be adapting to the remarriage of the custodial parent or parents, a point we shall return to in our discussion of potential mediators and intervention foci.

Thus, divorce is a significant social problem affecting over two million adults and one million children per year. Given the scope of the problem and the ease and reliability of identifying this population, parental divorce can certainly be viewed as a life transition around which preventive programs should be organized (Bloom, 1979). We will now turn to an examination of studies of its potential consequences.

Impact of Marital Disruption on Children

A number of studies have attempted to clarify the impact of parental separation/divorce on children. Investigators in this area have focused primarily on children's self-concept, sex role identification pattern, levels and types of behavioral disturbance, and academic performance. The general paradigm employed has been to compare children from homes where parental separation/divorce has occurred to those from intact families or from families that have experienced family disruption due to the death of a parent. The impact of parental divorce on a child's self-concept and sex role development has been examined in several studies with equivocal results. Hetherington (1972) compared adolescent girls from homes broken by the father's death or parental divorce to those from intact families. She reported that adolescent girls who had experienced either parental divorce or death displayed significantly more difficulties in their interactions with males than did girls from intact families. Girls who experienced parental divorce displayed more attention-seeking behavior, while those from families disrupted by the father's death tended to be more inhibited, rigid, avoidant, and restrained. Using an older subject population and somewhat different measures, Hainline and Feig (1978) failed to replicate these findings. Not only were no differences found between girls from these different types of family backgrounds in their interactions with males, but no significant differences were found in self-image, amount of anxiety, or feelings of control over their environment.

Young and Parish (1977) report that adolescent girls who had lost fathers through death or divorce had significantly more negative self-concepts and were more insecure than those from intact families. These differences did not exist, however, when the mother had remarried. Similar findings are reported by Parish and Taylor (in press) for males and females in grades three through eight. Berg and Kelly (1979) also found no differences in self-concept between boys age nine through 15 who experienced parental divorce and boys from intact families. They concluded that a simple relationship between divorce and self-concept has not been established, and suggest looking at such variables as family relationships and existing custodial arrangements to clarify this relationship.

A well-known series of studies by Wallerstein and Kelly (Kelly & Wallerstein, 1976; Wallerstein, 1977; Wallerstein & Kelly, 1974, 1975, 1976), using clinical interviews and school reports, have investigated the responses of children of divorce of different age groups, ranging from preschool through adolescence. They report that preschool children exhibited significant behavioral changes following parental divorce, including heightened anxiety and aggression. While some behavioral regression was evident in the majority of preschool children, this change was particularly dramatic for the youngest children in this group (Wallerstein & Kelly, 1975). Early latency children were seen to exhibit pervasive feelings of sadness, fear, and depression immediately following parental separation, but the intensity of these feelings had significantly diminished at a one-year follow-up (Kelly & Wallerstein, 1976). These authors found intense feelings of anger and loneliness as well as somatic symptoms to be characteristic of later latency-age children (Wallerstein & Kelly, 1976). Again, at the one-year follow-up, many of these effects had subsided. Adolescents in their sample (Wallerstein & Kelly, 1974) displayed anxiety and concern for their own future as marital partners.

Despite the richness of these findings, caution must be exercised in extrapolating too heavily from them. Wallerstein and Kelly rely primarily on clinical data for their statements rather than employing any systematic quantitative analyses. Frequently, case vignettes are used to substantiate assertions. Moreover, no comparison groups from intact or other types of broken families were observed, and almost all of their subjects came from middle-class families. Finally, small sample sizes were generally employed. For example, in a study examining differences between children who experienced negative outcomes following divorce and those who did not display negative effects, there were only four "good copers" and five "poor copers" in the early preschool age sample (Wallerstein, 1977). Similarly, small sample sizes were employed throughout the various age ranges, with the largest group comparison consisting of a total of 14 "good" and "poor" copers. These limitations notwithstanding, this work is important for helping to guide future preventive efforts by highlighting the potential role of the child's developmental level as a mediator of his or her response to parental divorce.

Increased "acting-out," antisocial, aggressive behavior is perhaps the most consistently found effect of parental divorce. A number of studies focusing on children of divorce (Hetherington et al., 1978a; McDermott, 1968, 1970; Wallerstein & Kelly, 1975) have reported high levels of aggressive behavior in children who have experienced parental divorce. More importantly, in attempting to clarify the impact of divorce per se, rather than the more general case of marital disruption or parental absence, several studies have shown differences between children from divorced homes and those from homes where a parental death had occurred. Glueck and Glueck (1950) reported that a significantly higher proportion of delinquent boys came from homes disrupted by parental divorce than from homes broken by parental death. Hetherington (1972) found adolescent daughters of divorce engaged in significantly more sexual acting-out behaviors, while those whose fathers had died were more shy and withdrawn. A similar pattern of results was found in a series of studies concerned with the school adjustment problems of primary grade children conducted by the senior author of this chapter and his colleagues (Felner, 1977; Felner et al., 1975, in press). Teachers reported that children from divorced homes had significantly more aggression and acting-out problems than did children from either intact families or families with parental death. By contrast, children with histories of parental death were more shy and anxious than those from intact families or those broken by parental divorce. In addition, comparisons of teacher reports of behavioral competencies of these groups revealed that children of divorce exhibited lower levels of frustration tolerance and more difficulty in following rules. These results were replicated across referred and nonreferred samples and urban/suburban and rural populations.

Despite this relationship between parental divorce and acting-out problems in children, it is clear that the search for a constellation of general effects of divorce on children is not the most productive approach. Differences in the responses of children due to psychological and situational mediating factors may well work to obscure such general patterns. A more fruitful approach, particularly for those concerned with developing preventive efforts, is to focus on the differential impact of divorce on children as a function of these psychological and situational variables. Moreover, if we are truly concerned with informing preventive efforts, we should not confine our attention to the negative consequences of divorce. Rather, we should broaden our focus to include those factors which facilitate successful, healthy postseparation/postdivorce adjustment in children. With such knowledge we will be able to develop programs that enhance adaptation and are truly preventive in nature rather than merely reconstructive. Let us now turn to an examination of those factors which may serve to mediate the impact of divorce on the child.

Mediating Factors

Characteristics of the Child

Two of the most obvious characteristics of the child which may influence his or her adjustment to divorce, both directly and in interaction with other mediators, are the child's age and sex. The studies by Wallerstein and Kelly (Kelly & Wallerstein, 1976; Wallerstein & Kelly, 1974, 1975, 1976) clearly demonstrate the need to consider the child's age at the time of the divorce as a mediating factor in postdivorce adjustment. Longfellow (1979) argues that key factors underlying differential reactions of children of different ages to divorce are the parallel changes in the child's social and cognitive development, which in turn affect the child's perception and understanding of the divorce situation. Such a position is consistent with that of Lazarus and Launier (1978), who emphasize the individual's cognitive appraisal of an event as an important determinant of coping efforts. The association of differential patterns of postdivorce adjustment and the child's age reported in a number of other studies (e.g., Jacobson, 1978a, 1978b; Santrock, 1970, 1972) provides further evidence of the importance of the child's age as a mediating factor.

The sex of the child also appears to play an important role in determining his or her response to divorce (Hetherington et al., 1978a; Wallerstein & Kelly, 1975). Unfortunately, the fact that these studies have employed primarily families in which the mother was the custodial parent severely limits their interpretation. Before anything definitive can be said about the influence of the child's sex on his or her postdivorce adjustment, further data must be gathered comparing differential outcomes in children living under mother custody, father custody, and joint custody arrangements. This failure to consider nonmaternal custodial arrangements is, perhaps, one of the greatest limitations of the majority of current studies of the impact of divorce on children. We shall consider this topic in greater detail below when we examine the influence of various custodial arrangements.

Only minimal work currently exists concerning the reactions to divorce of children from different ethnic groups. Several authors have raised this issue. Nieto (1972) argues that due to the more common extended family structure of Puerto Rican children, they may not suffer from the same emotional difficulties encountered by "Anglo" children from disrupted families. Campos (1972) has pointed to the prevalence of separation over divorce in Hispanic families and notes that there is no existing literature comparing adaptation to divorce between Hispanic and "Anglo" or black children. Indeed, the fact that almost all published studies have employed primarily white, middle-class populations has made such comparisons impossible. Clearly, this is an area deserving of further investigation.

In general, then, the child's age, cognitive and emotional development, sex, and, to a lesser extent, ethnic background have been the primary characteristics considered by researchers in their investigations of the impact of parental divorce. Recent literature on the process of coping with stressful life events (Bloom, 1979; Dohrenwend, 1978) points to several other salient child characteristics which may serve as mediators and thus which need to be attended to in future work. Such variables include the child's social competencies and available coping repertoire as well as previous experiences with similar life events.

Situational Mediators

With the notable exception of the work of Hetherington et al. (1978a), relatively little attention has been directed to the identification of situational factors which might influence the child's postseparation/postdivorce adjustment. Hetherington and her colleagues conducted an extensive two-year longitudinal study of white, middle-class intact and divorced families with nursery school age children in which custody had been awarded to the mother. While the limitations of such a select sample are apparent, their findings have led to an increased recognition that adaptation to divorce is a process that may extend over a period of time lasting two or more years. It has thus encouraged a greater focus on divorce-associated stressors, tasks, and environmental resources as potential factors mediating the differential vulnerability found in individuals experiencing divorce. Among those variables suggested as important in the mitigation or exacerbation of the negative consequences of divorce for children are changes in family stressors, level of family functioning, stability of household routines, parents' emotional health, legal process and custodial/visitation arrangements, number of other life changes which follow the divorce, and the nature and quality of social support available to family members (Felner et al., 1975, 1979; Hetherington et al., 1978a; Longfellow, 1979; Felner et al., Note 1). Indeed, Longfellow (1979) concludes that "knowledge of the major changes that accompany divorce would enable us to make a more accurate prediction of its impact on children" (p. 292). The remainder of this section will examine empirical studies of the influence of these and other variables on the adjustment of children of divorce.

Parental conflict surrounding the divorce and the extent to which the child is drawn into that conflict appear to have a pronounced impact on the coping efforts of children. Jacobson (1978b) found that there was a significant association between the amount of parental hostility both before and after the separation and the postseparation adjustment of children aged three through 13. This relationship was found to be stronger for children seven to 13 years old than those three through six. Wallerstein (1977) noted that one factor which seemed to differentiate children in her study considered "good" or "poor" copers was the capacity of parents to keep their conflicts separate from their relationships with their children. Hetherington et al. (1978a) reported that parental conflict and anger decreased over the two-year period following divorce, but was frequently reactivated by the remarriage of one of the spouses. They noted that anger by the mother almost invariably accompanied remarriage of the ex-husband. This anger often took the form of reopening conflicts about visitation or was directed at the children, especially around the issue of split loyalties. Certainly, these are not circumstances which would facilitate a child's efforts at adjustment.

Research concerning parental conflict and postdivorce adjustment of children has profound implications both for those who maintain the myth that the family should stay together for the good of the child and for proponents of joint custody. Rutter (1971), in a review of previous research, concluded that parental separation did not necessarily have a negative impact on a child's adjustment, but parental conflict did. An early study of adolescents by Nye (1957) found that children in single-parent families reported less psychosomatic illness, less delinquent behavior, and better adjustment to parents than those in unhappy, intact homes. Zill's (Note 2) recent survey of over 2000 children from a variety of family types reported that adjustment was poorest among those children from families with high degrees of parental conflict—that is, children from both high-conflict intact and divorced families. Raschke and Raschke (Note 3) found no differences in measured self-concepts of sixth or ninth graders from intact, single-parent, or reconstituted families. However, in homes where parental conflict was high, the child's self-concept was significantly lower. These studies, taken together, suggest that situations which perpetuate conflict between parents or in which the child remains embroiled are more detrimental in some instances to the child's well-being than if he or she lived with a single parent. We will return to the implication of this issue in our discussion of the adjudication process and visitation and custodial arrangements both as mediators of children's adjustment and as foci for preventive intervention efforts.

Another set of variables which may serve as important mediators of the child's coping efforts are the nature and quality of the parent-child relationship. Studies focusing on these variables may be broadly classified into two groups: those examining the impact of parental absence on the child and those studying the quality of the relationship between the parent and the child per se.

Research investigating the effects of parental absence has considered almost exclusively the situation in which the father is the noncustodial parent. Since this literature has been reviewed in detail elsewhere (Herzog & Sudia, 1973; Hetherington et al., 1978b) we will simply highlight some of the major issues relating to a child's attempts to cope with divorce. Hetherington et al. (1978b) point out that there may be some disruptions in sex-typing in children who have experienced father absence as well as deficits in cognitive performance which emerge with increasing age. Other authors investigating the effects of father absence have reported similar problems in sex-role behavior and sex typing (Biller, 1969, 1976; Biller & Bahm, 1971; Hetherington, 1972) and impaired academic performance and adjustment (Sutton-Smith et al., 1968; Tuckman & Regan, 1966; Felner, 1977; Felner et al., 1975, in press). However, Herzog and Sudia (1973) find little support for the claim that it is the father's absence from the home itself which accounts for problems displayed by children in such families. Rather, they argue that it is a variety of factors, such as deficits in the quality of custodial parent-child interaction following the divorce, which lead to such problems. Longfellow (1979), in her critique of the father absence literature, notes that most studies have "found no differences between the adjustment of children with no father and those with stepfathers" (p. 289). Moreover, the differential reactions of children who have lost a parent due to either death or divorce (Felner, 1977; Felner et al., 1975, in press; Glueck & Glueck, 1950; Hetherington, 1972) further substantiate the argument that father absence per se is an insufficient explanation of the child's response to divorce.

Studies of the impact of the quality of the parent-child relationship further support this position. Hetherington et al. (1978a) report that, following divorce, changes occurred in both the quality and the quantity of parent-child interaction. These changes were particularly evident in the marked inconsistency of parental control over the child, which, in turn, was associated with heightened levels of undesirable and coersive behavior in children. An important point raised by their findings is that the process of adjusting to divorce is a prolonged one. That is, the efficacy of parental management of child behavior reached a low point approximately one year following the divorce but showed noticeable improvement by the end of the second year. Furthermore, the potential interaction of the quality of parent-child relationships with the level of parental conflict or social support to mediate the impact of divorce on children is well illustrated by the finding that parental effectiveness in child rearing was related to the amount of agreement and support between divorced spouses on disciplinary practices (Hetherington et al., 1978a).

A number of other studies of divorce have investigated the quality of the parent-child relationship within divorcing families. Felner et al. (Note 1) found that elementary school children whose parents had divorced were rated by teachers as experiencing greater parental rejection and less educational stimulation than those from families in which a parent had died or those from intact families. It has also been reported that divorced parents tended to be less affectionate, less communicative, and more overprotective than parents in intact homes (Hetherington, 1972; Hetherington et al., 1978a). In a more positive vein, Jacobson (1978c) reported that children of divorce receiving greater amounts of parental attention and encouragement to discuss the divorce had significantly less behavioral problems and were rated as better adapted by clinical observers than children lacking such parental attention and encouragement.

Additional situational mediators which have been cited as potentially influencing the child's postdivorce adjustment are changes in family organization and routine, economic stress experienced by the custodial parent, the parent's emotional well-being, and the additional life change events associated with divorce (Hetherington et al., 1978a; Longfellow, 1979; Felner et al., Note 1).

Divorce is often accompanied by a considerable degree of family disorganization and disruption of daily routines. Recent work has shown that the maintenance or reestablishment of family organization and stable household routines may significantly enhance a child's postdivorce adaptation (Hetherington et al., 1978a; Wallerstein, 1977).

Bane (1979) has argued that the increased economic stress experienced by families undergoing divorce should be of central concern to those involved in developing preventive efforts. She states that "economic problems ought to be the main concern of policy makers who worry about the children of marital disruption" (p. 286). In this same vein, Herzog and Sudia (1973) argue that many of the negative consequences of a father's absence on children would be mitigated if economic stability was provided for the single-parent mother. The fact that economic stress is a correlate of marital disruption has been established by a number of studies (Eshlemann, 1969; Felner, 1977; Hetherington et al., 1978a; LeMasters, 1971; Wolff, 1969; Felner et al., Note 1). The work by Hetherington et al. (1978a) attempted to clarify the relationship between reported feelings of economic stress by parents and children's adjustment and failed to obtain significant results. They noted, however, that the high level and limited range of income of their subjects may have precluded detecting such effects. Thus, for the present, the potential impact of economic stress on children of divorce remains unclear.

The emotional well-being of parents following divorce has also been recognized as bearing on the child's differential coping ability. Bloom, Asher, and White (1978) point to the increased vulnerability of divorced adults to mental health problems. Several studies have examined this issue. Zill (Note 2) found that children whose mothers were psychologically troubled were more likely to feel rejected and unhappy than those whose mothers were psychologically healthy. Furthermore, mothers who were the most frequently depressed in this study were either single or unhappily married. Hetherington et al. (1978a) found that divorced parents had lower self-concepts, were more depressed, and exhibited poorer emotional adjustment than did married parents. Interestingly, these authors raise the question, "Who is doing what to whom?" (p. 170) when considering the causal relationship between parents' and children's emotional well-being. Their findings showed mothers' feelings of confidence, self-esteem, state anxiety, and level of depression to be synchronously correlated with children's frequency of noxious and aggressive behavior. Cross-lagged panel correlations indicated that the behavior of children, particularly the sons, influenced the affective responses of the mothers. A similar set of findings was reported by Patterson (Note 4), who concluded that children and their parents often become involved in a vicious cycle of coersion with the mother's and child's responses inextricably intertwined. Thus, the relationship between the emotional well-being of the parent and child is a complex one which, when finally unraveled, indicates that preventive efforts aimed exclusively at one or the other group may be shortsighted.

For many children, a number of other life changes may accompany divorce which, in their own right, are considered to be stressful life events and which may confound and exacerbate the impact of the divorce. For example, changes in economic circumstances or residential relocation of the custodial parent may force a child to change schools. School transfer has been shown to have potentially negative consequences and is thus considered another prime target of preventive efforts for children (Bloom, 1978; Bogat et al., Note 5; Primavera et al., Note 6). Another life change commonly experienced by children of divorce involves the custodial parent going to work for the first time or after a long time at home, which may, in effect, constitute an additional loss for the child (Hetherington et al., 1978a).

Parental remarriage and adaptation to a new family system constitute another set of major life changes and tasks which the child of divorce often confronts. Surprisingly little information is available concerning the impact of remarriage, and what little data exist present an unclear picture. The reason for the paucity of studies investigating the impact of remarriage on children is unclear. One may speculate, however, that it may be due to the unstated assumption that remarriage constitutes a "positive" life event with minimal negative consequences. Whatever the case, several authors have examined the adjustment of children in reconstituted families. Parish and Taylor (in press) and Burchinal (1964) found that young children and adolescents from reconstituted homes had more favorable self-concepts and attitudes toward school than those from homes where the custodial parent had not remarried. In contrast, Kalter (1977) and Zill (Note 2) found children in reconstituted families to have more behavioral difficulties than those in single-parent or intact homes. One possible explanation for the difference in the results of these studies may be the differing adjustment criteria employed, a frequent problem encountered in the postdivorce adjustment literature in general. However, despite the mixed nature of these results, it is clear that remarriage is an event which may generate additional difficulties and stressors for the child and markedly affect later adjustment.

Although the potential influence of social support and social networks on a child's postdivorce adjustment has been pointed to by several authors (Felner et al., in press; Hetherington et al., 1978a; Longfellow, 1979),

little empirical data exist. What little work has been done focuses on the
social support available to the parent and its indirect effect on the child.
Hetherington et al. (1978a) found that the quality of the parent-child
relationship was significantly enhanced by the support of the ex-spouse or
persons outside the family. Since the parent often serves as the primary
source of support for the child, it may be argued that studies concerned
with the quality of the child's relationship with his or her parent are, in
fact, investigating the influence of social support on the child. A great deal
of work remains to be done examining the utilization and impact of
parental and other sources of informal and formal support by the child
and how this may vary as a function of age or sex (Cauce et al., Note 7).
For example, while the family may serve as the major source of social
support for a five-year-old, as the child matures, peers and other adults
outside the home increasingly may assume greater supportive roles. If this
assumption is true, parent-child relationships, while still important, may be
less salient in influencing an older child's ability to adapt to the divorce.
Clearly, this is only speculation, and much work needs to be done to
explain the role of social support as a situational mediator for children of
various ages experiencing parental divorce.

Of all the factors which may serve to mediate the child's postdivorce
adjustment, the custodial and visitation arrangements are certainly among
the most important. However, almost no research exists which directly
examines this question. Studies of divorce, instead, have typically utilized
families in which the mother was the sole custodial parent. Those studies
which do exist investigating paternal or joint custody have tended to focus
almost exclusively on the impact of these custodial arrangements on the
parents themselves (Gersick, 1979; Greif, 1979; Orthner et al., 1976).
Authors in this area have argued strongly, though based on little empirical
data, for either single-parent custody (Goldstein et al., 1973) or joint
custody (Roman & Haddad, 1978) to be the operating legal presumption
of the courts. A recent review of this issue (Felner et al., 1979) has
emphasized the need to develop useful information to ensure the best fit
between a particular family system and the specific custody and visitation
arrangements. It is not enough to ask in the abstract what custodial
arrangement is best for a particular child without considering what family
circumstances are necessary for that arrangement to work. Since the ideal
circumstances are not always available, the question of which "trade off"
is better for a child often needs to be answered. For example, is it better
to have two antagonistic parents involved with the child or to have a
single, overburdened parent who may provide a semblance of consistency?

How does the age and sex of the child and sex of the custodial parent change this answer? The need for more research on the influence of custodial arrangements on the child and its interaction with other mediating factors is clear. As Weiss (1979: 336) states:

We do not know nearly enough about the implications for children and their parents of different approaches to the management of custody and visitation after parental separation and divorce. . . . It would be most useful if custody decisions could be informed by empirical findings on the consequences of various arrangements.

Taken together, the studies discussed above provide preliminary evidence that a number of variables may serve to mediate the child's post-divorce level of adjustment. Even more sharply demonstrated is that divorce is not a unitary stressful event with which a child must cope. Indeed, the stress of the separation itself may be only one of a myriad of stressors and changes set in motion by the parents' divorce with the actual process of adaptation extending over a period of several years (Hetherington et al., 1978a). It remains for future research to determine the ways in which the stressors and tasks confronted by the child following divorce interact and the degree to which the situational and psychological resources available serve to facilitate or impede the success of his or her coping efforts. Furthermore, such relationships need to be clarified as they relate to children of different ages, sexes, and socioeconomic and ethnic backgrounds. Results from this type of research will be especially helpful in the targeting and tailoring of effective preventive efforts by illustrating which factors may constitute the necessary and sufficient ingredients of such efforts for particular children.

Interventions with
Children of Divorce

Given the extent of research on the impact of divorce on children, documentation of the existence of intervention efforts directed at such children is surprisingly scarce. The majority of programs reported, however, are generally much closer in design and orientation to traditional reconstructive models of service delivery rather than being primarily preventive in nature.

The Children of Divorce project of Wallerstein and Kelly (1977) offers counseling to children and parents within a time-limited psychotherapy model. Based on their clinical impression, they note that the optimal period for intervention with children appears to be one to six months following the divorce. However, no systematic evaluation of the success of their project has been conducted.

Several authors have explored the utility of school-based intervention programs for children of divorce. Felner, Ginter, Boike, and Cowen (Note 8; Felner, 1977) demonstrated that secondary prevention programs which attempt to intervene with children of divorce who may already be displaying school maladaptation are not particularly effective. While such efforts appear to prevent the development of further difficulties, they had only minimal success in ameliorating existing ones. Cantor (1977) described a school-based support group for nine children whose parents were recently divorced and reported that parents and teachers saw little behavioral change in such children. The senior author of this chapter and his colleagues in Rochester, New York (Felner et al., Note 9), developed a school-based primary prevention program for primary-grade children who had displayed no previous school maladaptation but who, within the preceding eight weeks, had experienced a major stressful life event. Children were seen twice weekly for six weeks by nonprofessionals who were trained in crisis intervention techniques. During one and a half years, 57 children were seen in the program, 31 of whom were experiencing parental separation or divorce. Comparisons of pre and post ratings of child behavior and measures of anxiety showed a significant reduction in state anxiety and shy, anxious behavior as well as increases in adaptive, assertive behavior. An important sidelight of this project is its illustration of a problem in developing controlled studies of intervention with children experiencing stressful life events. Originally, a demographically matched waiting list control group had been planned. However, mental health personnel in the participating schools perceived that such a control group was an unjust denial of what they felt was an important clinical service. Additional personnel resources were allocated to the program so that perspective control children could be seen. Thus, ultimately, clinical needs within the program settings outweighted research considerations. This issue must be grappled with by all who would develop such preventive efforts.

Social support groups have also been employed for children of divorce. Guerney and Jordon (1979) developed a community-based support program for nine children aged nine through thirteen who had experienced parental separation approximately one and one-half years earlier. Group leaders were parents drawn from the community, and there was a community-based board of directors. Based on positive, impressionistic feedback from parents and children, two new groups have been started for pre- and early adolescents. Guerney and Jordon further note that those involved in the program expressed the need for the initiation of groups in earlier stages of divorce. Again, however, no systematic evaluation efforts have been carried out.

Finally, a number of recommendations have been made for interventions through the legal system. Several authors have advocated more careful collaboration between the courts and mental health professionals in developing guidelines and procedures for custody decision-making to facilitate the fit between the family and the adjudicated custodial arrangement, as well as to minimize the strife between the parents throughout the divorce process (Derdeyn, 1975; Felner et al., 1979). The levels of intervention recommended range from those which involve mental health consultation to lawyers or court personnel (Benedek et al., 1977; Elkin, 1977; Felner et al., 1979; Sheffner & Suarez, 1975; Woody, 1978) to those which advocate interdisciplinary collaboration between mental health professionals and those in the legal system toward the development of a more prevention-oriented and informed social policy for arriving at child custody decisions (Felner et al., 1979). While cooperation between the legal system and mental health professionals is in its early stages, its need is clearly demonstrated by the work of Spanier and Anderson (Note 10), who report that frequently, as part of the adversarial nature of the divorce process, lawyers may actually increase the strife and conflict between parents, which may result in additional stress for children.

In summary, although some productive starts have been made toward developing preventive programs for children of divorce and identifying future directions, the current lack of systematic evaluation of such efforts makes it difficult to assess their utility for designing future programs. Indeed, it may be that before great quantities of energy and resources are expended in developing and evaluating numerous programs, many of which may have minimal success, further attention should be paid to understanding the ways the factors discussed in the preceding section facilitate postdivorce adjustment for different subpopulations of children. Such knowledge will ensure the most efficient expenditure of limited manpower and financial resources.

Summary and Concluding Comments

This chapter has examined the impact of parental separation and divorce on children through a stressful life events framework. An examination of the literature demonstrated that children vary markedly in their adjustment to such an event as a function of a number of stressors, life changes, and tasks precipitated by the divorce process, as well as the psychological and situational resources that may be utilized in their coping efforts. However, studies in this area are, at best, preliminary in nature and suffer from a number of serious design and sampling problems. Future research must focus on (1) the investigation of those stressors and individual and family coping resources which lead to differential adaptive outcomes in children experiencing parental divorce; and (2) the clarification of how the presence and impact of these mediators vary due to the child's age, sex, ethnic, and socioeconomic background, as well as type of custodial arrangement.

Our review of preventive interventions for children of divorce showed them to be preliminary in nature, suffering from a great deal of rhetoric and little systematic data. This paucity of work may not be as puzzling as it first appears, however, given the lack of a sound knowledge base upon which to develop such programs. Indeed, recent calls to initiate such preventive efforts (Bloom et al., 1978) may be premature for children of divorce, and until many of the questions raised in this chapter concerning mediating factors are answered, those developing such programs may too often be "shooting in the dark."

The appropriateness of a stressful life events framework for understanding the impact of divorce on children must also be questioned. While this model is useful in calling attention to mediating factors, it may result in too narrow a focus by those concerned with the investigation of the consequences of divorce and the development of preventive programs. The data make it clear that a perspective which views divorce as a unitary stressful event is, at best, misleading. It appears far more helpful to focus not only on the brief period surrounding that "event," but also on its aftermath and the repercussions it precipitates in the lives of family members which may continue to engender new stressors and changes and demand new adaptations for some time to come. Thus, a framework which focuses on the entire period of transition may be more beneficial for understanding the consequences of divorce and organizing preventive efforts. This approach, emphasizing the transitional nature of a child's adjustment to a divorce, better mirrors the quality of the divorce experience reported in the literature where new divorce-related "life transitions" continue to occur for several years following the event. Changes and tasks arising from the divorce include the reconstruction of support systems, the reorganization of the family's daily life, residential or school changes, the development of new skills, and the restructuring of parent-child interactions. Such a readaptation process certainly takes far longer than the six to eight weeks hypothesized by Caplan (1964) for crisis resolution. Indeed, the findings of Hetherington et al. (1978a) demonstrate that the process can extend over several years.

In summary, the work reviewed indicates that parental divorce may be the precipitant of a transitional period in children's lives in which they are confronted by a number of stressors, tasks, and life changes. Future research needs to focus on these factors as they influence the ability of the child and his or her family system to successfully negotiate this transition. Only when we have a more comprehensive understanding of this life transition and the skills and resources it requires can we develop effective preventive programs for children of divorce.

Reference Notes

1. Felner, R.D., Ginter, M.A., Farber, S.S., Boike, M.F., & Cowen, E.L. *Marital Dissolution: Related Family Stresses.* Manuscript submitted for publication, 1979.

2. Zill, N. Divorce, marital happiness and the mental health of children: Findings from the Foundation for Child Development National Survey of Children. Prepared for National Institute of Mental Health Workshop on Divorce and Children, Bethesda, Maryland, 1978.

3. Raschke, H.J., & Raschke, V.J. Family conflict and children's self concepts: A comparison of intact and single parent families. Presented at the 72nd Annual Meeting of the American Sociological Association, September, 1977.

4. Patterson, G. Mothers: The unacknowledged victims. Presented at the Society for Research in Child Development meeting, Oakland, California, April, 1976.

5. Bogat, G.A., Jones, J.W., & Jason, L.A. School transitions: Preventive intervention following elementary school closing. Presented at the 87th Annual Meeting of the American Psychological Association, New York, September, 1979.

6. Primavera, J., Felner, R.D., Ginter, M.A., & Cauce, A.M. School transitions: A focus for preventive efforts. Presented at the 87th Annual Meeting of the American Psychological Association, New York, September, 1979.

7. Cauce, A.M., Felner, R.D., Ginter, M.A., & Primavera, J. Social support systems in adolescents: A structural and functional analysis. Presented at the 87th Annual Meeting of the American Psychological Association, New York, September, 1979.

8. Felner, R.D., Ginter, M.A., Boike, M.F., & Cowen, E.L. *Parental Death or Divorce in Childhood: Problems, Interventions and Outcomes in a School-Based Mental Health Project.* Manuscript submitted for publication, 1979.

9. Felner, 'R.D., Norton, P., Boike, M.F., & Cowen, E.L. *An Evaluation of Crisis Intervention with Primary Grade Children.* Unpublished manuscript, 1979. (Available from R.D. Felner, Department of Psychology, Yale University, New Haven, CT)

10. Spanier, G.B., & Anderson, E.A. The impact of the legal system on adjustment to marital separation. Presented at the meeting of the American Association of Marriage and Family Counselors, New York, March, 1978.

References

Albee, G.W. *Mental Health Manpower Trends.* New York: Basic Books, 1959.

Bane, M.J. Marital disruption and the lives of children. In G. Levinger & O.C. Moles (Eds.), *Divorce and Separation: Context, Causes and Consequences.* New York: Basic Books, 1979.

Benedek, R.S., DelCampo, R.L., & Benedek, E.P. Michigan's Friends of the Court: Creative programs for children of divorce. *The Family Coordinator,* 1977, *16,* 447-450.

Berg, B., & Kelly, R. Measured self-esteem of children from broken, rejected, and accepted families. *Journal of Divorce,* 1979, *2,* 363-370.

Biller, H.B. Father absence, maternal encouragement, and sex role development in kindergarten-age boys. *Child Development,* 1969, *40,* 539-546.

Biller, H.B. The father and personality development: Paternal deprivation and sex-role development. In M.E. Lamb (Ed.), *The Role of the Father in Child Development.* New York: John Wiley, 1976.

Biller, H.B., & Bahm, R.M. Father absence, perceived maternal behavior, and masculinity of self-concept among junior high boys. *Developmental Psychology,* 1971, *4,* 178-181.

Bloom, B.L. Marital disruption as a stressor. In D.G. Forgays (Ed.), *Primary Prevention of Psychopathology. Volume II. Environmental Influences.* Hanover, NH: University Press of New England, 1978.

Bloom, B.L. Prevention of mental disorders: Recent advances in theory and practice. *Community Mental Health Journal,* 1979, *15,* 179-191.

Bloom, B.L., Asher, S.J., & White, S.W. Marital disruption as a stressor: A review and analysis. *Psychological Bulletin,* 1978, *85,* 867-894.

Burchinal, L.G. Characteristics of adolescents from unbroken, broken and reconstituted families. *Journal of Marriage and the Family,* 1964, *26,* 44-51.

Campos, L.P. The Spanish-American child. In I.R. Stuart and L.E. Abt (eds.), *Children of Separation and Divorce.* New York: Grossman, 1972.

Cantor, D.W. School-based groups for children of divorce. *Journal of Divorce,* 1977, *1,* 183-187.

Caplan, G. *Principles of Preventive Psychiatry.* New York: Basic Books, 1964.

Coddington, R.D. The significance of life events as etiological factors in the diseases of children. I. A survey of professional workers. *Journal of Psychosomatic Research,* 1972, *16,* 7-18.

Cowen, E.L. Demystifying primary prevention. In D.G. Forgays (Ed.), *Primary Prevention of Psychopathology. Volume II. Environmental Influences.* Hanover, NH: University Press of New England, 1978.

Cowen, E.L. The wooing of primary prevention: Foreplay and beyond. *American Journal of Community Psychology,* in press.

Cowen, E.L., Gardner, E.A., & Zax, M. *Emergent Approaches to Mental Health Problems.* New York: Appleton-Century-Crofts, 1967.

Derdeyn, A.P. Child custody consultation. *American Journal of Orthopsychiatry,* 1975, *45,* 791-801.

Dohrenwend, B. Social stress and community psychology. *American Journal of Community Psychology,* 1978, *6,* 1-14.

Elkin, M. Post-divorce counseling in a conciliation court. *Journal of Divorce,* 1977, *1,* 55-65.

Eshlemann, J.R. Perspectives in marriage and the family. In P. Glasser and E. Navarre (Eds.), *Structural Problems of the One Parent Family.* Boston: Allyn & Bacon, 1969.

Felner, R.D. *An Investigation of Crisis in Childhood: Effects and Outcomes in Children Experiencing Parental Death or Divorce.* Doctoral dissertation, University of Rochester, 1977. (unpublished)

Felner, R.D., Farber, S.S., & Kent, J.S. Toward the development of a social policy for child custody: A multidisciplinary framework. *Connecticut Bar Journal,* 1979, *53,* 301-309.

Felner, R.D., Ginter, M.A., Boike, M.F., & Cowen, E.L. Parental death or divorce and the school adjustment of young children. *American Journal of Community Psychology,* in press.

Felner, R.D., Stolberg A., & Cowen, E.L. Crisis events and school mental health referral patterns of young children. *Journal of Consulting and Clinical Psychology,* 1975, *43,* 305-310.

Gersick, K.E. Fathers by choice: Divorced men who receive custody of their children. In G. Levinger and O.C. Moles (Eds.), *Divorce and Separation: Context, Causes and Consequences.* New York: Basic Books, 1979.

Glick, P.C., & Norton, A.J. Marrying, divorcing, and living together in the U.S. today. *Population Bulletin,* 1977, *32* (5).

Glueck, S., & Glueck, E. *Unraveling Juvenile Delinquency.* Cambridge, MA: Harvard University Press, 1950.

Goldstein, J., Freud, A., & Solnit, A.A. *Beyond the Best Interests of the Child.* New York: Free Press, 1973.

Goldston, S.E. An overview of primary prevention programming. In D.C. Klein and S.E. Goldston (Eds.), *Primary Prevention: An Idea Whose Time Has Come.* Washington, DC: U.S. Government Printing Office, 1977. (a)

Goldston, S.E. Defining primary prevention. In G.W. Albee & J.M. Joffe (Eds.), *Primary Prevention of Psychopathology. Volume I. The Issues.* Hanover, NH: University Press of New England, 1977. (b)

Goldston, S.E. A national perspective. In D.G. Forgays (Ed.), *Primary Prevention of Psychopathology. Volume II. Environmental Influences.* Hanover, NH: University Press of New England, 1978.

Gottlieb, B.H., & Hall, A. Social networks and the utilization of preventive mental health services: A research framework. In R.H. Price, R.F. Ketterer, B.C. Bader, and J. Monahan (Eds.), *Prevention in Mental Health: Research, Policy, and Practice.* Beverly Hills, CA: Sage, 1980.

Greif, J.B. Fathers, children, and joint custody. *American Journal of Orthopsychiatry,* 1979, *49,* 311-319.

Guerney, L., & Jordon, L. Children of divorce: A community support group. *Journal of Divorce,* 1979, *2,* 283-294.

Hainline, L., & Feig, E. The correlates of childhood father absence in college-aged women. *Child Development*, 1978, *49*, 37-42.

Heller, K. The effects of social support: Prevention and treatment implications. In A.P. Goldstein and F.H. Kanfer (Eds.), *Maximizing Treatment Gains*. New York: Academic Press, 1979.

Herzog, E., & Sudia, C.E. Children in fatherless families. In B.M. Caldwell & H.N. Ricciuti (Eds.), *Child Development and Social Policy*. Chicago: University of Chicago Press, 1973.

Hetherington, E.M. Effects of father absence on personality development in adolescent daughters. *Developmental Psychology*, 1972, *7*, 313-326.

Hetherington, E.M., Cox, M., & Cox, R. The aftermath of divorce. In J.H. Stevens, Jr. & M. Mathews (Eds.), *Mother/Child Father/Child Relationships*. Washington, DC: National Association for the Education of Young Children, 1978. (a)

Hetherington, E.M., Cox, M., & Cox, R. The development of children in mother-headed families. In H. Hoffman and D. Reiss (Eds.), *The American Family: Dying or Developing*. New York: Plenum Press, 1978. (b)

Holmes, T.H., & Masuda, M. Life change and illness susceptibility. In B.S. Dohrenwend & B.P. Dohrenwend (Eds.), *Stressful Life Events: Their Nature and Effects*. New York: John Wiley, 1974.

Holmes, R.H., & Rahe, R.H. The social readjustment rating scale. *Journal of Psychosomatic Research*, 1967, *11*, 213-218.

Hough, R.L., Fairbank, D.T., & Garcia, A.M. Problems in the ratio measurement of life stress. *Journal of Health and Social Behavior*, 1976, *17*, 70-82.

Jacobson, D.S. The impact of marital separation/divorce on children: I. Parent-child separation and child adjustment. *Journal of Divorce*, 1978, *1*, 341-360. (a)

Jacobson, D.S. The impact of marital separation/divorce on children: II. Interparent hostility and child adjustment. *Journal of Divorce*, 1978, *2*, 8-19. (b)

Jacobson, D.S. The impact of marital separation/divorce on children: III. Parent-child communication and child adjustment, and regression analysis of findings from overall study. *Journal of Divorce*, 1978, *2*, 175-194. (c)

Kalter, N. Children of divorce in an outpatient psychiatric population. *American Journal of Orthopsychiatry*, 1977, *47*, 40-51.

Kelly, J.B., & Wallerstein, J.S. The effects of parental divorce: Experiences of the child in early latency. *American Journal of Orthopsychiatry*, 1976, *46*, 20-32.

Kobasa, S.C. Personality and resistance to illness. *American Journal of Community Psychology*, 1979, *7*, 413-424.

Lazarus, R.C., & Cohen, J.B. Environmental stress. In I. Altman and J. Wohlwill (Eds.), *Human Behavior and Environment*. Volume 1. New York: Plenum Press, 1977.

Lazarus, R.S., & Launier, R. Stress-related transactions between person and environment. In L.A. Pervin and M. Lewis (Eds.), *Perspectives in Interactional Psychology*. New York: Plenum Press, 1978.

LeMasters, E.E. Parents without partners. In A.S. Skolnick and J.H. Skolnick (Eds.), *Family in Transition*. Boston: Little, Brown, 1971.

Lindemann, E. The meaning of crisis in individual and family living. *Teachers' College Record*, 1956, *57*, 310-315.

Longfellow, C. Divorce in context: Its impact on children. In G. Levinger and O.C. Moles (Eds.), *Divorce and Separation: Context, Causes and Consequences*. New York: Basic Books, 1979.

McDermott, J.F., Jr. Parental divorce in early childhood. *American Journal of Psychiatry*, 1968, *124*, 118-126.

McDermott, J.F., Jr. Divorce and its psychiatric sequelae in children. *Archives of General Psychiatry*, 1970, *23*, 421-427.

Monaghan, J.H., Robinson, J.O., & Dodge, J.A. The children's life events inventory. *Journal of Psychosomatic Research*, 1979, *23*, 63-68.

National Center for Health Statistics. *Summary Report, Final Divorce Statistics, 1975.* (Monthly vital statistics report, 26:2, Supplement). Washington, DC: U.S. Government Printing Office, 1977.

Nieto, J. The Puerto Rican child. In I.R. Stuart and L.E. Abt (Eds.), *Children of Separation and Divorce.* New York: Grossman, 1972.

Norton, A.J., & Glick, P.C. Marital instability in America: Past, present and future. In G. Levinger and O.C. Moles (Eds.), *Divorce and Separation: Context, Causes, and Consequences.* New York: Basic Books, 1979.

Nye, F.I. Child adjustment in broken and in unhappy, unbroken homes. *Marriage and Family Living*, 1957, *19*, 356-361.

Orthner, D.K., Brown, R., & Ferguson, D. Single-parent fatherhood: An emerging life style. *Family Coordinator*, 1976, *25*, 429-438.

Parish, T.S., & Taylor, J.C. The impact of divorce and subsequent father absence on children's and adolescent's self-concepts. *Journal of Youth & Adolescence*, in press.

Rabkin, J.G., & Streuning, E.L. Life events, stress and illness. *Science*, 1976, *194*, 1013-1020.

Roman, M., & Haddad, W. *The Disposable Parent: The Case for Joint Custody.* New York: Holt, Rinehart & Winston, 1978.

Rutter, M. Parent-child separation: Psychological effects on the children. *Journal of Child Psychology and Psychiatry*, 1971, *12*, 233-260.

Santrock, J.W. Influence of onset and type of paternal absence on the first four Eriksonian crises. *Developmental Psychology*, 1970, *3*, 273-274.

Santrock, J.W. Relation of type of onset of father absence to cognitive development. *Child Development*, 1972, *43*, 455-469.

Sarason, I.G., Johnson, J.H., & Siegel, J.M. Assessing the impact of life change: Development of the life experiences survey. *Journal of Consulting and Clinical Psychology*, 1978, *46*, 932-946.

Sheffner, D.J., & Suarez, J.M. The post-divorce clinic. *American Journal of Psychiatry*, 1975, *132*, 442-444.

Sutton-Smith, B., Rosenberg, B.G., & Landy, F. Father absence effects in families of different sibling compositions. *Child Development*, 1968, *39*, 1213-1221.

Tuckman J., & Regan, R.A. Intactness of the home and behavioral problems in children. *Journal of Child Psychology and Psychiatry*, 1966, *7*, 225-233.

Turk, D.C. Factors influencing the adaptive process with chronic illness: Implications for intervention. In I.G. Sarason and C.D. Spielberger (Eds.), *Stress and anxiety.* Volume 6. Washington, DC: Hemisphere Publishing, 1979.

Wallerstein, J.S. Responses of the preschool child to divorce: Those who cope. In M.F. McMillan and S. Henas (Eds.), *Child Psychiatry: Treatment & Research.* New York: Brunner/Mazel, 1977.

Wallerstein, J.S., & Kelly, J.B. The effects of parental divorce: The adolescent experience. In E.J. Anthony and C. Koupernik (Eds.), *The Child in His Family: Children at Psychiatric Risk.* Volume 3. New York: John Wiley, 1974.

Wallerstein, J.S., & Kelly, J.B. The effects of parental divorce: The experiences of the preschool child. *Journal of American Academy of Child Psychiatry,* 1975, *14,* 600-616.

Wallerstein, J.S., & Kelly, J.B. The effects of parental divorce: Experiences of the child in later latency. *American Journal of Orthopsychiatry,* 1976, *46,* 256-269.

Wallerstein, J.S., & Kelly, J.B. Divorce counseling: A community service for families in the midst of divorce. *American Journal of Orthopsychiatry,* 1977, *47,* 4-22.

Weiss, R.S. The emotional impact of marital separation. In G. Levinger & O.C. Moles (Eds.), *Divorce and Separation: Context, Causes and Consequences.* New York: Basic Books, 1979.

Wolff, S. *Children under Stress.* New York: Basic Books, 1969.

Woody, J.D. Preventive intervention for children of divorce. *Social Casework,* 1978, *59,* 537-544.

Young, E.R., & Parish T.S. Impact of father absence during childhood on the psychological adjustment of college females. *Sex Roles,* 1977, *3,* 217-227.

6

Prevention in the Schools
Behavioral Approaches

Leonard A. Jason
DePaul University

The purpose of this chapter is to articulate a coherent, conceptual system for behavioral preventive interventions in schools and to provide concrete examples of this approach (many of these interventions were implemented by a team of investigators at DePaul University). The first section is devoted to explicitly defining models of mental health service delivery; that is, the traditional, community mental health, and community psychology approaches. The subsequent section delineates specific, person-centered, primary preventive approaches and a range of compatible behavioral technologies. Switching from person-centered approaches, the next section focuses on the relatively unexplored potential of preventive environmental interventions. It is hoped that the presentation of several conceptual models and schemas will elucidate a field which has, unfortunately, been characterized as confusing, contradictory, and abstruse. Finally, there is a discussion of critical issues germane to primary prevention in the schools, including the feasibility of utilizing support systems and larger-scale interventions, receptivity for preventive services among school personnel, prospective barriers in obtaining requisite funds for these projects, and cost-effectiveness of preventive interventions.

Defining Terms

Numerous behavioral studies were implemented in the schools in the 1960s and 1970s; however, the vast majority focused on individual young-

My thanks to Louise Ferone, David Glenwick, Edwin Zolik, Frank Dinello, and the many graduate students at DePaul University who helped me conceptualize the issues presented in this chapter. I am particularly grateful to Anne Bogat, who suggested the subtype by period schema presented in the bottom section of Figure 6.1.

sters who manifested moderate to serious behavioral or academic problems. This orientation typified behavioral mental health professionals who
unwittingly operated out of a traditional service delivery model
(MacDonald et al., 1974; Nietzel et al., 1977). More specifically, behavioral practitioners extended services based on a one-to-one service
delivery model, a late treatment focus, and a passive-receptive position
(Jason & Glenwick, 1980a). Jason (1977) presented a heuristic schema
(top section of Figure 6.1) to differentiate traditional from other mental
health service delivery models. In this model, the vertical axis refers to
time points in the unravelling of a dysfunction, during which an intervention is mounted (that is, primary, secondary, and tertiary), and the
horizontal axis specifies targets at which an intervention is directed (that
is, individual, group, organization, community, society). Traditional
approaches would occupy cells intersecting the late secondary and tertiary
time points, and individual and group target points. As an example of this
approach, a school psychologist might identify a child with well-
entrenched behavioral and academic problems and refer the youngster for
individual behavior therapy.

There are two slightly different ideologies encompassing a community
approach: a community mental health and a community orientation.
Those behavioral practitioners adopting a community mental health model
implement interventions at the individual or group target points and the
secondary and tertiary time points; surprisingly, the same target and time
points as advocates of a traditional model. In contrast to traditional
adherents, community mental health psychologists actively enter school
settings to identify and treat youngsters with incipient behavioral or social
difficulties, or geometrically extend the reach of services through use of
paraprofessionals or consultation (Jason, 1977). Their emphasis is exclusively on those with identified problems and on helping individuals better
adjust to their environment.

The community model incorporates time and target domains not within
the purview of the traditional and community mental health models.
Community adherents implement interventions at the primary preventive
time points and the organizational, community, or societal target points.
When adopting a behavioral conceptual orientation, primary preventive
interventions might employ classical conditioning, operant, modeling, or
cognitive restructuring strategies. In person-centered interventions, these
behavioral strategies are directed toward (a) preventing the onset of
specific disorders, (b) ensuring that children from high-risk populations do
not succumb to disorders, (c) strengthening competencies to enable chil-

FIGURE 6.1   Person-Centered Behavioral Primary Prevention Approach

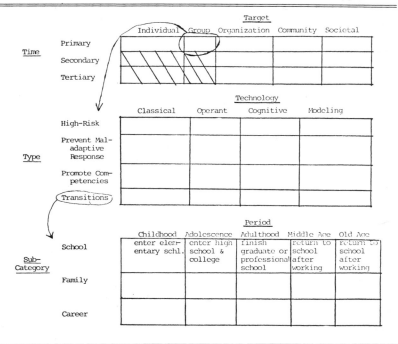

dren to withstand later school and life stresses, and (d) helping youngsters cope with major milestone transitions. When community psychologists operate at an organizational level, they attempt to change (a) the inanimate environment, (b) characteristics of individuals inhabiting settings, (c) interactions between individuals and the inanimate environment, or (d) the social climate (Jason & Glenwick, 1980b). In the subsequent sections, these concepts are explicitly articulated and interventions illustrating these principles are provided.

Person-Centered Approaches

Following the model sketched in Figure 6.1, the behavioral community interventions described below can be primarily conceptualized as involving the cell intersecting the group target dimension and the primary time point. Within this cell, it is possible to insert another matrix delineated in the middle portion of Figure 6.1, the horizontal axis specifying the type of preventive program (that is, high-risk, prevent maladaptive response, promote competencies, transitions) and the horizontal axis referring to the behavioral technology employed (that is, classical, operant, modeling, cognitive). In the subsequent paragraphs, each of those dimensions is explicitly articulated.

Four distinct *types* of primary prevention programs can be differentiated. The first type of approach involves preventing vulnerable populations from succumbing to disorders (Poser & Hartman, 1979). High-risk target groups might include children having one or two schizophrenic parents (Garmezy, 1971), children of alcoholics and drug addicts, youngsters experiencing the death of a parent, and children with physical handicaps. À potential iatrogenic hazard in this approach might involve inadvertently labeling or stigmatizing normal functioning children as being marginally adjusted.

A second type focuses on preventing the onset of carefully defined target disorders (Plunkett & Gordon, 1960). Interventions attempting to prevent poisonings from lead-based paints, infections (such as syphillis), genetic diseases (such as P.K.U.), nutritional diseases (for example, pellegra; Goldston, 1977), school phobias, or addictive behaviors (such as smoking) illustrate this approach. The potency of this approach is a direct function of the extent to which these behaviors or disorders are associated with short-term as well as long-term debilitating psychological and physical conditions.

Another type of prevention program switches the emphasis from preventing unfortunate, deficit-oriented end-states to promoting and enhancing adaptivity and healthy functioning. Building or strengthening low-probability competencies in affective (for example, social skills), cognitive (such as problem-solving abilities), or behavioral (for example, peer-tutoring skills) modalities typifies this orientation. Attractive features of this approach include focusing on salutary goals and precluding unintentional stigmatization.

The final type of preventive intervention provides individuals with experiences to ease the impact of traumatic milestone, transitional events in three areas: school (for example, school entrance), family life (for example, marriage), and work (as in the first job; Bogat, Note 1). Strategic placement of these types of positive educational interventions might represent the most economical and efficient approach for enhancing coping skills to successfully navigate stressful life experiences.

The behavioral technologies utilized in the actual interventions are based on either classical conditioning, operant strategies, cognitive tactics, or modeling procedures. A preventive model based on classical conditioning has been proposed by Poser (1970). He coined the term "antecedent systematic desensitization," which involves providing individuals graduated preexposure to anxiety-arousing situations to prevent the establishment of conditioned-avoidant responses. For example, overprotected children about to enter nursery school might first be provided a tour of the school with their parents accompanying them to prevent the establishment of school phobias. Poser and King's (1975) pioneering investigations with this model have involved immunizing children to dental visits and snake phobias.

Operant techniques focus on strengthening or establishing behaviors which might build adaptive skills to immunize youngsters against future stressful situations. This approach is illustrated by interventions which teach disadvantaged children mainstream linguistic and academic skills prior to school entry (Jason, 1975), train parents in child management skills before the birth of their first child (Matese et al., in press), or establish parenting skills prior to the identification of behavior problems in their children (Sirbu et al., 1978). School-based preventive operant approaches might focus on entire classrooms of youngsters in order to prevent initial manifestation of problems (Jason et al., 1979), build positive interactions (Strain et al., 1976), establish social skills (Kirschenbaum, 1979), foster creativity (Glover & Gary, 1976), or strengthen problem-solving capacities (Allen et al., 1976).

A third preventive behavioral strategy involves cognitive restructuring (that is, modifying the internal statements which people say to themselves). These techniques have been successfully applied to a wide range of clinical problems (Goldfried & Merbaum, 1973). Meichenbaum and Turk (1976), two prominent theorists in this area, have proposed a stress-inoculation training model which enables clients to apply cognitive restructuring techniques to deal effectively with present as well as future stressful situations. By changing negative self-statements to positive ones and engaging in internal dialogue to facilitate emission of adaptive behavior, the individual is provided with the internal coping skills to handle disparate stressful situations and problems. By shifting the emphasis from clinical to normal populations, this approach has limitless possibilities for primary prevention. For example, those prone to anger might imagine themselves being provoked and then cognitively rehearse coping skills for effectively dealing with the situation (Jaremko, 1979).

The last behavioral approach involves the use of modeling procedures. Bandura (1971) has written extensively on the use of such procedures in establishing and strengthening pro-social behaviors and decreasing maladaptive fearful responses. In order to imitate, a client must attend to the target behavior, employ verbal and imagery labeling (which facilitates later imitation when modeling cues are not present), have requisite motor reproduction abilities, and obtain reinforcement (if the performance is to be maintained over time). Modeling techniques have been successfully employed to treat individuals with phobias and test anxiety, to alleviate dental-medical stresses, and to establish interpersonal skills (Thelen et al., 1979). Such techniques might profitably be extended to engineering in strengths and competencies prior to problem onset in primary prevention-type activities.

In addition to selecting the type of prevention program and the behavioral technology to be utilized, an investigator needs to specify precisely the subcategory of the intervention as well as the period in which the project is implemented (see the bottom section of Figure 6.1). For example, the transition interventions can be broken down into school, career, and family life categories. Specific preventive transition interventions could occur during childhood, adolescence, adulthood, middle age, and old age. Specification of style of service delivery, conceptual orientation (that is, behavioral, humanistic, psychoanalytic, and so on), time and target points, preventive-type and behavioral technology, and subcategory and period might serve a heuristic function by imposing a structural order to the area of primary prevention in the schools.

Over the last few years, a team of investigators at DePaul University has been devising and evaluating person-centered, primary preventive interventions in Chicago schools (primary time points, group target points). These behavioral-community interventions utilized various behavioral technologies to prevent the development of specific maladaptive responses, to establish and build competencies, and to help youngsters navigate through milestone developmental transitions.

The first series of group-centered, primary prevention programs to be described involved preventing the establishment of a maladaptive behavior using primarily operant and modeling behavioral technologies. The specific response involved smoking and the period focused on adolescents. The rationale for the intervention was derived from the fact that there are patent health hazards associated with smoking, and over 3000 youngsters start smoking each day (Garell, 1976). In the first year of the program, support groups of ninth-grade smokers and nonsmokers were brought together for weekly meetings which focused on building assertive responses to resist pressures or urges to smoke (Jason, Note 2). At program end, nonsmokers remained abstinent, cigarette smoking had declined for smokers, and the youngsters were unanimous in their praise of the program. In the subsequent year, several entire ninth-grade health classes were involved in the project. In the actual intervention, the children role-played various scenes involving resisting peer pressure and being afflicted with illnesses due to smoking. At school end, fewer children in the treatment condition began to smoke than those in the control groups. In addition, at postpoint and a three-month follow-up, 67 percent of smokers in the two treatment classes had stopped smoking (Spitzzeri & Jason, 1979). The following year, all ninth graders in a high school (n = 149) participated in a smoking prevention program featuring discussion and role-playing (Jason & Mollica, Note 3). In the treatment conditions, 59 percent of smokers were abstinent at a three-month follow-up; only 10 percent of those in a control school were abstinent. Among program youngsters who smoked more than ten cigarettes a day, no reductions in cigarettes were noted. Dramatic reductions, however, were observed for program children who smoked less than ten cigarettes a day; rates increased for control smokers (see Figure 6.2). These secondary preventive findings indicate the need for early efforts to prevent youngsters from acquiring intractable, maladaptive behavior patterns.

The next primary preventive group interventions focused on developing competencies and employed operant techniques. All children in a first- and third-grade classroom were taught peer-tutoring skills in order to transform the learning experience from a passive to an active process (Jason et al., 1979). During this twice-weekly program, the classrooms were restructured so that all youngsters had a chance to serve as tutors and students. Student teachers taught their pupils by presenting flash cards of either vocabulary or arthmetic problems. Using a multiple baseline design, the children were systematically prompted first to give corrective feedback, then re-present the question, and finally use contingent praise. In addition to acquiring peer-tutoring skills, the youngsters manifested increases in appropriate classroom behavior during nonproject times, earned higher math and spelling grades, and 50 percent of the students indicated they used the peer-tutoring game during nonproject times with friends and relatives. During the subsequent year, peer-tutoring skills were again established; the children demonstrated significant gains in academic achievement tests; and the program youngsters were rated by the teacher as evidencing significant improvements in overall adjustment (Jason &

FIGURE 6.2 Number of Cigarettes Smoked for E and C Experimenting (Smoking less than 10 per day) Smokers Across Pre, Post, and Follow-Up Periods

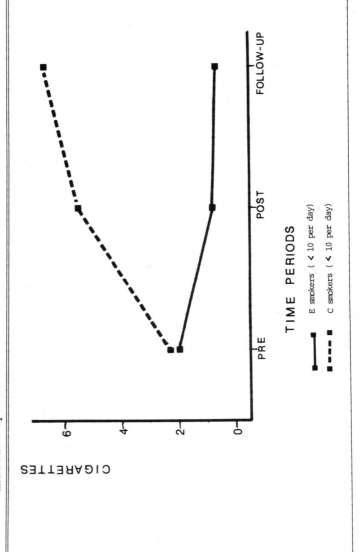

Frasure, Note 4). In addition, a group of eighth graders was taught to teach the first graders how to play the tutoring game. Figure 6.3 depicts the teaching behaviors of the eighth graders over time. When the eighth graders were prompted by university students to teach a tutoring behavior, the eighth graders manifested dramatic increases in the specific behavior. When the eighth graders were taught how to score interactions during the second-to-last phase, they continued to prompt accurately without feedback in the last experimental phase. By training personnel within the school system to monitor and supervise the intervention, the school was provided the skilled resources to independently implement the tutoring project.

The next primary prevention, group-oriented intervention involved promoting competencies through cognitive restructuring techniques. Focusing on a class of fourth-grade youngsters, Press, Alvarez, Jason, and Cotler (Note 5) identified and enhanced critical components in the problem-solving process. Previous investigators have used complex treatment packages in enhancing problem-solving skills and have not systematically documented behaviors accelerated in the interventions (Spivack & Shure, 1976). In the Press et al. study, the children demonstrated elevated levels of two problem-solving skills (correctly identifying emotions and labeling appropriate consequences of one's actions) during the baseline condition. Following this assessment, an intervention succeeded in increasing the children's abilities to generate alternative solutions to interpersonal problems. By initially conceptualizing active ingredients in the problem-solving process and then assessing extant levels of proficiency, investigators are able to target their intervention toward those behaviors judged below criterion levels.

The last series of group-centered, primary preventive interventions focused on transitions and utilized operant, cognitive restructuring, and modeling behavioral techniques. In the first project, operant techniques were extended to a first-time teacher who was experiencing some difficulties in managing her classroom of first graders (Douglas & Jason, 1979). The teacher was taught how to implement a home note system; that is, children were given a positive note which they could bring home to their parents contingent upon meeting daily criteria in behavioral and academic areas. With implementation of this home note procedure, youngsters' appropriate behavior increased from 59 to 82 percent (gains were maintained during a follow-up period). Significant improvements were also found on standardized achievement tests. The study indicated that a first-time teacher could effectively implement an operant strategy to

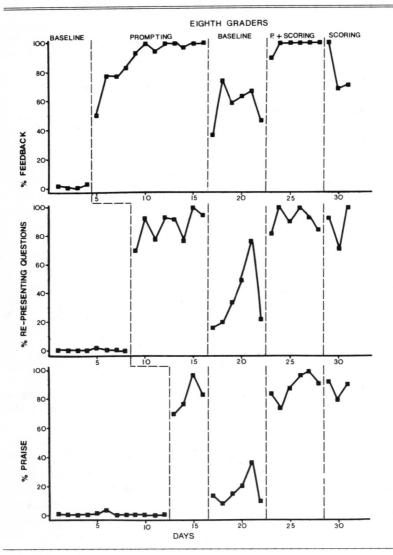

promote adaptive behaviors in first-grade children. The time spent in implementing the project may continue to reap benefits for the teacher with other classes of youngsters and for the students as they face future transition points.

The next transition project compared two behavioral techniques, classical conditioning and cognitive restructuring. The intervention was geared toward enhancing public speaking skills in adolescents entering high school, a time when more oral presentations are required by school personnel. In the actual program, children were exposed to six sessions of systematic desensitization or cognitive rehearsal (Cradock et al., 1978). The cognitive rehearsal intervention provided the youngsters with strategies for mastering 18 hierarchical steps in presenting a speech (for each step, the children imagined the situation and attempted several coping strategies). Compared with a control group, only the youngsters provided cognitive rehearsal showed a significant improvement in self-confidence in a public speaking situation. The study succeeded in assessing the differential effectiveness of disparate behavioral techniques in enhancing children's confidence in mastering a transitional event.

Another transition intervention employed cognitive restructuring as well as modeling components. The program focused on elementary-age children who were forced to attend a public school following the closing of their parochial school. The two-day preventive orientation program occurred one week prior to the beginning of school (Bogat et al., in press). During the intervention, target youngsters were provided tours of the new school, peer-led discussion groups, and information concerning school rules and regulations. The children involved in the intervention scored significantly higher than did the controls in terms of self-esteem related to peer relationships, knowledge of school rules, and teacher conduct ratings. The findings suggest that the brief, economical orientation intervention was successful in helping transfer students adjust to a new school environment.

A preventive transitional intervention currently being planned involves providing twelfth graders with cognitive restructuring techniques to handle transitions. Following graduation from high school, adolescents separate from parents, siblings, and close friends; obtain greater autonomy in making important decisions; establish new friendships; experience pressures for greater intimacy and sexuality; and deal with new intellectual challenges. In the planned study, youngsters about to graduate from high school will be provided graded crisis experiences to work through under circumstances which favor successful outcomes in order to facilitate the acquisition of competencies to better handle later transitions. Borrowing from the stress inoculation and problem-solving procedures, youngsters will be taught how to lower elevated levels of physiological arousal, alter self-defeating cognitive interpretations of stress, and expand behavioral alternatives for dealing with stressful events. In addition, the adolescents will be taught procedures to identify and gain entry into informal and formal support systems (social supports might facilitate optimal functioning of adolescent coping behaviors). This broad-based preventive intervention will focus on equipping youngsters with coping responses to handle milestone life transitions.

Environmental Interventions

The behavioral interventions described in the above section exclusively focused on persons as opposed to environmental components directly or tangentially affecting individuals. Figure 6.1 shows that environmental interventions occur at the organizational, community, or societal target levels, where efforts are initiated to conceptualize and construct new settings or to participate via advocacy or consultation in the modification of structural-environmental features in already existing settings. At a more micro level of analysis, changes in school organizations can occur at four levels: (a) the inanimate environment (that is, physical design, resources, or ambient conditions); (b) characteristics of individuals inhabiting the settings; (c) interactions between the individuals and their environments; and (d) the settings' social climates. Each of these constructs is delineated below.

The Inanimate Environment

Physical Design

A burgeoning body of research has identified physical design elements (such as seating patterns, furniture arrangement, and architecture) as potently affecting children's behaviors. As an example, Sommer (1969) noted that students participated more when they sat in front rows in classrooms as opposed to rear rows. O'Neill (1976) found creative girls had higher self-esteem in open classrooms (that is, classes with the flexible educational format of open space), whereas those with less creative abilities had higher self-esteem within closed, conventional classrooms.

Another physical design variable pertains to the size of a setting. In Barker's (1976) classic seminal research, students in small high schools participated in responsible positions in an average of 3.7 school behavior settings, whereas those in large schools participated in only .6 of these settings. Of most importance was that academically marginal students received almost five times as many deviation-countering measures (that is, forces toward participation) in smaller as opposed to larger schools. Jason and Nelson (1980) investigated the influence of two children's positions in several classroom ecological niches (that is, teacher present, a large unsupervised group, and a large, teacher-supervised group). Figure 6.4 depicts a child naturalistically observed in these three classroom structural units. The highest rates of misbehavior were evident in the unstructured large group, whereas less problem behaviors were noted in the supervised large and small groups. Another child's classroom behavior is shown in Figure 6.5. This study employed an ABAB design, with the A condition specifying the large unsupervised group and the B condition indicating a large teacher-supervised group. The data indicate that misbehaviors increased during phase A (unsupervised large group) and decreased during phase B (supervised large group). These studies suggest that strategic placement of some children in highly structured and supervised behavior settings might facilitate their ability to more adequately follow classroom rules.

Resources

Another aspect of the inanimate environment involves the resource materials used in play or instruction. Several investigators have documented the substantial influence of inanimate play materials on children's behavior and development. For example, Wargo, Campeau, and Tallmadge (Note 6) described a project by Levenstein who found increases in intellectual development after placing educational materials and toys in homes of disadvantaged children. Quilitch and Risley (1973) reported that seven-year-olds engaged in social play 85 percent of the time when social toys (toys designed for use by several youngsters at a time) were available, and only 10 percent of the time when isolate toys (toys designed for use by one child at a time) were used. Robson, Lipshutz, and Jason's (Note 7) experiment used an ABA design to investigate the relationships between the relative quantity of play materials and sharing behaviors in four groups of elementary-school-age children (see Figure 6.6). The children were initially provided with a restricted number of play materials in order to facilitate sharing among the youngsters during the first baseline condition. During the next phase, when each child was supplied with all play materials, sharing behaviors were eliminated in all groups. When the

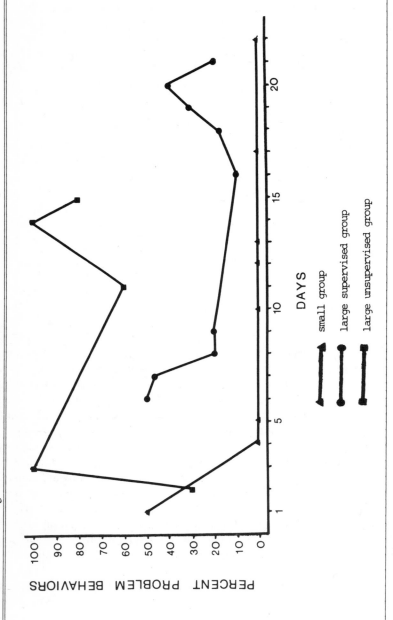

FIGURE 6.4   Percentage of Problem Behaviors over Time

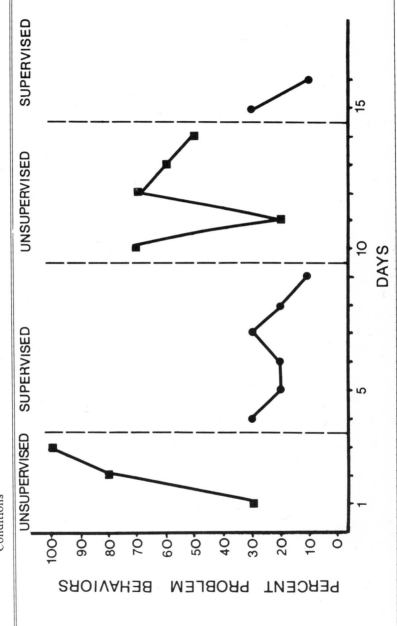

FIGURE 6.5 Percentage of Disruptive Behaviors over Experimental Conditions

FIGURE 6.6 Sharing Behaviors Across Experimental Conditions

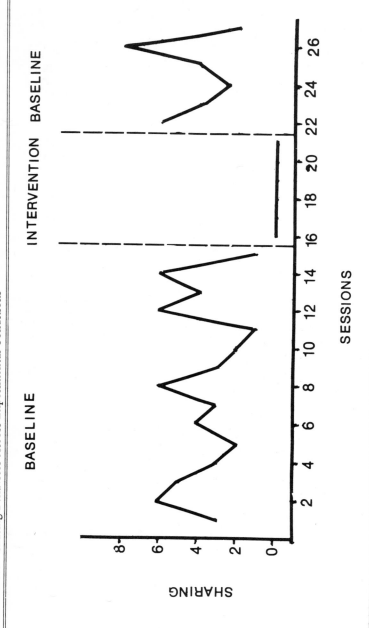

124

children were again provided limited access to materials, sharing interactions were again documented among all program youngsters. These latter studies indicate that the quality and quantity of available play materials have the potential to enhance or impede critical, pro-social, interactional patterns among school-age children.

Ambient Conditions

Ambient conditions (such as noise, lighting, and temperature) represent yet another component of the inanimate environment. High sound levels, one of the most noticeable, ubiquitous irritants in areas of high density, have been negatively correlated with the psychological development of infants and toddlers (Wachs et al., 1971). Meyers, Artz, and Craighead (1976) operationalized this ambient condition and successfully reduced aversive noise levels in a college dormitory by providing instructions and setting up rewards which were contingent on acceptable noise levels. In regard to lighting, Mayron et al. (1974) found decreases in children's hyperactive behavior when full-spectrum illumination replaced conventional fluorescent lighting. Finally, Russell and Bernal (1977) conducted a study involving temperatures and observed more inappropriate child behaviors on cold days and fewer deviant behaviors on rainy days.

As a group, these studies suggest that inanimate properties of settings exert strong influences upon disparate behaviors. Modification of such environmental properties might beneficially alter the stimulus qualities of settings and prospectively engender long-term changes.

Inhabitants of Settings

Pervasive environmental influences are also exerted by inhabitants of a setting—that is, the number of members (setting density), the client or staff turnover (member stability), and demographic and personality characteristics of the inhabitants of a behavior setting. In regard to setting density, Dawe (1934) found that as the number of students in classes increased, the remarks of kindergarten children decreased. As for member stability, Kelly (1969) has reported that youngsters in a stable school (one with low student turnover) were generally unresponsive to outsiders and tended to ostracize nonconforming members. In addition, high exploratory behaviors were labeled deviant in this setting. In marked contrast, children in fluid schools (those with high student turnover) helped newcomers adjust to their settings via an informal welcoming committee, and exploratory behavior was accepted and valued.

Inhabitant characteristics also exert shaping influences on behavior. DeCoster (1966), for example, found that when high-ability students were concentrated in certain resident halls, their academic achievement was higher than that of similar high-ability students who were randomly assigned to several resident halls. Member density and stability as well as characteristics of neighbors, friends, family members, and personnel who staff agencies represent another pervasive environmental dimension which can be documented and potentially modified.

Interactions

The inanimate environment and its inhabitants enhance or moderate the display of certain behaviors. As a corollary to this principle, some interactions between the environment and its inhabitants are beneficial, while others are detrimental. Rather than intervening directly with remediating person-centered dysfunctions, mental health professionals might function as behavioral matchmakers by identifying youngsters desiring behavior change and linking them with salutary settings analyzed previously as potentially facilitating those specific changes. As an example of this approach, Suomi (1979) found that monkeys which had become socially incompetent after being reared alone from six months to one year overcame their debilitating conditions following exposure to younger, socially competent infant monkeys. Using this animal experiment as a model, Hartup (1979) exposed socially withdrawn preschoolers to younger competent children. Children in this treatment group, compared with controls, evidenced significant improvements in sociability. In another study employing this behavioral matchmaker approach, Jason and Smith (in press) created peer-led support groups of college undergraduates, some of whom had been successful and others unsuccessful in ameliorating personal, observable, behavioral problems. During the group sessions, the more successful students provided the others with behavioral strategies which frequently succeeded in modifying previously recalcitrant problems. Jason, Ferone, and Soucy (in press) identified a behavior setting in a classroom (that is, a group of three children) where high rates of sharing behaviors were manifested. When an isolated child was placed in this setting, the child's rate of sharing increased exponentially. In an attempt to replicate and expand upon this study, Jason, Robson, and Lipshutz (in press) identified groups of high and low sharers in first- and third-grade classrooms (see Figure 6.7). In Figure 6.7, the lined bars indicate the rates of sharing for the combined high sharers and the open bars for low sharers

FIGURE 6.7 Overall Sharing Averages for Low Sharers Placed in High Sharing Groups

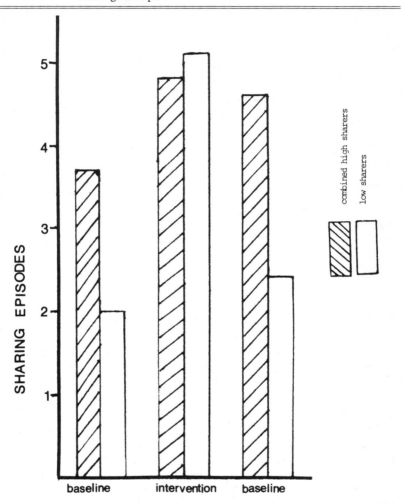

during the baseline phase. When children evidencing low rates of sharing were placed in groups of two high sharers during the treatment phase, the low sharers evidenced significant increases in sharing behaviors. During the subsequent phase, when the original groups were reconstituted, sharing once again decreased for the low sharers. These findings suggest that pro-social behaviors might be modified by careful placement of children in behavior settings analyzed as conducing specific behavioral change.

Social Climate

The last construct, social climate, is concerned with the perceptions and feelings of individuals with respect to their environments. Moos (1975) has indicated that a setting's social climate has important influences on mood; behavior; health; sense of well-being; and social, personal, and intellectual development. In schools, students are more satisfied when there are personal student-teacher relationships, innovative teacher methods, student involvement, and clarity regarding rules (Trickett & Moos, 1974). Regrettably, many schools can be characterized as having a vitiating social climate, one which dampens group spirit and discourages autonomy, independence, and leadership. There is a patent need to precisely document these social-climate variables and to devise behavioral interventions which systematically alter the social climate within school systems.

Conclusion

The principal purpose of this chapter was to provide a theoretical model for conceptualizing primary preventive interventions in schools and to illustrate this approach with interventive programs implemented in school settings. Prior to initiating interventions, investigators might profit from explicitly identifying which theoretical models their programs can be subsumed under (that is, the style of service delivery: community psychology, community mental health, or traditional; conceptual orientation: behavioral, humanistic, or psychoanalytic; target and time dimensions). In addition, when implementing person-centered preventive interventions, intervenors would also benefit considerably from precisely specifying the selected behavioral technology, the type and subtype of preventive intervention, and the period when implemented. Shifting to environmental approaches, the author hopes that delineation of a four-part heuristic schema for organizational-level interventions (that is, the inanimate environment, characteristics of inhabitants, interactions, and social climate), concretized an oft-neglected area which undoubtedly deserves more attention from behavioral investigators. Due to space considerations, only selective investigations illustrating this behavioral-community approach were included in this chapter. Many topics germane to this approach, including self-control procedures, behavioral rehearsal, cognitive variables, antecedent stimuli (Drabman & Furman, 1980), curriculum development, racial integration, children as agents of change, and issues of generalization and dissemination (Nietzel et al., 1977), were either excluded or dealt with in a cursory fashion.

Given that the thrust of this chapter was devoted to school preventive programs, the environmental interventions discussed focused exclusively on organizational as opposed to community- or societal-level targets. It is possible, however, for behaviorists to begin actively experimenting with change at the community or societal levels through adoption of a conflict (that is, action-oriented and confrontative, using strategies to directly challenge those holding power) or consultation approach (documenting the existence of problems and working cooperatively with different parties in problem resolution). Behavioral community psychologists might utilize either activist or consultative approaches to stimulate the creation of new support systems for schools or to collaborate with organized or informal support systems in the community. Exemplifying an activist strategy, Iscoe (1974) worked with a group of Chicano parents who brought a million-dollar suit against a school system for employing discriminative techniques in evaluating and teaching minority children. With the threat of a lawsuit, the school officials capitulated to the parental demands and subsequently involved the parents in the planning of a new school. At more societal levels, behavioral psychologists might begin efforts at evaluating the impact of prospective legislative enactments (for example, negative income tax—Wright & Wright, 1975; direct grants to purchase public housing—Second Annual Report of the Experimental Housing Allowance Program, 1974) on the short- and long-term psychological and behavioral development of children and adolescents.

A pertinent question concerns the receptivity for preventive-community services among school personnel. In an attempt to gather data on this issue, Jason and Glenwick (1979) surveyed rural and urban school-based mental health professionals' interest in receiving myriad school-based mental health services. In general, traditional mental health services were rated as more desirable than community mental health or community-oriented programs. One implication of these findings is that mental health professionals might need to inform and educate school personnel of potential advantages inherent in primary preventive interventions. In a separate publication, Jason and Ferone (in press) found school personnel extremely receptive to a series of preventive interventions implemented in nine separate inner-city school systems. More than likely, primary prevention interventions will be valued and adopted when school administrators and teachers perceive a need for the services; when the programs, training, and evaluation are explicitly described; and when the projects are portrayed as positive, educational, competency-enhancing experiences.

Funding for primary prevention interventions remains precarious at best and nonexistent at worst. Youngsters with entrenched, dysfunctional behavior patterns continue to capture the attention of mental health professionals and the public, as well as federal, state, and local bureaucrats. While some state and federal offices of prevention have been established, their funding levels are minuscule compared with the amounts allocated for more traditional modalities of treatment. At the present time, primary prevention programs are often implemented by persistent investigators committed to this orientation in spite of severe funding obstacles. (Whether such quixotic efforts will continue in the future is a moot question.) Future funding of such preventive efforts might be contingent on an evolving public's perception which construes this approach as more humane, efficient, and cost-effective than current styles of delivering mental health services.

In regard to evaluation of primary prevention programs, some of the more egregious methodological flaws have included failure to specify active intervention ingredients, nonrandom assignment of participants to treatment groups, inadequate sample sizes, and lack of follow-up data. Even though these interventions are implemented in nonlaboratory settings, there is a need to employ the most sophisticated experimental designs possible in order to both document treatment effects and persuade colleagues of the scientific viability of this emerging field. Critical unmet information needs in this area include demonstrating whether primary preventive interventions are more efficient and cost-effective than secondary or tertiary interventions. Until quintessential long-term follow-up data are available and analyzed, conducting research in the area of primary prevention remains an act of faith. It is hoped that future research will validate the usefulness and effectiveness of the community paradigm (Kuhn, 1962).

Exciting, relatively unexplored possibilities are inherent within the entire field of school preventive programs. In part, an emerging renaissance in this area is the result of the confluence of deductive theoretical formulations on primary prevention and environmental interventions by community psychologists, and inductive empirical research conducted by behavior analysts. As behavioral and community psychologists solidify their mutually reinforcing collaborative relationship, it is hoped that more research will be directed toward investigating the differential effectiveness of interventions based on different styles of service delivery, ascertaining the most efficacious target and time points for implementing interventions, and specifying which behavioral technologies are most effective with which types and subtypes of prevention programs during specific developmental periods.

Reference Notes

1. Bogat, A. *Life Transitions: Applications for Community Psychology.* Unpublished manuscript, 1979. (Available from Anne Bogat, Psychology Department, DePaul University, Chicago, IL 60614.)

2. Jason, L.A. Research collaboration between academia and the real world. Presented at the meeting of the American Psychological Association, San Francisco, August, 1977.

3. Jason, L.A., & Mollica, M. Comparative effectiveness of smoking prevention programs. Presented at the meeting of the American Psychological Association, New York, September, 1979.

4. Jason, L.A., & Frasure, S. Establishing supervising behaviors in eighth graders and peer-tutoring behaviors in first graders. Presented at the meeting of the Midwestern Psychological Association, Chicago, May, 1979.

5. Press, S., Alvarez, J., Jason, L.A., & Cotler, S. Developing a behavioral problem solving program in a school setting. Manuscript submitted for publication, 1980.

6. Wargo, M.J., Campeau, P.L., & Tallmadge, G.K. *Further Examination of Exemplary Programs for Educating Disadvantaged Children.* Final report, U. S. Department of Health, Education and Welfare, 1971, ED 055 128.

7. Robson, S.D., Lipshutz, S.A., & Jason, L.A. *Altering Sharing Interactions Through Stimulus Control.* Presented at the meeting of the Association for Behavior Analysis, Dearborn, Michigan, May 1980.

References

Allen, G.J., Chinsky, J.M., Larcen, S.W., Lochman, J.E., & Selinger, H.V. *Community Psychology and the Schools: A Behaviorally Oriented Approach.* Hillsdale, NJ: Lawrence Erlbaum, 1976.

Bandura, A. Psychotherapy based upon modeling procedures. In A.E. Bergin and S.L. Garfield (Eds.), *Handbook of Psychotherapy and Behavior Change.* New York: John Wiley, 1971.

Barker, R.G. On the nature of the environment. In H.M. Proshansky, W.H. Ittelson and L.G. Rivlin (Eds.), *Environmental Psychology.* New York: Holt, Rinehart & Winston, 1976.

Bogat, G.A., Jones, J.W., & Jason, L.A. School transitions: Preventive intervention following an elementary school closing. *Journal of Community Psychology,* in press.

Cradock, C., Cotler, S., & Jason, L.A. Primary prevention: Immunization of children for speech anxiety. *Cognitive Therapy and Research,* 1978, *2,* 389-396.

Dawe, H.C. The influence of size of kindergarten group upon performance. *Child Development,* 1934, *5,* 295-303.

DeCoster, D. Housing assignments for high ability students. *Journal of College Student Personnel,* 1966, *7,* 10-22.

Douglas, J.A., & Jason, L.A. Transitions: Utilizing behavioral technology to facilitate entry into a school and an occupation. *Crisis Intervention,* 1979, *10,* 68-79.

Drabman, R.S., & Furman, W. Behavioral procedures in the classroom. In D.S. Glenwick and L.A. Jason (Eds.), *Behavioral Community Psychology: Progress and Prospects.* New York: Praeger, 1980.

Garell, D.C. A new approach to teen-age smoking. *Pediatrics,* 1976, *57,* 465-466.

Garmezy, N. Vulnerability research and the issue of primary prevention. *American Journal of Orthopsychiatry,* 1971, *41,* 101-116.

Glover, J., & Gary, A.L. Procedures to increase some aspects of creativity. *Journal of Applied Behavior Analysis,* 1976, *9,* 79-84.

Goldfried, M.R., & Merbaum, M. (Eds.). *Behavior Change Through Self-Control.* New York: Holt, Rinehart & Winston, 1973.

Goldston, S.E. An overview of primary prevention programing. In D.C. Klein and S.E. Goldston (Eds.), *Primary Prevention: An Idea Whose Time Has Come.* Rockville, MD: Department of Health, Education and Welfare, 1977.

Hartup, W.W. Peer relations and the growth of social competence. In M.W. Kent and J.E. Rolf (eds.), *Primary Prevention of Psychopathology. Volume III. Social Competence in Children.* Hanover, NH: University Press of New England, 1979.

Iscoe, I. Community psychology and the competent community. *American Psychologist,* 1974, *29,* 607-613.

Jaremko, M.E. A component analysis of stress inoculation: Review and prospectus. *Cognitive Therapy and Research,* 1979, *3,* 35-48.

Jason, L.A. Early secondary prevention with disadvantaged preschool children. *American Journal of Community Psychology,* 1975, *3,* 33-46.

Jason, L.A. Behavioral community psychology: Conceptualizations and applications. *Journal of Community Psychology,* 1977, *5,* 303-312.

Jason, L.A., Ferone, L., & Soucy, G. Teaching peer-tutoring behaviors in first and third grade classrooms. *Psychology in the Schools,* 1979, *16,* 261-269.

Jason, L.A., & Ferone, L. From early secondary to primary preventive interventions in schools. *Journal of Prevention,* in press.

Jason, L.A., & Glenwick, D.S. An overview of behavioral community psychology. In D.S. Glenwick and L.A. Jason (eds.), *Behavioral Community Psychology: Progress and Prospects.* New York: Praeger, 1980. (a)

Jason, L.A., & Glenwick, D.S. Future directions: A critical look at the behavioral community approach. In D.S. Glenwick and L.A. Jason (Eds.), *Behavioral Community Psychology: Progress and Prospects.* New York: Praeger, 1980. (b)

Jason, L.A., & Glenwick, D.S. Urban and rural perspectives towards traditional and community-oriented mental health services in the schools: An initial investigation. *Journal of Community Psychology,* 1979, *7,* 50-52.

Jason, L.A., & Nelson, T. Investigating relationships between problem behaviors and environmental design. *Corrective and Social Psychiatry,* 1980, *26,* 53-57.

Jason, L.A., & Smith, T. The behavioral ecological matchmaker. *Teaching of Psychology,* in press.

Jason, L.A., Robson, S.D., & Lipshutz, S.A. Enhancing sharing behaviors through the use of naturalistic contingencies. *Journal of Community Psychology,* in press.

Jason, L.A., Soucy, G.P., & Ferone, L. Open field investigation in enhancing children's social skills. *Group,* in press.

Kelly, J.G. Naturalistic observations in contrasting social environments. In E.P. Willems and H.L. Raush (Eds.), *Naturalistic Viewpoints in Psychological Research*. New York: Holt, Rinehart & Winston, 1969.

Kirschenbaum, D.S. Social competence and evaluation in the inner-city: Cincinnati's social skills development program. *Journal of Consulting and Clinical Psychology*, 1979, *47*, 778-780.

Kuhn, T.S. *The Structure of Scientific Revolutions*. Chicago: University of Chicago Press, 1962.

MacDonald, K.R., Hedberg, A.G., & Campbell, L.M. A behavioral revolution in community mental health. *Community Mental Health Journal*, 1974, *10*, 228-235.

Matese, F., Shorr, S., & Jason, L.A. Behavioral and community interventions during transitions to parenthood. In A. Jeger and R. Slotnick (Eds.), *Community Mental Health: A Behavioral-Ecological Perspective*. New York: Plenum, in press.

Mayron, L.W., Ott, J., Nations, R., & Mayron, E. Light, radiation and academic behavior: Initial studies on the effects of full-spectrum lighting and radiation shielding on behavior and academic performance on school children. *Academic Therapy*, 1974, *10*, 33-47.

Meichenbaum, D.H. & Turk, D. The cognitive-behavioral management of anxiety, anger and pain. In P.O. Davidson (Ed.), *The Behavioral Management of Anxiety, depression, and Pain*. New York: Brunner/Mazel, 1976.

Meyers, A.W., Artz, L.M., & Craighead, W.E. The effects of instructions, incentive, and feedback on a community problem: Dormitory noise. *Journal of Applied Behavior Analysis*, 1976, *9*, 445-457.

Moos, R.H. *Evaluating Correctional and Community Settings*. New York: John Wiley, 1975.

Nietzel, M.T., Winett, R.A., MacDonald, M.L. & Davidson, W.C. *Behavioral Approaches to Community Psychology*. New York: Pergamon Press, 1977.

O'Neill, P. Educating divergent thinkers: An ecological investigation. *American Journal of Community Psychology*, 1976, *4*, 99-107.

Plunkett, R.J. & Gordon, J.E. *Epidemiology and Mental Illness*. New York: Basic Books, 1960.

Poser, E.G. Toward a theory of behavioral prophylaxis. *Journal of Behavior Therapy and Experimental Psychiatry*, 1970, *1*, 39-45.

Poser, E.G., & Hartman, L.M. Issues in behavioral prevention: Empirical findings. *Advances in Behavior Research and Therapy*, 1979, *2*, 1-25.

Poser, E.G., & King, M. Strategies for the prevention of maladaptive fear responses. *Canadian Journal of Behavioral Science*, 1975, *7*, 279-294.

Quilitch, H.R., & Risley, T.R. The effects of play materials on social play. *Journal of Applied Behavior Analysis*, 1973, *6*, 573-578.

Russell, M.B., & Bernal, M.E. Temporal and climatic variables in naturalistic observation. *Journal of Applied Behavior Analysis*, 1977, *10*, 399-405.

Second Annual Report of the Experimental Housing Allowance Program. U. S. Department of Housing and Urban Development. Washington, DC: Office of Policy Development and Research, 1974.

Sirbu, W., Cotler, S., & Jason, L.A. Primary prevention: Teaching parents behavioral child rearing skills. *Family Therapy*, 1978, *5*, 163-170.

Sommer, R. *Personal Space: The Behavioral Basis of Design.* Englewood Cliffs, NJ: Prentice-Hall, 1969.

Spitzzeri, A., & Jason, L.A. Prevention and treatment of smoking in school age children. *Journal of Drug Education,* 1979, *9,* 285-296.

Spivack, G., & Shure, M.B. *Social Adjustment of Young Children.* San Francisco: Jossey-Bass, 1976.

Strain, P.S., Shores, R.E., & Kerr, M.M. An experimental analysis of "spillover" effects on the social interaction of behaviorally handicapped preschool children. *Journal of Applied Behavior Analysis,* 1976, *9,* 31-40.

Suomi, S.J. Peers, play and primary prevention in primates. In M.W. Kent and J.E. Rolf (Eds.), *Primary Prevention of Psychopathology. Volume III. Social Competence in Children.* Hanover, NH: University Press of New England, 1979.

Thelen, M.H., Fry, R.A., Fehrenbach, P.A., & Frautchi, N.M. Therapeutic videotape and film modelling: A review. *Psychological Bulletin,* 1979, *86,* 701-720.

Trickett, E., & Moos, R. Personal correlates of contrasting environments: Student satisfaction in high school classrooms. *American Journal of Community Psychology,* 1974, *2,* 1-12.

Wachs, T.D., Uzgiris, I.C., & Hunt, J.M. Cognitive development in infants of different age levels and from different environmental backgrounds: An explanatory investigation. *Merrill-Palmer Quarterly,* 1971, *17,* 283-318.

Wright, S.R., & Wright, J.D. Income maintenance and work behavior. *Social Policy,* 1975, *6,* 24-32.

7

Delinquency Prevention Programs
Mental Health and the Law

Gary R. VandenBos
American Psychological Association
Michael O. Miller
University of Michigan

Within the interface of mental health and the law, the most common type of preventive efforts has been the secondary prevention of juvenile delinquency. These efforts have been labeled "diversion programs." They attempt to change the behavior of youths after they have had some contact with the juvenile justice system as an alternative to further processing within the justice system. Such programs were recommended by the Task Force on Juvenile Delinquency of the President's Commission on Law Enforcement and Administration of Justice (1967), which had recognized the basic ineffectiveness (and potential harm) of involving juveniles who manifest primarily social and emotional problems in the justice system. Interest in and development of diversion programs for youth was spurred by this increasing recognition of the limits of rehabilitation in "correctional" institutions.

This is not the first time that a shift in the place and focus of "rehabilitative" efforts with youthful offenders has occurred. Ironically, the juvenile justice authority itself was established to prevent abuse to youth within the traditional adult justice system. The first juvenile court was founded in Chicago in 1899 because of the awareness of harm done to children who were subjected to the same procedures and punishments as adults (although an alternative explanation has been offered by Platt, 1969). The goals and motivations of current diversion advocates are similar to those of the reformers at the turn of the century. Both have sought to avoid the ineffective and potentially harmful effects of legal processing of juveniles by changing the names, location, focus, and procedures used. These new programs will be subject to the same dangers involving coercion, stigmatization, and ineffectiveness, unless careful attention is given to the design, implementation, evaluation, and modification of diversion programs (Campbell, 1969).

In this chapter we will selectively examine the literature on delinquency, focusing upon the problem of predicting it and the effectiveness of diversion programs. We will then consider some illustrative examples of diversion programs that are well designed, both clinically and from a research standpoint. We will conclude by noting features we believe are critical to effective diversion programming.

Juvenile Delinquency and
Juvenile Diversion

Primary prevention efforts within the mental health/law interface have been very limited. This is related to the fact that there are many interesting and plausible, yet unproven, accounts of delinquency causation. Theories concerning delinquency have ranged from psychoanalytic explanations (Aichhorn, [1925] 1963) to sociological theories based on the negative correlations between rates of delinquency and socioeconomic status (Shaw & McKay, 1942), to mixed theories which incorporate many diverse views (Cohen, 1955; Hirschi, 1969; Gold & Mann, 1972). Lacking a comprehensive theory *and* empirical proof, it has been nearly impossible to identify "high risk" children by isolating the social or psychological pathogens that "cause" delinquency.

However, major attempts have been made to identify predictor variables. Glueck and Glueck (1950) undertook a massive study in which 500 urban delinquents were compared with 500 nondelinquents on several hundred variables. Selected "predictor" variables were then put into tabular form (Glueck & Glueck, 1959) to predict later delinquency. Unfortunately, longitudinal studies have demonstrated many problems with this approach (Lundman & Scarpitti, 1978). A recent review by Rappaport, Lamiell, and Seidman (in press) did not find any more conclusive research.

A central research problem of equal importance to program administrators and evaluators concerns the definition of the target population(s). It is well illustrated in the Rappaport et al. (in press) review. They reviewed all of the delinquency prediction studies reported over the past decade in the *Journal of Abnormal Psychology* and the *Journal of Consulting and Clinical Psychology*. Of the 20 studies, 16 defined "delinquents" as juveniles who had been so labeled by virtue of court action and "nondelinquents" as juveniles not involved with the courts. The distinction between the two groups, however, is far from clear, as seen by studies by Gold (1970; Williams & Gold, 1972) and others (Erickson & Empey, 1963) which have demonstrated that "nondelinquents" report numerous anti-social behaviors which could have brought them to the attention of the juvenile justice system. Thus, studies utilizing a "delinquent" versus "non-delinquent" design, based on official definitions, may actually be mea-suring variables which make an offender "visible" to the police and others, rather than the antecedents of delinquent behavior itself. Moreover, re-search has shown that socioeconomic, racial, and sexual biases influence the handling of delinquency cases (Black & Reiss, 1970; Arnold, 1971).

All 20 studies reviewed by Rappaport et al. involved the contrasting group technique of comparing scores obtained by a "delinquency" group and by a "nondelinquency" group on various measures. The research examines the relative presence in each group of such attributes as demo-graphic and socioeconomic characteristics, ego development, problem-solving ability, discrimination-learning ability, verbal mediation skills, fu-ture time perspective, or some combination of these. The level of dis-crimination between the groups was typically quite small. In the absence of perfect predictors, the danger of identifying and serving "false posi-tives" (children predicted to become delinquent but who will not, in fact, become delinquent) is high (Toby, 1968). It has been argued, in fact, that rather than diverting children who would have been brought into the legal system, diversion programs are bringing into the quasi-legal diversion programs children who would have been previously excluded from the legal system (Rutherford & McDermott, 1976; Fo & O'Donnell, 1975).

This is not to say that delinquency research has been without clinical value. It simply does not help us predict who will or will not become a "delinquent" in the future. Since there is a distinct risk in any program that labels children as delinquent or predelinquent (Schur, 1973), it seems to us that the use of any marginally valid prediction instrument is ques-tionable. The clinical value of earlier research attempting to predict delin-quency relates to the "clues" it provides about the type of emotional and/or cognitive differences between populations varying in their degree of penetration into the legal system. This research suggests the types of interpersonal and communication skill training that might be helpful with alienated adolescents, and can be used in designing intervention programs for youths who engage in frequent delinquent behavior. Of course, the effectiveness of such programs must be empirically evaluated (Gold, 1974).

There have been many summaries of diversion approaches (Dixon & Wright, 1975; O'Brien, 1977; Rovner-Piecznik, 1974; Wright & Dixon,

1977), as well as examples of individual projects (Carter & Klein, 1976; Davidson et al., 1977; Lemert, 1971; Shepherd & Rothenberger, 1978). There is also a growing literature skeptical of the overall value and effectiveness of diversion (Bullington et al., 1978; Klein, 1975, 1976; Lundman, 1976; Lundman et al., 1976; Rutherford & McDermott, 1976; Scari & Hassenfeld, 1976; Vinter, 1976). Bullington et al. (1978), for example, contend that current programs cannot avoid stigmatizing and are basically incompatible with due process ideals. Lundman, McFarlane, and Scarpitti (1976) reviewed 22 years of delinquency prevention projects and found that few of them had any demonstrable beneficial impact. Lundman and Scarpitti (1978) offer a set of recommendations to guide future efforts: (a) an expectation of minimal effect or failure, (b) evaluations which utilize several objective measures within an experimental design, and (c) increased protection of the clients. Such realistic suggestions are similar to Campbell's (1969) observations in reference to any social service delivery system. Administrators must emphasize the importance of the problem and the need to conduct many "false" trials, rather than investing themselves in one cure-all approach.

From a policy perspective, we must consider what these reveiws represent. They are normative. They tell us what is reasonable to expect of the average program. They do not tell us what is possible. They do not tell us what the critical factors are which determine whether or not a given program is effective. For this we must examine programs which demonstrate some effectiveness *and* a degree of scientific credibility, and evaluate them in light of knowledge of the populations they attempt to serve and with an understanding of clinical technique.

Illustrative Effective
Delinquency Prevention Programs

The Sacramento Diversion Project (Baron et al., 1976; Baron & Feeney, 1976) operated under the aegis of the juvenile court. The overall study included all status offense and minor criminal offense cases. The diversion component utilized intensive short-term family counseling provided by specially trained probation officers.

The probation staff volunteered to participate in the diversion project. Project staff were selected on the basis of expressed interest and perceived aptitude. Half of the probation department staff worked on the project and half served as the "control" staff. The diversion project staff consisted of eight professionals (a supervisor and seven counselors). All had college educations, and their experience in working with populations similar to the project population ranged from zero to ten years (with the mean appearing to be between three and four years). The "control" staff consisted of nine professionals (a supervisor and eight counselors). All had college degrees, and they had comparable experience with adolescent delinquent populations.

Initial training and ongoing in-service training and supervision were a major feature of this diversion project. The diversion staff received one week of intensive training and orientation from experienced family therapists, which included psychologists, psychiatrists, and other family therapy specialists. In-service training and ongoing supervision continued throughout the project.

Lectures on family processes and family counseling techniques were given, but they generally preceded actual demonstrations by the lecturer, and the demonstration was followed by a discussion of the lecture and observed clinical work. Considerable use was made of role-playing. Trainees, under the observation of the rest of the training group, role-played counselors, adolescents, and family members, and then discussed the experience. Understanding of communication patterns and interactional patterns was taught by examining them as they developed within the training group. A norm regarding the value of self-understanding and its relation to being an effective family counselor was established. This included using one's own family and co-workers to understand the dynamics of interpersonal communication and interaction in general and one's own patterns in particular.

Trainees in this project worked as co-therapists with an experienced family therapist and had their independent work with families observed by an experienced family therapist. In addition, their independent work with families was videotaped for later supervision with an experienced therapist (with other trainees present), and individual consultations with experienced family therapists were arranged. As would be expected, trainees found observation of others and role-playing to be the least threatening and supervision in a group setting and the analysis of training group processes the most threatening aspect of the program. The specific training and treatment procedures are described in detail by Baron and Feeney (1976).

The design of the study required that intake procedures at the court be modified. All cases involving status offenses (truants, runaways, and incorrigibles) and minor "criminal" offenses (fighting or possession of alcohol were included, but drug possession was excluded) were part of the study.

All such cases were randomly assigned to either the diversion project or routine court processing. Out of 2438 referrals, 1361 met their criteria; 803 cases were assigned to the diversion project, and 558 cases were assigned to the comparison condition.

If the case was assigned to the diversion project, a family session was scheduled for the same day (staff were available from 8:00 a.m. to 2:00 a.m.). Such sessions could be as long as necessary, and varied from one hour to two and a half hours in length. The counselor discussed the "problems" and suggested that they could best be handled if they were addressed by the family as a whole. All sessions after the first session were completely voluntary. The maximum number of sessions that could be provided was five. If the family chose not to continue, a telephone follow-up was made to assess its functioning.

If the case was assigned for routine handling, interviews with various individuals were scheduled over the course of several weeks, and placements out of the home, case investigation, and informal and formal hearings were begun, as necessary. Consultation with and/or referral to community agencies and schools occurred.

The researchers found that only 3.7 percent of the diversion cases had to be petitioned to the juvenile court, whereas 19.8 percent of the control cases required petitioning. Only 13.9 percent of the diversion cases required initial out-of-home placement, whereas 55.5 percent of the control cases required such placement. Diversion cases required fewer subsequent out-of-home placements than controls, and the length of placement in all cases were shorter for diversion than for control cases. Rebooking, multiple booking, and booking for serious offenses were all significantly lower for the diversion cases than for control cases. The average total cost per diversion case was $274 compared with $562 for control cases.

A second family-counseling-type diversion program attempted to evaluate the effectiveness of a more behaviorally oriented family intervention program (Alexander & Parsons, 1973; Klein et al., 1977). The goal of the treatment was to modify the interactions within the "deviant" families so that they would approximate the interactions within families considered to be better adjusted. The specific interactions focused on were derived from the findings of Patterson and Reid (1970): families of delinquents differ from families of "normals" in that they (a) talk infrequently, (b) are less active, (c) respond to each other in unequal ways, and (d) generally have few positive interactions. The therapists attempted to reduce maladaptive family behavior by actively modeling, prompting, and reinforcing (a) clear communication of substantive concerns as well as feelings, (b) clear presentations of "demands" and alternative solutions, and (c) negotiation among family members regarding privileges and responsibilities, based on the principles of contingency contracting.

Ninety-nine families that came into contact with the juvenile court because of status offenses were referred to the program. Forty-six families were randomly assigned to the treatment program. The behaviorally oriented family therapy was provided by 18 first- and second-year graduate students in clinical psychology who were participating in a practicum emphasizing family treatment and were supervised by the two authors. The treatment group (Group I) was compared with three comparison groups: (a) court-provided, client-centered family counseling by newly trained therapists (Group II); (b) eclectic, psychodynamically oriented family therapy provided upon referral of clergymen through a church-sponsored program (Group III); and (c) a "no-treatment" control group which had been released from court jurisdiction (Group IV).

The data suggest that the short-term behavioral family intervention (Group I) was superior on several measures. Recidivism (reappearance in juvenile court) for Group I was 26 percent compared with 50 percent for no-treatment controls (Group IV), and compared with 47 percent for Group II and 73 percent for Goup III. A further follow-up study found a difference in the percentage of siblings referred to the court in the two to three years after termination of treatment. Only 20 percent of the siblings of Group I subjects were referred, while 40 percent of the Group IV (no-treatment controls) were referred, and 59 percent of Group II and 63 percent of Group III were referred. These latter findings suggest that treatment effects can extend beyond the individuals originally seen as the focus of the intervention.

There have been some relatively successful tertiary treatment programs for delinquents which provide information relevant to planning and implementing a diversion program. The California Youth Authority authorized random placement of criminally delinquent youths into intensive community placement programs and/or intensive small-residential centers (Palmer, 1971, 1974). Youths placed in the community were provided differential treatment based upon their level of ego-functioning, as defined by a precise set of diagnostic procedures. A central ingredient of the program was the pairing of the youth and the probation officer, matching agents who were especially adept in working with particular types of youths with such adolescents. A second phase of the investigation involved placement of specifically designated youths into small residential centers before they were released to the community. In both phases community treatment was found to be effective and less costly than traditional residential placement.

A second program (Persons, 1966, 1967) was administered within a traditional correctional school. It offered an intensive therapeutic program involving both group therapy and individual therapy. Forty-one adolescents received treatment and were compared with 41 matched controls. The first-year rate of return to a penal institution among the treated group was 32 percent compared with 61 percent for the comparison group. The recidivism rate of those judged before release to be "successfully treated" treatment cases (n = 30) was also compared with that of the "unsuccessfully treated" treatment cases (n = 11). The "unsuccessfully treated" treatment cases had a recidivism rate higher than that of the controls. In addition, the therapy failures were more "spectacular" failures: they included armed robbery and murder.

These two programs illustrate several points. First, any single intervention program with delinquent youth will be ineffective with a certain percentage of the population. Second, moderately accurate indicators can be developed (from combined program evaluation and clinical evaluation) to improve clinical effectiveness. Third, generally effective programs may have a negative impact on some clients. The worst failures (defined by later serious—and possibly violent—behavior) are overrepresented in "treated" groups. Unfortunately, the design of these and other studies does not permit a determination of whether the later criminal behavior was "caused" by the program or whether the assessment and treatment were simply inadequate. (A more general discussion of negative effects in psychotherapy is given by Strupp and Hadley, 1977).

Prevention programs for seriously alienated adolescents do not have to be based in a hospital, clinic, or youth services agency. A comprehensive, vocationally oriented, psychotherapeutic demonstration project, which did not utilize a centralized office or center, has been reported (Massimo & Shore, 1963, 1967). This project has been the subject of long-term evaluation (Shore & Massimo, 1966, 1969, 1973, 1979).

Twenty "antisocial" adolescent males were selected for study. Each subject met the following criteria: (a) between 15 and 17 years old; (b) an IQ between 85 and 110, (c) a long-standing history of difficulty with school, peers, and authority, including a history of overt aggression; (d) suspension from or voluntary dropping out of school attributable to poor school performance combined with antisocial behavior; (e) no gross observable psychotic behavior; and (f) no previous psychotherapy for the boy or any members of his family. The 20 adolescents were randomly assigned to either the treatment program or a "no-contact" control group.

Services of the treatment program were initiated at a crisis point in the life of the adolescent—premature exits from school, generally with little choice and with little regret. The original contact with the adolescent was in the form of an "outreach," wherein the worker offered help oriented toward concrete issues such as getting a job, filling out application forms, or visiting potential employers. After an initial meeting, the service was voluntary. Service was available for 10 months, provided on a one-to-one basis, and was flexible and individualized for the particular adolescent. The "therapist" purposely identified his independence of the school, court, or other authoritarian agencies by "accidental" mispronunciation of the name of the adolescent's truant officer and meeting in such settings as bowling alleys and public buildings. It was recognized that alienated adolescents often reject assistance because of their poor experiences with and mistrust of authority figures (including parents and "helping" professionals). Initial discussions never involved "return to school" invitations or other obvious "do what I want you to" initiatives. The initial direction of service was determined by what the adolescent wanted or selected from a casually mentioned list of examples of how the worker might be helpful. Remedial education was provided on an informal basis, usually in response to a specific real-life difficulty. Employment served as the main catalyst or vehicle for exploring educational, familial, and interpersonal issues. As contact continued, it included vocational counseling, advocacy, remedial education, and psychotherapy—all provided by the same professional, not through "fragmenting" referrals. The program is well described by Massimo and Shore (1963), and an excellent description of alienated adolescents and the experience of working with them is provided in a later publication by the same authors (1967).

Four follow-up studies of the 20 adolescents have been conducted over the last 15 years (Shore & Massimo, 1966, 1969, 1973, 1979). In each instance, the treatment group has been found to be functioning at a significantly higher level than the control group. This difference is evident in better work histories (including higher pay, higher levels of employment, and more stable employment), better interpersonal relations (including higher rates of marriage and more stable marriages), and less likelihood of later legal difficulties (including lower rates of contact with legal authorities and less serious contact when it does occur). There is also evidence that significant psychological changes occurred—first in self-esteem, next in impulse control (including improved ability to verbalize and solve problems rather than "act-out"), and finally in attitude toward others, particularly authority figures. Not every case was successful, but the differences between the two groups is dramatic.

Another vocationally oriented program is richly described in *Build Me A Mountain: Youth, Poverty, and the Creation of New Settings* (Goldenberg, 1971). Twenty-nine inner-city youths with frequent law violations were "treated" by indigenous workers who lived with them. Workers were selected on the basis of their commitment to others and mild dissatisfaction with traditional agencies and intervention methods. The treated youths, as compared with the controls, at the end of one year had higher employment rates, better "attitudes," and lower rates of legal difficulties.

Elements Related to the
Effectiveness of Diversion Programs

A genuine interest in and commitment to the adolescents. All of the effective juvenile diversion programs we have reviewed in the literature or reviewed as consultants have involved staff with a clear primary goal of being helpful to the adolescents to whom they were assigned. This often means that the therapist sees agency paperwork and procedures as "necessary evils" that the therapist, not the adolescent, must endure and must not let get in the way of being helpful to the adolescent. It requires having the adolescent's interest and needs foremost in one's mind, rather than the agency's image in the community, or expectations of the adolescent's family.

A nonjudgmental helpful orientation. Adolescents, particularly the type of alienated adolescent who comes through the juvenile court, will "disappoint" their therapists. A genuine commitment is needed to tolerate the many disappointments caused by minor "wrongs" and a few major unacceptable acts by such adolescents. Such a commitment involves being willing to help the adolescents deal with any situation they have gotten into without telling them it is their own fault and without making them feel unnecessarily guilty. The availability of help cannot be dependent on "being good" or "obeying the therapist." A commitment to being helpful involves communicating that the therapist can understand and accept the feelings and impulses which prompted the youths' actions, while making it clear that he or she does not approve the behavior—and helping them to think of better solutions for similar situations they will face in the future.

Multiple foci of problem resolution. The problems of the adolescents who come through the juvenile court are both interpersonal and intrapersonal. The effective therapist must acknowledge that the problems of the alienated adolescent reflect a complex intertwining of "reality" problems and psychological problems. Both should be addressed, but the first step generally will be with "real world" problems. This is typically the area of the adolescents' lives with which they want and see help as needed. They want "action." The adolescent may need help in dealing with family, school, police, or employers. At first the therapist will often need to intervene on the adolescent's behalf with these individuals, because the adolescent will have little status and poor credibility. Effective diversion programs always involve the therapist acting in part as the advocate for the adolescent, in one form or another, at some point. The therapist should help the adolescent get back into school if that is what he or she wants, or to get a job now if the youth does not want to go to school. Over time, the therapist will be able to help the adolescent begin to anticipate difficult situations, think them through in advance, and plan how to handle them—and realize that only half the time will things work out as planned.

Tailoring the system to the adolescent, not the adolescent to the system. Alienated adolescents are in legal difficulty because they do not "obey the rules." They do not obey rules because rules have rarely gotten them anything they wanted. Most adolescents who come through the juvenile court system see "doing what someone else wants" to mean losing, giving in, and being ineffective. It is also boring. Effective diversion programs start by proving to the adolescent that "the system" can deliver something. The first step for the therapist who wishes to be effective is to find something that the adolescent wants or wants help with (and which is reasonable and appropriate to provide) and provide it. This might mean help with a boss, teacher, parent, or friend. But it always involves considering first what the adolescent says he or she needs, not what others think the adolescent needs. Often, the adolescent's perceived needs involve the desire to be respected by his or her peers. The therapist can acknowledge this desire and help the adolescent to find alternative ways to earn that respect.

Flexible programming that delivers help when it is needed. Effective diversion programs do not operate on a nine-to-five basis with rigidly scheduled appointment hours. Nor do they wait for the adolescent to come to them. Effective diversion programs have strong "outreach" components. They operate in a timely fashion. Someone is always available—

perhaps not ｒthe person the adolescent has regular contact with, but someone.ｒ Effective diversion programs keep reaching out. When the adolescent does not show up when expected, the therapist calls to find out what happened and does this in a nonjudgmental manner. Resources and contact should be most intensively provided in the first few days or weeks of contact. This is the point at which the therapist "proves" to the adolescent that he or she can be helpful. This cannot be done when meetings are for one hour each week. After the adolescent knows that working with the therapist is useful, meetings can be scheduled on a routine basis once or twice a week, but even then there must be mechanisms for emergencies.

Strong training components. Work with alienated adolescents is tiring. Since young therapists tend to be more energetic than older therapists, successful diversion programs generally have a majority of the staff under 30 years old. "Burn-out" is an ever-present staff problem. Effective diversion generally involves some mechanism for continually examining one's clinical work as one way of preventing the buildup of frustration and resulting ineffective clinical functioning. Effective diversion programs have as a program norm that it is valuable to continue to learn—to learn more about yourself and to learn more about helping others. Diversion programs that do not emphasize staff growth do not generally encourage client growth.

Ongoing and meaningful program evaluation. Effective diversion programs monitor their clinical operation and program effectiveness and use the information to improve the program. Clinical supervision and some type of management information system are needed, but these are only a small part of useful program monitoring. A range of clinically meaningful data on the clients served should be gathered throughout the contact with youth. This does *not* mean an "intake" in which someone asks a series of questions and fills out a form. Rather, the therapist should know the type of information routinely needed and gather it as the opportunity arises, recording it later. There should be regular staff meetings to discuss their interactions with clients. Psychological and behavioral assessments can provide data which is useful in both treatment planning and later program evaluation. However, a large battery should rarely be used (except for formal research projects), and a specific rationale should exist for using particular tests. Some type of end-of-service assessment should be made, and follow-up data (reassessment, school performance, work performance, legal contacts, and so on) should be collected at standard intervals. The entire staff should be involved in reviewing the data, and it should be examined from several perspectives—including clinical ones. On the basis of evaluation data, the referral system, intake process, client assignment procedures, treatment procedures, program structure, training and supervision, administration, and program evaluation should be altered if indicated.

Summary

Only limited mental health prevention initiatives have taken place within the legal system. Most such interventions with adolescents have been "secondary" prevention efforts, involving diversion programs which direct juveniles away from legal involvement and into more psychotherapeutically oriented service programs. Many of these juvenile diversion programs, in our opinion, have been poorly conceptualized and/or poorly implemented. An examination of some programs with documentation of effectiveness suggests several key ingredients which should be incorporated in developing future programs of this type.

References

Aichhorn, A. *Wayward Youth.* New York: Viking Press, [1925] 1963.

Alexander, J.F., & Parsons, B.V. Short-term behavioral intervention with delinquent families: Impact on family process and recidivism. *Journal of Abnormal Psychology,* 1973, *81,* 219-225.

Arnold, W. Race and ethnicity relative to other factors in juvenile court dispositions. *American Journal of Sociology,* 1971, 77, 211-227.

Baron, R., & Feeney, F. *Juvenile Diversion Through Family Counseling.* Washington, DC: National Institute of Law Enforcement and Criminal Justice (LEAA), 1976.

Baron, R., Feeney, F., & Thornton, W. Preventing delinquency through diversion. In R.M. Carter and M.W. Klein (Eds.), *Back on the Street: The Diversion of Juvenile Offenders.* Englewood Cliffs, NJ: Prentice-Hall, 1976.

Black, D., & Reiss, J., Jr. Control of juveniles. *American Sociological Review,* 1970, *35,* 63-77.

Bullington, B., Sprowls, J., Katkin, D., & Phillips, M. A critique of diversionary juvenile justice. *Crime and Delinquency,* 1978, *24,* 59-71.

Campbell, D.T. Reforms as experiments. *American Psychologist,* 1969, *24,* 409-429.

Carter, R.M., & Klein, M.W. (Eds.). *Back on the Street: The Diversion of Juvenile Offenders.* Englewood Cliffs, NJ: Prentice-Hall, 1976.

Cohen, A. *Delinquent Boys.* New York: Free Press, 1955.

Davidson, W.S., Rappaport, J., Seidman, E., Berck, P., Rapp, C., Rhodes, W., & Herring, J. A diversion program for juvenile offenders. *Social Work Research and Abstracts,* 1977, *1,* 47-56.

Dixon, M.C., & Wright, W.E. *Juvenile Delinquency Prevention Programs: An Evaluation of Policy Related Research on the Effectiveness of Prevention Programs.* Nashville, TN: Peabody College for Teachers, Office of Educational Services, 1975.

Erickson, M., & Empey, L.M. Court records, undetected delinquency and decision-making. *Journal of Criminal Law, Criminology and Police Science,* 1963, *54,* 456-469.

Fo, W.S.O., & O'Donnell, C.R. The buddy system: Effect of community intervention on delinquent offenses. *Behavior Therapy,* 1975, *6,* 522-524.

Glueck, S., & Glueck, E. *Unraveling Juvenile Delinquency.* Cambridge, MA: Harvard University Press, 1950.

Glueck, S., & Glueck, E. *Predicting Delinquency and Crime.* Cambridge, MA: Harvard University Press, 1959.

Gold, M. *Delinquent Behavior in an American City.* Belmont, CA: Brooks/Cole Publishing, 1970.

Gold, M. A time for skepticism. *Crime and Delinquency,* 1974, *20,* 20-24.

Gold, M., & Mann, D. Delinquency as defense. *American Journal of Orthopsychiatry,* 1972, *42,* 463-479.

Goldenberg, I.I. *Build Me a Mountain: Youth, Poverty and the Creation of New Settings.* Cambridge: MIT Press, 1971.

Hirschi, T. *Causes of Delinquency.* Berkeley: University of California Press, 1969.

Klein, M.W. Issues and realities in police diversion programs. *Crime and Delinquency,* 1975, *22,* 421-427.

Klein, M.W. Issues in police diversion of juvenile offenders. In R.M. Carter and M.W. Klein (Eds.), *Back on the Street: The Diversion of Juvenile Offenders.* Englewood Cliffs, NJ: Prentice-Hall, 1976.

Klein, N.C., Alexander, J.D., & Parsons, B.V. Impact of family systems intervention on recidivism and sibling delinquency: A model of primary prevention and program evaluation. *Journal of Consulting and Clinical Psychology,* 1977, *45,* 469-474.

Lemert, E. Instead of court: Diversion in juvenile justice. Chevy Chase, MD: National Institute of Mental Health, Center for Studies of Crime and Delinquency, 1971.

Lundman, R.J. Will diversion reduce delinquency? *Crime and Delinquency,* 1976, *22,* 428-437.

Lundman, R.J., McFarlane, P.T., & Scarpitti, F.R. Delinquency prevention: A description and assessment of projects reported in the professional literature. *Crime and Delinquency,* 1976, *22,* 297-308.

Lundman, R.J., & Scarpitti, F.R. Delinquency prevention: Recommendations for future projects. *Crime and Delinquency,* 1978, *24,* 207-220.

Massimo, J., & Shore, M. The effectiveness of a comprehensive vocationally oriented psychotherapy program for adolescent delinquent boys. *American Journal of Orthopsychiatry,* 1963, *33,* 634-643.

Massimo, J., & Shore, M. Comprehensive vocationally oriented psychotherapy: A new treatment technique for lower class adolescent delinquent youth. *Psychiatry,* 1967, *30,* 229-236.

O'Brien, K.E. *Juvenile Diversion, Second Edition. A Selected Bibliography.* Washington, DC: National Institute of Law Enforcement and Criminal Justice, 1977.

Palmer, T. California's community treatment program for delinquent adolescents. *Journal of Research in Crime and Delinquency,* 1971, *8,* 74-92.

Palmer, T. The Youth Authority's treatment project. *Federal Probation,* 1974, *38,* 3-14.

Patterson, G.R., & Reid, J.B. Reciprocity and coercion: Two facts of social systems. In C. Neuringer and J. Michael (Eds.), *Behavior Modification in Clinical Psychology.* New York: Appleton-Century-Crofts, 1970.

Persons, R.W. Psychological and behavioral change in delinquents following psychotherapy. *Journal of Clinical Psychology,* 1966, *22,* 337-340.

Persons, R.W. Relationship between psychotherapy with institutionalized boys and subsequent community adjustment. *Journal of Consulting Psychology,* 1967, *31,* 137-141.

Platt, A. *The Child Savers.* Chicago, IL: University of Chicago Press, 1969.

President's Commission on Law Enforcement and Administration of Justice. *The Challenge of Crime in a Free Society.* Washington, DC: U.S. Government Printing Office, 1967.

Rappaport, J., Lamiell, J., & Seidman, E. Ethical issues for psychologists in the juvenile justice system: Know and tell. In J. Monahan (Ed.), *Who is the Client? The Ethics of Psychological Intervention in the Criminal Justice System.* Washington, DC: American Psychological Association, in press.

Rovner-Pieczenik, R. *Pretrial Intervention Strategies: An Evaluation of Policy-Related Research and Policymaker Perceptions.* Washington, DC: National Pretrial Intervention Service Center, American Bar Association, 1974.

Rutherford, A., & McDermott, R. *National Evaluation Program. Juvenile Diversion Phase 1 Summary Report.* Washington, DC: National Institute of Law Enforcement and Criminal Justice, 1976.

Scari, R., & Hassenfeld, Y. (Eds.). *Brought to Justice? Juveniles, the Courts and the Law.* Ann Arbor, MI: National Assessment of Juvenile Corrections, 1976.

Schur, E.M. *Radical Non-Intervention: Rethinking the Delinquency Problem.* Englewood Cliffs, NJ: Prentice-Hall, 1973.

Shaw, C., & McKay, H. *Juvenile Delinquency and Urban Areas.* Chicago: University of Chicago Press, 1942.

Shepherd, J., & Rothenberger, D. *Police-Juvenile Diversion: An Alternative to Prosecution.* East Lansing: Michigan State Police, 1978.

Shore, M., & Massimo, J. Comprehensive vocationally oriented psychotherapy for adolescent delinquent boys: A follow-up study. *American Journal of Orthopsychiatry,* 1966, *36,* 609-616.

Shore, M., & Massimo, J. Five years later: A follow-up study of comprehensive vocationally oriented psychotherapy. *American Journal of Orthopsychiatry,* 1969, *39,* 769-774.

Shore, M., & Massimo, J. After ten years: A follow-up study of comprehensive vocationally oriented psychotherapy. *American Journal of Orthopsychiatry,* 1973, *43,* 128-132.

Shore, M., & Massimo, J. Fifteen years after treatment: A follow-up study of comprehensive vocationally oriented psychotherapy. *American Journal of Orthopsychiatry,* 1979, *49,* 240-245.

Strupp, H.H., & Hadley, S.W. A tripartite model of mental health and therapeutic outcome: With special reference to negative effects in psychotherapy. *American Psychologist,* 1977, *32,* 187-196.

Task Force on Juvenile Delinquency. The President's Commission on Law Enforcement and Administration of Justice. *Report: Juvenile Delinquency and Youth Crime*. Washington, DC: U.S. Government Printing Office, 1967.

Toby, J. An evaluation of early identification and intensive treatment programs for predelinquents. In J. Stratton and R. Terry (Eds.), *Prevention of Juvenile Delinquency*. New York: Macmillan, 1968.

Vinter, R.D. (Ed.). *Time Out: A National Study of Juvenile Corrections Programs*. Ann Arbor, MI: National Assessment of Juvenile Corrections, 1976.

Williams, J., & Gold, M. From delinquent behavior to official delinquency. *Social Problems*, 1972, *20*, 209-229.

Wright, W.E., & Dixon, M.C. Community prevention and treatment of juvenile delinquency. A review of evaluation studies. *Journal of Research in Crime and Delinquency*, 1977, *14*, 35-67.

8

Prevention in Industrial Settings

The Employee Assistance Program

Andrea Foote
John C. Erfurt

*Worker Health Program, Institute of Labor and
Industrial Relations, University of Michigan—
Wayne State University*

The literature on prevention of health problems attempts to distinguish between primary prevention (prevention of the development of any health risk factors—that is, encouragement of healthful practices), and secondary prevention (treatment or amelioration of risk factors in order to prevent the development of disease). Primary prevention is often emphasized over secondary prevention because it attempts to intervene before problems develop, and therefore may be more effective in improving health or reducing illness. This can only happen, however, if there exists an effective technology for primary prevention. To the extent that the technology is ineffective or nonexistent, secondary prevention will be necessary if serious illness or disease is to be prevented.

In order to examine the effectiveness of a prevention technology, one must be able to specify what is to be prevented and to measure the degree to which the technology in fact prevented it. Since secondary prevention is aimed at a specific health problem, technologies or methodologies for intervening are easier to design, test, and evaluate than are technologies for primary prevention, in which the outcomes to be measured are often vague at best.

The existence of empirically effective technologies for primary prevention in the health field is questionable. In addition to the question of effectiveness, however, there is the question of cost. An intervention that attempts primary prevention must be aimed at everyone, or everyone who is statistically at risk. Secondary prevention, on the other hand, focuses on a subgroup of people who have a specific risk factor, and thus it involves a smaller target group. The choice between intervention methodologies requires information on both cost and effectiveness.

The Role of Industry
in Prevention

All intervention activities incur a cost. A decision regarding who will implement a certain activity should take into account who has incentives for the activity to be successful—in other words, who loses if the activity is not successful and/or gains if it is. Community mental health activities have been governmentally funded because mental health is a common good; the "community" gains or loses.

A community is more than an aggregate of individuals who reside within a bounded area. It is organized and stratified in various ways, and an attempt to reach the "community" will fail to the extent that it ignores the community's organization. Industry has commonly been left out of discussions of community mental health, and yet industry is not only an integral part of the larger community; each industrial organization is in fact a functioning subcommunity.

There are a number of significant points about industry in relation to health care, both physical and mental. First, industry has a captive population that includes a majority of adults for about half of their waking hours. There is no more effective way to reach these people than at the work site.

Second, not only are employed people available in a predictable location, but they are also monitored. Each employer maintains certain standards of work performance for employees and can enforce these through disciplinary procedures. Thus, the employer is not only likely to be aware of personal problems that affect people's performance at the work site, but also has considerable leverage over employees whose performance is unsatisfactory. Consequently, an employer can identify employees who may be in need of help for personal problems; and he can also make a recommendation to the employee regarding a course of action with the expectation that the employee will at least consider the recommendation seriously.

Third, industry feels the impact of personal problems in the work force through deficiencies in work performance and through the impact in high health care costs. Industry pays, either directly (to health care providers or insurance carriers) or indirectly (through wages to employees) for health care. Industry therefore has an incentive to undertake prevention activities if such activities will result in a reduction in costs sufficient to pay for themselves.

These points suggest that work sites may not be especially good locations for conducting primary prevention activities; such activities can take place at the work site, but they can take place equally well elsewhere. The special advantages of the work site favor secondary prevention activities—that is, activities focused on the identification of people who exhibit certain symptoms or risk factors that may interfere with job performance and/or increase costs to the company. The company is not only in a better position than a community agency to identify these individuals; it also has a strong incentive to help them resolve their difficulties as well as leverage to induce employees with substandard performance to take appropriate action.

Employee Assistance Programs in Industry

Industrial organizations have long been aware that certain types of personal problems result in significant decreases in productivity and/or increases in operating costs (Trice and Roman, 1972; Threatt, 1976). Alcoholism is the most commonly identified problem, costing industry billions of dollars annually in absenteeism, lost production, health care costs, and the like (Pell and D'Alonzo, 1970; Seidel, 1970). In response, many organizations set up employee alcoholism programs designed to identify and confront employees whose work performance suffers due to alcoholism and to assist them in getting to a source of care and controlling their problem (Schramm and DeFillippi, 1975).

As these programs were established, employers began to gear their problem identification, or case-finding, efforts toward objective criteria of work performance, for several reasons (Von Wiegand, 1972). First, the employer has no right to interfere with an employee's personal life off the job. If an employee has a drinking problem which does *not* interfere with his work performance, the employer has no right to interfere. Second, in the absence of objective criteria, a search for alcoholics in the work site can result in protection of friends who have an alcohol problem and mislabeling of foes who do not. Third, most people within a work force are not qualified to make a diagnosis of alcoholism, but supervisors should be qualified to identify poor work performance. In addition, work performance measures provide the program with a certain leverage in confronting employees and inducing them to take appropriate action (Roman and Trice, 1969).

The programs therefore found that they were not in the business of finding alcoholics, but of finding employees whose work performance was substandard for one or more reasons (for example, excessive absenteeism, scrap production, interpersonal problems, and violation of rules). Using work performance measures as the criteria, the programs found that while they were identifying people with alcohol problems, they were also identifying people with many other types of problems, including abuse of other drugs, emotional problems, and marital and family problems. The person with an alcohol problem was often the most obvious, especially in the later stages of the disease, but other personal/emotional problems were found to be causing equally serious problems in work performance, and the programs needed to be able to deal with those problems also (Schmidt, 1976).

Thus, occupational alcohol programs tended to broaden their focus and become employee assistance programs,[1] while maintaining a strong emphasis on the identification and treatment of alcoholism. The National Institute on Alcohol Abuse and Alcoholism estimated that, by mid-1977, some 2,400 American businesses had established such programs.

Employers are not alone in recognizing the negative consequences to employees of alcoholism and other personal problems. Labor as well has become highly involved in employee assistance programming, in part because of labor's historical concerns over the welfare of workers and in part to ensure that programs established by management do not jeopardize employees' rights. Some programs are largely or entirely labor-sponsored (Tucker, 1974), and many programs are based upon a joint union-management agreement and include both union and management representatives on the program team (Foote et al., 1980). Labor has also become involved to some extent in the establishment and/or support of appropriate treatment facilities (Schramm et al., 1978).

Structure and Functions of
Employee Assistance Programs

Because employee assistance programs have largely developed internally, they show great diversity of structure and staffing arrangements. However, most programs perform a similar set of functions. Figure 8.1 describes diagrammatically the functions performed by occupational

FIGURE 8.1   An Occupational Program: The Integration of 3 Systems

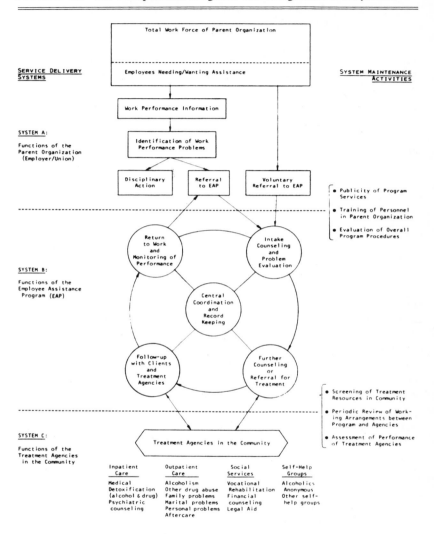

SOURCE: Erfurt and Foote (1977).

employee assistance programs. (For a more detailed discussion of this diagram and its components, see Erfurt and Foote, 1977.)

The figure is divided into three service delivery systems, each comprising a set of activities. The first system (System A) is embedded in the parent organization (the employer and/or union). This system exists to some extent in all work organizations, regardless of whether or not they operate an employee assistance program. This is the system which monitors and evaluates work performance and intervenes with remedial or disciplinary action when performance falls below minimum standards.

In the context of an employee assistance program, then, System A is responsible for identifying employees who need or want assistance, and for referring them to System B, which is the employee assistance program proper. Note that System A may generate voluntary referrals to System B that are not based on work performance problems. This is done through publicity about the services being offered by the program.

The activities of System A can be carried out by almost anyone in the work force—supervisors, medical department staff, personnel staff, labor union representatives, and co-workers. The activities are carried out as part of their normal duties. However, special training is required in how to confront employees with their job performance problems and how to make a referral to System B, and also in differentiating between the proper roles of System A and System B (Beyer and Trice, 1978).

System B—the employee assistance program (EAP)—may be a component of the organization located in a labor union, company medical department, personnel department, or free-standing within the company; or it may be an external organization that performs central diagnostic and referral functions. Normally the EAP is internal for organizations of sufficient size (for example, more than 1000 employees). Central diagnostic and referral agencies (CDRs) most often work with a number of small employers who cannot afford to staff their own programs, or, in some cases, with employers who do not want it known that they have employees with such problems.

System B (the EAP) is the critical system, in that it provides the link between the work context and the community treatment resources. This system includes (a) intake counseling and problem evaluation, (b) further counseling or referral to a treatment agency if indicated, (c) follow-up activities with program clients and treatment agencies, (d) helping clients return to work and sometimes monitoring their performance after reentry, and (e) central coordination and record-keeping.

The third system (System C) represents the range of treatment resources available in the community, including inpatient and outpatient care for a variety of problems, self-help resources, and various types of social services.

There are two different types of linkages between these three systems. The first type involves direct service linkages—the referral and follow-up activities. Thus, System B accepts referrals from System A and provides feedback information when required about the status of the clients. System B also *makes* referrals to System C (that is, to the treatment agencies which the EAP staff feel are the best treatment resources for specific clients), and receives follow-up information from System C about the progress of clients.

The type of feedback given by the EAP to the referring agent in System A is limited to need-to-know information and does not normally include the diagnosis or treatment information, except as this affects the employee's ability to work. Likewise, the feedback given by the treatment agency to the EAP is based on a consent form signed by the client and is normally limited to general information about treatment participation and progress.

The second type of linkage between Systems A and B and between Systems B and C focuses on system maintenance rather than client service. These linkages are shown along the righthand side of Figure 8.1. Between Systems A and B there are three distinct system maintenance activities: (1) general publicity to the work force about the services being offered by the EAP, how they are obtained, for whom, and so on; (2) training of various people within the work force to carry out the System A activities (that is, how to make referrals to the EAP, how to make use of the EAP staff, and so on); and (3) evaluation of the activities of both systems.

Between Systems B and C there are also three types of system maintenance linkages. The first involves screening of community treatment resources and routine updating of information about the range of resources available. The second involves a periodic review of the working arrangements that the program has made with the various treatment resources it uses in the community. This is especially important for treatment agencies that have a relatively high turnover of treatment personnel. The third linkage consists of routine evaluation of the effectiveness of agencies that are utilized, including assessment of relative cost.

The EAP and Prevention

The extent to which an employee assistance program delivers preventive services depends upon the definition of what is to be prevented. The primary impetus for the establishment of EAPs is the amelioration of certain health and mental health problems and prevention of further deterioration. In addition, however, many programs attempt early intervention, prior to the development of any serious health problem or work deterioration (Holden, 1973).

Early intervention strategies cannot rely on case-finding through work performance measures, since an attempt is being made to intervene prior to work deterioration. These programs must therefore rely on more informal methods of case-finding in which the company (System A) takes no formal action to intervene with a worker, but rather provides sufficient information and channels of communication so that employees can seek help on their own (with co-workers or family members perhaps encouraging the employees to seek help at early stages).

The degree to which EAPs actually accomplish early intervention is difficult to establish. Some programs use the number of self-referrals as an indicator of early intervention, but this is not an accurate measure; an examination of self-referrals shows that many of them have experienced a significant deterioration in work performance (Foote et al., 1978). Some self-referrals may have come to the program before the formal case-finding system identified them (thus representing failures of the work performance monitoring system); others may in fact have been referred formally, but preferred to indicate that they came on their own.

Furthermore, it is impossible to tell, without good normative data about what happens in work-site populations, whether self-referrals who do not show work performance problems would in fact have developed such problems in the absence of an EAP. This is, of course, a critical problem in the evaluation of prevention programs. The only means of determining whether an event has been prevented is to count the number of similar events that did occur and compare this with the number that was expected to occur in the absence of the prevention program.

Occupational programs are not able to do this with any degree of confidence. First, estimates of the number of "problems" in a plant are only guesses. For example, if one wants to prevent employee alcoholism, there is no reliable estimate of the incidence or prevalence of alcoholism in a given work force. If the range of "problems" to be prevented is broadened to include mental/emotional problems, estimates of incidence and prevalence are even more difficult.

However, if EAPs attempt to prevent substandard work performance in the plant, they are in a better position. Work performance measures can be identified, standards set, and a count made of the number of employees whose work is substandard during a given time period. A prevention program can then be evaluated in terms of the reduction in number of employees whose performance is judged substandard.

Employee assistance programs typically have not been evaluated in these terms, for several reasons. Most EAPs were not designed as prevention programs in this sense. As noted above, they were designed to intervene with people who already exhibit symptoms reflected in their work performance; it is only in this context that they can intervene directly with an employee. EAPs were not designed for broad prevention activities that attempt to educate the work force (although some programs do undertake this type of activity), and there is no demonstrably effective methodology for conducting such activities.

To the extent that the client-focused program design is effective at early intervention, it can be expected to result in reduction of the incidence and prevalence of work performance problems. However, most EAPs have not been staffed at a level that allows enough clients to be seen to make an impact on these overall measures.

Consider a plant with 5000 employees which hires one full-time program counselor (a staff/employee ratio considerably higher than exists in a great many programs). Suppose that the counselor is able to work with 250 clients each year, a figure that may be too high to allow for appropriate follow-up activities. This is 5 percent of the work force. However, it is estimated that more than 15 percent of the work force has an alcohol problem (National Council on Alcoholism, 1968), and at least an equivalent number have other types of personal/emotional problems that interfere with work performance (Foote et al., 1978).

In this case the counselor may be able to reach the persons exhibiting such problems over a two- or three-year period. However, work force turnover will add cases annually, and new problems will develop at an unknown rate. Furthermore, it will be necessary to provide follow-up with many clients for a period of years, so that the counselor will not be able to take on new cases at the same rate in subsequent years and continue to do an adequate job. Staff members of employee assistance programs are normally overwhelmed with the number of employees referred to them who exhibit symptoms, and they have little time for outreach to employees who do not.

If we consider the prevalence of work performance problems, rather than behavioral/medical problems, we are likely to find that reviews of work and absenteeism records show considerably more than five percent of the work force to be exhibiting problems. Furthermore, many of these job performance problems are not caused by any kind of health problem. Some employees who are chronically poor performers are referred to the EAP but are found by the EAP staff to have no underlying problem for which a source of help can be found. Many of these employees simply do not wish to work the expected five days a week.

In summary, the following points may be noted regarding the ability of employee assistance programs to undertake primary prevention or early intervention:

(1) Most programs are unable to attempt primary prevention because they are overwhelmed with employee problems that have already developed.

(2) The proportion of the work force that an EAP is able to serve is not usually large enough to make much of an impact on overall plantwide performance figures.

(3) EAPs are structured to provide a range of treatment services for which technologies exist, and are not structured for primary prevention for which the technology is unknown.

(4) Prevention of work performance problems is beyond the scope of an EAP to the extent that such problems are not caused by underlying health problems that the programs are equipped to address.

In terms of secondary prevention, however, most employee assistance programs feel they are quite successful. The available studies generally show considerable reduction in certain key work performance problems (absenteeism, use of sick leave benefits, disciplinary actions, and the like), and it is argued that these reductions are the result of program intervention. Controlled studies to test this argument are not available, and there are serious questions as to the ethical issues that would be involved in such studies. EAPs argue, however, that in the case of alcoholism there is at least clinical evidence that their interventions speed the recovery process.

In any case, employee assistance programs have the ability to provide a particularly powerful incentive to employees to take action that will improve their work performance if it is substandard: job security. Strictly speaking, that incentive is not provided by the EAP (System B) but by the employer (system A) when the employee is confronted with his or her job problem(s) and offered a referral to the EAP for help. That is, an employee is accountable to the employer (not to the EAP) for performing according to the terms of the work agreement. However, the EAP staff are normally able to reinforce the message and work with the employee to identify the problems contributing to poor work performance.

Relationship of EAPs to the
Community Mental Health Field

Community mental health agencies have become considerably more interested in reaching employed populations as third-party payment has become more common. In the past, employed persons who needed help with behavioral/medical problems have been assumed to seek help from private sources (psychiatrists or psychologists). Publicly funded mental health agencies were organized primarily to provide service to those who could not afford private sources. However, the availability of third-party payments created an incentive for CMHCs to move into a new area. Thus, the mental health community began to be aware that employed persons are a part of the general community, that from time to time they need mental health services (which in some cases can be paid for by third parties), and that employee assistance programs are good links to the industrial population.

This recognition is very useful to EAPs. To the extent that community treatment facilities (System C) recognize that EAPs have a considerable influence over the selection of agencies to which employees will go for treatment, they are likely to make an effort to adapt their procedures to meet the needs of the programs. EAPs are likely to send fewer and fewer referrals to those treatment agencies that (1) cannot take new patients within a reasonable amount of time (immediately if necessary, and within a few days otherwise), (2) keep patients in inpatient therapy for inordinate amounts of time, (3) set treatment protocols geared to the length of the third-party payment period, (4) refuse to provide the program with adequate feedback, or (5) ultimately do not provide treatment that helps the employees. Industry is in the unique position of being able to evaluate the effectiveness of the agencies because, as described above, industry has a captive population that is subject to routine monitoring.

An important issue for EAP staff is the qualifications of personnel in community agencies who provide services to employees. Because of the frequency of alcohol-related problems in the work force, EAP staff look for expertise in treating alcohol problems. In general, EAP staff who refer a person for treatment of an alcohol problem will want that problem given primary attention, and will be unlikely to use an agency that does not do this. Agencies that are organized for the treatment of mental health problems are not normally organized and staffed for the treatment of alcoholism and will be unlikely to receive such referrals from industry.

As mental health professionals become interested in employee assistance programs, they need to be aware that they will, in general, need additional training in order to do this type of work. A staff member in an employee assistance program needs, in addition to counseling skills and skills in assessment of personal/emotional problems, two other sets of skills: (1) in assessment of alcohol and other drug problems, including skills in confronting employees with these problems; and (2) in working within an industrial community, including organizational knowledge about both labor and management, and ability to utilize documented information about employees in the process of confrontation.

The effective EAP staff member requires specialized knowledge and experience in all of the above areas. These staff tend to come from two different sources. Some are identified within the company, appointed to the EAP program because of their experience, and then develop additional knowledge through workshops and short courses. These include both labor and management representatives. Other staff train in professional programs such as schools of social work; gain additional experience through internships in industry; and are subsequently hired, usually by management, as professional program staff.

In fact, the diversity of skills and experience required to operate employee assistance programs is not often found in a single individual. Professionally trained individuals seldom have a solid understanding of union-management relations or of work site operations. While professionally trained staff are likely to be better equipped to assess and work with community treatment facilities, nonprofessional personnel within the organization (such as labor union or personnel department representatives) are better equipped to assess what is happening inside the work force and to make judgments about work site operations that may be affecting employees. Many organizations establish a program team that includes both types of personnel, thus utilizing the special capabilities of staff with both types of backgrounds and also, in most cases, providing a balance between labor and management interests in the program (Foote et al., 1980).

Despite the need, professional training programs are only just beginning to recognize the market for mental health professionals in industry, and very few have developed curricula that include both the full range of knowledge that is necessary and sufficient training experience within industrial settings. At this time, therefore, the relationship between community mental health centers and employee assistance programs in industry is primarily the relationship between System B and System C: Community mental health centers represent one group of agencies that is available to treat EAP clients.

Some community agencies, recognizing the largely untapped group of potential clients who work in industry, have set up organizational components which work with employers in setting up employee assistance programs. In some cases the agencies establish central diagnostic and referral services (CDRs) and request that area employers send employees there for assessment rather than setting up EAPs within the company. In other cases the agencies offer to assist the companies in establishing EAPs. In either case, the agencies may offer to help establish System A (that is, the mechanism by which employees are identified and referred to System B), often including training of supervisors and union personnel.

Agencies offering these types of services need to recognize that they are dealing with more than an untapped population to which they can offer mental health services. When community agencies possess the capacity to treat alcoholism and other addictive disorders and understand industrial procedures and incentives, they are most likely to show success in working with industry.

Mental health agencies are relative newcomers to the field of occupational programming. Two other groups have much greater experience in assisting industry to establish such programs. In 1972 the National Institute on Alcohol Abuse and Alcoholism (NIAAA) established the position of occupational program consultant (OPC) and funded two such positions in each of the 50 states. These 100 people were charged with assisting industry to establish programs to identify and treat alcoholism. Federal funding for these positions has been discontinued, but in most cases the states have continued the programs, supporting a large staff of OPCs who work throughout the state.

The second group that has been highly involved in occupational programming is the National Council on Alcoholism (NCA) and its local affiliates (Von Wiegand, 1971). Both of these groups have been more attuned to the problem of alcoholism and its treatment than have mental health agencies. They have had a stronger impact on industry than has the mental health field, due both to their earlier recognition of the industrial setting as an appropriate intervention site and to industry's recognition of the cost of alcoholism to the company. As industrial programs expand to include problems other than alcoholism, the skills available through community mental health agencies should take on greater importance, and a team approach that utilizes both sets of expertise should become more effective.

Summtary

The community mental health movement has been slow to recognize employed people as part of the community, particularly in their role as workers. Employees are a substantial proportion of any community. But beyond that, employers (that is, the industrial community) are a significant part of the community structure in terms of the influence they exert over community affairs and the financial base they provide for the community.

When a significant amount of income from employment is being lost because of preventable or treatable problems, the community suffers in several ways. First, workers with problems are a part of the community, and along with their families they suffer directly. Second, money that is lost because of (a) lowered productivity and (b) preventable health care cost could have been spent in ways more beneficial to the community (for example, as higher wages). Finally, when people become unemployed because of their problems, the community suffers additional costs.

Community mental health agencies must recognize the important position of employers who routinely monitor the performance of large numbers of people. Workers whose behavior becomes erratic or inappropriate due to personal or health problems can be identified relatively easily. Furthermore, employers are in a better position to motivate people to seek treatment than are most other community organizations (barring the legal system), because they hold both a carrot and a stick. The carrot is improved health and greater income; the stick is the threat to job security if work performance is not satisfactory. Community mental health staff committed to preventive efforts in industry must develop the specialized skills which will enable them effectively to link with employee assistance programs.

Note

1. The label "employee assistance program" has come into general use because (a) it is nonstigmatic (a label that includes such words as "alcohol," "drug abuse," or

"mental health" is likely to scare some people off) and (b) it is difficult to coin a more precise phrase that describes the range of problems these programs address. There are, of course, "employee assistance programs" that assist employees with entirely different types of problems than alcoholism and other personal difficulties that interfere with work performance. These programs do not normally use the label "employee assistance program," but are more likely to use a title more descriptive of their program focus (for example, the "Blood Pressure Control Program").

References

Beyer, J.M., & Trice, H.M. *Implementing Change: Alcoholism Policies in Work Organizations.* New York: Free Press, 1978.

Erfurt, J.C, & Foote, A. *Occupational Employee Assistance Programs for Substance Abuse and Mental Health Problems.* Ann Arbor: Institute of Labor and Industrial Relations, University of Michigan, 1977.

Foote, A., Erfurt, J.C, & Austin, R. Staffing occupational employee assistance programs: The General Motors experience. *Alcohol Health and Research World,* 1980, *4,* 22-31.

Foote, A., Erfurt, J.C, Strauch, P.A., & Guzzardo, T.L. *Cost-Effectiveness of Occupational Employee Assistance Programs: Test of an Evaluation Method.* Ann Arbor: Institute of Labor and Industrial Relations, University of Michigan, 1978.

Holden, C. Alcoholism: On-the-job referrals mean early detection, treatment. *Science,* 1973, *179,* 363-365, 413-415.

National Council on Alcoholism. *Prevalence of Alcoholism Among Employees.* New York: Author, 1968.

Pell, S., & D'Alonzo, C.A. Sickness absenteeism of alcoholics. *Journal of Occupational Medicine,* 1970, *12,* 198-210.

Roman, P.M., & Trice, H.M. The sick role, labelling theory and the deviant drinker. *International Journal of Social Psychiatry,* 1969, *14,* 245-251.

Schmidt, R.T. Safety and the problem employee. *Journal of Occupational Medicine,* 1976, *18,* 763-766.

Schramm, C.J., & DeFillippi, R.J. Characteristics of successful alcoholism treatment programs for American workers. *British Journal of Addiction, 1975, 70,* 271-275.

Schramm, C.J., Mandell, W., & Archer, J. *Workers Who Drink.* Lexington, MA: D.C. Heath, 1978.

Seidel, L.E. Industry's $4 billion albatross: Alcoholism. *Textile Industries,* 1970, *134,* 55-71.

Threatt, R.M. The influence of alcohol on work performance. Raleigh, NC: The Human Ecology Institute, February, 1976.

Trice, H.M., & Roman, P.M. *Spirits and Demons at Work: Alcohol and Other Drugs on the Job.* Ithaca, NY: New York State School of Industrial and Labor Relations, Cornell University, 1972.

Tucker, J.R. A worker-oriented alcoholism and "troubled employee" program: A union approach. *Industrial Gerontology,* 1974, *Fall,* 20-24.

Von Wiegand, R.A. The problem of alcoholism. *Environmental Control and Safety Management,* 1971, *March.*

Von Wiegand, R.A. Alcoholism in industry (U.S.A.). *British Journal of Addiction,* 1972, *67,* 181-187.

9

Social Networks and
the Utilization of
Preventive Mental Health Services

Benjamin H. Gottlieb
Alan Hall
University of Guelph

As the community mental health movement gained momentum in the late 1960s, a number of new practice principles were articulated, principles which were then used to guide the planning and placement of services which might be capable of reaching the poor. This emphasis on programs for the poor was only one part of a larger movement aimed at reducing poverty and promoting the rights and opportunities of ethnic minorities. The mental health field invested considerable energy and funds to improve the availability and acceptability of mental health services to all segments of society. However, the high priority placed on serving the needs of low-income and minority populations has yielded few results. There is still much evidence indicating that these populations continue to be the least likely to use mental health services. Kelly, Snowden, and Munoz (1977) make this point in their annual review of "Social and Community Interventions":

> One of the most important characteristics of SCI is that they take into account and work with diverse societal groups. The YAVIS client—young, attractive, verbal, intelligent, and successful (Schofield, 1964)—is no longer our sole preoccupation. Active efforts to work with people who are old, of low status, working class, uneducated and poor have begun. . . . Though very recent data show some improvement (Bloom, 1975), the general picture has been one of under-utilization of services [Kelly et al., 1977: 329].

At the same time, principles of preventive mental health practice were also introduced to and accepted by the mental health field. Within a period of 10 years an impressive array of prevention services and concepts have been developed (Albee and Joffe, 1977). However, the mandate to extend prevention programs to the community has, if anything, compounded the underutilization problem because it has been found that the poor are even more unlikely to use preventive health services than treatment services (Bullough, 1972; Kraft and Chilman, 1966).

While several strategies of resolving the problem of underutilization have been proposed in the literature (see, for example, McKinlay's [1972] review), the majority of actual attempts to increase utilization rates have focused on either changing the attitudes of the poor toward service use or on changing aspects of the delivery system which were believed to discourage participation by the poor. In this chapter we present another means of analyzing and ameliorating the problem of service underutilization. We will attempt to show how social network concepts can be fruitfully brought to bear on this problem. Specifically, we will illustrate some of the dimensions of the underutilization problem by focusing on a particular case example concerning one agency's efforts to design and deliver prevention programs on behalf of low-income families in its catchment area.

The authors of this chapter were called in to consult with agency staff about the means of improving the agency's ability to reach low-income citizens. Hence, the chapter opens with a description of the historical context surrounding the agency's difficulties in extending a preventive mental health program to a low-income population. This first section describes the staff's unsuccessful efforts to foster program utilization by observing the dictums of community mental health practice. The body of the chapter describes a social network perspective which we introduced to our consultees in order to enlarge their appreciation of the manner in which the social world surrounding their potential clients might influence the latter's utilization behavior. While the basic elements of network analysis are only briefly introduced, detailed attention is given to three ways in which social networks might have an impact upon service utilization: First, they may be structured in such a way as to insulate members from information about the existence of social programs; second, depending on their structure and their norms, they may place great or very little pressure on members' decisions about whether or not to utilize a given social program; and third, they may influence utilization rates in accordance with their own abilities to generate resources and support on their members' behalf.

In short, this chapter focuses on the ways in which utilization rates of social programs are affected by social networks acting as communication systems, referral systems, and support systems. Throughout the chapter, we have also attempted to show how this evolving network perspective was applied to the particular problem faced by our consultees. The chapter closes with a research framework for the study of social network influences on service utilization.

A word about the current state of research on social networks and service utilization is in order here, since it may help to explain both the goals and the limits of this chapter. First, it is important that our readers understand that this is a first effort to specify a set of network variables which bear on the study of service utilization. While several researchers have suggested that social network analysis offers a promising new conceptual framework for systematically examining patterns of service use, the fact is that, to date, very little empirical work has been carried out. McKinlay (1972) makes this point on the basis of his review of the service utilization literature. He writes: "It is perhaps truistic to point out that the family, and its associated kin and friendship networks, are important influences on health and illness behavior, yet there have been remarkably few attempts to specify the nature of such influences" (p. 139). We believe that there are two major reasons for the dearth of such research on the topic of service utilization. First, as we will show in this chapter, social networks can be analyzed in terms of a large number of both structural properties and types of interpersonal transactions. However, there is little accumulated evidence of a hierarchy of network variables which influence utilization. Researchers therefore face the arduous and complex task of distilling this panel of network variables and identifying the subset which best predicts service utilization. The size of this task alone may discourage agency-based researchers from pursuing social network analyses. A second reason why so little network research has been performed by agency researchers has to do with the uncertainties surrounding the appropriate methodology to be used. Network research has been undertaken by university-based investigators from different disciplines, each favoring pathways to data which reflect his or her disciplinary biases. Anthropologists tend to engage in extended ethnographic studies which are both costly and time-consuming but which yield rich qualitative data with high ecological validity. Sociologists have tended to favor survey research approaches to the study of social networks, and while this means that they tend to hold their subjects at some distance and therefore fail to capture the social processes in the environment, they trade this off against the enormous yield of information they gain about the structural properties (for example, density, size, composition, and symmetry), of people's social orbits. Psychologists and social psychiatrists tend to study egocentric networks by concentrating especially on the nature of the links between people. They tend to rely on intensive interviewing of respondents and, in this context, they are best able to establish the sort of rapport which encourages people to disclose their feelings about their social intimates and about what resources are exchanged in these relationships. The diversity of approaches to the investigation of people's social surroundings is likely to discourage agency-based researchers from initiating utilization studies. While academicians and other researchers who are not pressed to deliver services to the hard-to-reach may see a "healthy tension" in this methodological diversity, agency personnel are unlikely to invest limited research resources in unproved methods of data collection.

In what follows, we try to provide greater clarity and more specific guidelines to agency-based researchers about the sort of network structures and network functions which ought to be investigated in the study of the use of services. Thus, this chapter concentrates on the task of sifting through the array of variables involved in social network analysis to identify the subset which may be most important in determining people's involvement in social programs. Our goal is to provide the reader with a more limited conceptual map of the terrain surrounding the study of social networks and service utilization. We hope that our attempt to generate this map, while maintaining a dialogue about the specific utilization problems faced by the staff of one agency, will help to tie theory to practice.

A Case Example of Service Underutilization

The authors were brought in as consultants to a children's center (CC) located in a catchment area which included a large number of public housing developments, composed largely of one-parent and new immigrant families. In the early 1970s, the center was steadily expanding its service offerings to include a variety of treatment programs designed to help emotionally disturbed children and their families. As the decade proceeded, however, it became increasingly evident to the CC's staff that the annual number of referrals to the agency was outpacing the agency's service capabilities. Recognizing that professional resources were limited and with a mind to stemming the tide of new cases, the CC took steps to develop a distinct prevention department which was to have as its mandate the reduction of the incidence and prevalence of emotional disturbance among children in the center's catchment area. This department's staff were much impressed by the research evidence which documented the critical role of the family in the development of social competence and intellectual skills among children (Freeburg & Payne, 1967; Gordon, 1970; Hunt, 1964; Rutter, 1974). Accordingly, a decision was made to place major emphasis on programs aimed at improving family functioning, and since parent education in particular has been enthusiastically promoted by a variety of authorities (Auerbach, 1968; Brim, 1965; Chilman, 1963; Hereford, 1963; Pickarts & Fargo, 1970), the staff chose this form of service to spearhead their department's preventive activities.

In organizing the service delivery efforts of this prevention department, the staff adhered to a number of key practice principles derived from community mental health theory. First, they recognized the need to involve community residents in the planning of services (Reissman, 1967). Accordingly, a steering committee comprised of "concerned" local residents was established to help map out the direction of the department. Second, rather than developing programs in isolation, the staff invested considerable effort in establishing collaborative relationships with various community, social, and educational organizations, including local school boards, hospitals, community centers, the public health department, and the police department. For example, the department developed a series of parent education programs in collaboration with the local school board. Such a collaborative relationship with the schools meant that (a) the programs could be advertised on a large scale via letters sent home with the students; (b) the programs could be located at local schools, thus making them easily accessible to large segments of the community; and (c) the sharing of program costs permitted the delivery of a large number of programs distributed across the entire community. In addition to developing programs collaboratively, the department hoped, over the long term, to turn increasing responsibility for the day-to-day running of various programs over to the collaborating agency. The basic principle was that once the "bugs" had been worked out of a particular program, the center would turn the operations of the program over to the "community" as represented by school boards, volunteer organizations, and various community groups. The department, meanwhile, could turn its energies to the development and evaluation of new service strategies.

A third operating principle established by the department, again derived from community mental health theory, was to ensure that lay persons play a major role in the delivery of services (Gershon & Biller, 1977). Recognizing that the delivery of large-scale prevention programs would involve considerable personnel resources, the department established a relatively rigorous training program for volunteers. Again, the intent of the department over the long term was to distribute increasing responsibilities to volunteers from the community.

Within three years of operation, the staff had developed a number of sophisticated prevention strategies of an educational sort. Parents and community care givers were the targets for these programs. Service strategies ranged from single-session seminars to mass media packages to home visit intervention programs. Most of the programs were oriented toward providing information on child development and management issues. Major emphasis was placed on services to the parents of preschool children. However, when it came time to evaluate these programs, it was found that they were reaching a relatively select segment of the community and that virtually no contact was being made with potentially high-risk populations, such as the low-income single-parent and immigrant families. The effect of these data was to convince the staff that they had to redouble their efforts to bend their programs to the needs and community situation of low-income residents. Alternative program formats were experimented with. For example, acting on Chilman's (1973) observations that many low-income mothers may not have the life-skills or confidence necessary to participate in group programs, the staff developed "low threat" programs, such as unstructured drop-in centers located in shopping centers and schools, and phone-in advice and crisis services. In addition to changing service formats to heighten program acceptability, the staff made increased efforts to improve accessibility by locating the services directly in the housing areas where single-parent and immigrant families resided. Furthermore, all financial barriers to program utilization were removed. Mass media efforts were intensified and greater efforts were made to establish connections with the leadership of various low-income and ethnic interest groups. For example, a review of the agency's steering committee members revealed that representatives of low-income and immigrant populations were absent. It also became clear that the department's volunteers were, without exception, well-educated, middle-class women. Attempts were therefore made to establish contacts with the "grass roots" leadership in low-income areas. The department hired a West Indian woman to act as a consultant with respect to services for West Indian immigrants.

Two years after all these program changes were effected, evaluative data showed that only little gain had been made in reaching high-risk populations. Efforts to follow the principles of community mental health practice had failed to ameliorate the problem. Outside help was called for, and the authors were brought in as consultants.

Network Analysis of Service Utilization

In the previous section we have attempted to reconstruct as faithfully as possible the events leading up to the CC's call for outside consultation. When we first convened with the staff of the agency's prevention unit, we were faced with a team of three professionals who had conscientiously followed the principles of community mental health practice, but who were nevertheless sorely frustrated by their inability to attract low-income residents. From their point of view, they had "bent over backwards" to make their programs as accessible and as acceptable as possible to the style of life of the low-income sector of their catchment area; they had attempted to seek counsel from indigenous citizens and to involve others in direct service delivery roles; and throughout all these efforts they had been zealous about cooperating with a consortium of other agencies and informal caregivers who also served this catchment area. Now they felt "burnt out," unappreciated, and in their frustration they were beginning to lay blame for the problem on the heads of those who were failing to use their programs, a defensive reaction which temporarily exonerated them from having to make any further adaptations in their program planning. Indeed, our knowledge of attribution theory helps us to understand this reaction, since, as outside observers, the agency staff tended to focus on the behavior of the target population, not on the circumstances which conditioned that behavior. They saw people who were failing to take advantage of a range of services, and attributed their inaction to the personalities, attitudes, and private motives of these people and tended to overlook environmental constraints. In the case of these three staff members, the situation was somewhat more complicated, however. It was clear that they had not started out by adopting this attributional bias, but had worked long and hard to modify the service environment with which low-income residents would come into contact. It was only now that these environmental modifications had failed to increase program utilization rates that they had permission to blame the problem on the dispositional characteristics of community residents.

In our consultation strategy, we focused precisely on the need to enlarge the staff's understanding of another field of environmental forces which might be operating in such a way as to keep low-income residents from availing themselves of the agency's services. Specifically, our first goal was to engage the staff in a discussion which probed their knowledge of local patterns of social organization and which focused on *how the natural social environment might interact with the service environment which they had created to jointly determine the utilization behaviors of local residents.* As this discussion began to unfold, we quickly realized that our consultees were unprepared to pursue such an analysis for two reasons. First, they did not know what sort of variables ought to be considered in assessing the social environments of their target population—they were unfamiliar with the parameters of social network analysis. Second, they felt that it was necessary to hedge their bets on this first venture into social network analysis by restricting their investigation to one segment of the low-income population which they were mandated to serve. If the network approach seemed promising in relation to this one group, it could then be extended to the situation of other low-income subgroups in their catchment area. We therefore agreed that the best initial approach to the work we would undertake together would be to limit attention to the one high-risk subgroup about which they and their colleagues in other agencies knew most—sole support mothers who lived in low-income housing projects. While our consultees had evidence showing that few of these women were attending the agency's preventive parenting programs, we consultants endorsed the choice of this population, recognizing that its vulnerability was jointly determined by the stressors associated with low-income status and the absence of a marital tie (see Bloom, 1975).

Our initial goal was to help our consultees appreciate the fact that, within the broad parameters of community life, most people inhabit smaller social worlds which set their standards for evaluating their lives and their environments, and which channel people's behavior. It is this smaller social context in which most people live which has been largely ignored by professional service providers but which plays an active part in funneling some people into professional services and keeping others outside the bounds of professional practice. In short, people in similar stressful circumstances will take different routes toward resolving their difficulties, and the paths they take will be determined in large part by the structure, norms and direct interventions of the primary groups in which they participate. While several of these avenues may eventually lead to the doors of professionals, some will not. Some people will be able to resolve their difficulties within the confines of their social networks; some may seek assistance there but use these connections to get help from lay persons who are one step removed from the help-seeker; some may begin "at home" but eventually find themselves at the doors of professionals;

and some may participate in a social network which immediately defines the help-seeker's situation as one requiring professional counsel. Regardless of which route is chosen, the underlying implication for human service agencies is that people's social networks are capable of exercising a good deal of control over professional practice, since they regulate matters affecting the number of people who seek professional help, the timing of their requests for help, and the expectations which people form about how they can best be helped.

While these propositions made intuitive sense to our consultees, they provided little more than a general orientation to the sociocultural context of potential service recipients. Our consultees needed more grounding in how network dynamics among sole support mothers could be studied and, ultimately, how their study could inform subsequent efforts to deliver services to this population. We were pressed by our consultees to specify the ways in which social networks might influence service utilization and to pinpoint the sort of network variables which might be implicated in the influence process. We agreed that such details were needed before any action research could be undertaken by the staff, and we returned some weeks later with a more precise framework to guide our discussion and with much-needed examples to illuminate the elements of this framework.

The Social Network: Structure and Functions

Much of the work in social network analysis has been conducted by anthropologists and urban sociologists who found that they could understand a great deal about the organization of social systems by focusing on discrete sets of actors who interact with one another and whose interaction patterns shape members' relations with the institutions of their society. Most individuals have a personal network which is made up of their ties to family members, friends, neighbors, workmates, casual acquaintances, and professionals in a variety of health, welfare, educational, legal, and commercial fields. One person's network will differ from another's in the proportion of certain of these categories of ties, depending on his or her involvement in different social settings and as a function of the breadth of his or her role relationships. Some persons may have a relatively large field of kinship ties, others may have networks which are heavily populated by work and recreational associates, while some people may recruit a large neighborhood sector to their network. Networks may be racially homogeneous and socioeconomically heterogeneous, or vice-versa. In short, people's networks can be characterized according to a great number of morphological variables, and these structural variations have been found to condition people's behavior toward a wide variety of institutions, to influence their attitudes toward diverse social phenomena, and to affect people's adaptation to cultural and social changes. Examples of how network analysis has been applied to these issues can be found in Whitten and Wolfe's (1974) excellent review.

Network research can be directed toward two kinds of analyses which Craven and Wellman (1973) describe as the "whole network" versus the "personal network" approaches. In the former case, all the links among all the persons in a given population are studied, while in the latter case, the focus of research is on a given individual and all the persons to whom he or she is tied. The latter approach is somewhat more common than the former, simply because it is more manageable; yet it, too, can reach a high level of complexity when attention is turned to the influence on behavior of an individual's indirect ties, which are those ties mediated through others. Elizabeth Bott's (1971) study of the effects of certain structural characteristics of a family's social network on conjugal role relations was one of the first anthropological ventures to document the radiating effects of interactions in one segment of a network on persons occupying other sectors. In the following quotation, Bott (1971) enunciates the two orders of analyses which she included in her study of family networks: "My aim was (and still is) to understand how the internal functioning of a group is affected not only by its relationship *with* the people and organizations of its environment, but also by the relationships *among* those people and organizations" (p. 249).

Regardless of whether any given study adopts the whole network strategy or the personal network approach, analysis focuses on the form and the functions of the linkages among sets of actors. When we speak of the form which is created by the linkages among sets of actors, we are talking about network structure. This structure can be broken down into a number of properties or dimensions, some of which include the network's size, its composition, its density or degree of connectedness, its clustering or extent of internal segmentation, and its demographic homogeneity. These structural properties can be invoked to characterize the entire network. It is also possible to characterize the nature of any individual's link with others in terms of a series of dimensions. For example, strong links are those characterized by frequent and mutual interactions of an affectively intense nature with long-standing social intimates. Weak ties are those which are only infrequently activated and which tend not to involve social intimates, or concern matters of significant emotional import to the participants. Considered together, analysis of the structural properties of networks and the dimensions which characterize the links among members provides a means of assessing the patterning of people's social environments.

We are now in a somewhat better position to launch our discussion of how the structure and the sorts of links to which people are tied affect their utilization behavior. Are some kinds of social networks more likely than others to encourage the use of health and welfare services? Are there social networks which function to insulate people from these sorts of institutional programs? We can begin to answer questions of this magnitude by partialling out three ways in which people's social networks can exercise an influence on service utilization patterns. First, they can be structured in such a way as to prevent certain information about social programs from reaching people. Second, even when information about social programs is available, the network may be structured in such a way as to deter people from using agency services, or it may be aligned to norms which do not favor participation. Third, the network itself may be providing its own forms of remedies to the kind of problems or needs which agency programs address and, hence, comes to define the agency's program as irrelevant or competitive with its own solutions. In short, when people are embedded in networks which either fail to transmit programmatic information to them or which counsel them away from formal programs, or when the network is deemed to have its own service capability, in any of these instances low service utilization may result. In what follows we review selected studies which have used network analysis to illuminate how people's social worlds condition their use of agency programs in each of these three ways.

Network Structure and Access to Information about Social Programs

What sort of network structure is most conducive to keeping people abreast of new and diverse information in the environment? Certainly, one measure of any human system's adaptive potential is its ability to quickly and accurately monitor information from the outside world and transmit that information to the subsystems which can use it. When networks are composed of people who participate in varied social settings, it follows naturally that there is a greater likelihood that the network will contain a greater diversity of information. But if the network is relatively closed—if all members face inward—the network will have little ability to monitor

changes in the environment which may affect the health of the collec-
tivity, and its adaptive potential will suffer. Furthermore, even when the
network contains a subsystem which monitors the external world, effective functioning of the network is highly dependent upon two factors: the
ability of the boundary spanners to distinguish between the sorts of
information which are most useful to the core members and information
which would make no contribution to their growth, and the effectiveness
of the system of radiating useful information from the boundary-spanning
members to the core members. In short, the network's system of communication must be structured to allow useful information to pass from those
at the boundary to all members and especially to members who do not
have direct contact with those occupying boundary positions. An example
may help to illustrate this issue.

In the undirected graph which appears in Figure 9.1, H can be seen as
occupying a boundary position between two fairly dense clusters of people
(cluster CDEF and cluster WXYZ). H may learn from X about a new
welfare program which C and D might be eligible for, and which might
meet certain of their family needs, but depending on H's frequency of
contact with E, C and D may never learn of this program. If H has heard
nothing from E about the life situation of her closest associates (C and D),
or if E fails to recognize that H's information environment could be of
more general use to C and D, then it is difficult to see how C and D would
ever learn of this new program unless it was announced to them through
the mass media or through a direct mailing.

Two research studies shed light on the relation between network
structure and the flow of communication. The first comments on what the
author refers to as the "strength of weak ties" (Granovetter, 1973),
signifying with this phrase the value of people's second-order contacts. The
second reveals the insulating effects which occur among people enmeshed
in tight knit sectors of social networks.

Granovetter (1973) was particularly interested in the role of weak ties
in any individual's social network. By "weak ties" he meant ties to persons
with whom there is little regular and intense interaction. These persons are
not themselves strongly connected to one another, and this also distin-
guishes them from the relatively dense character of the individual's strong
ties. For example, family members and close friends make up a tight-knit
primary group in the network, while a work associate, casual acquaintance
in a social club, and a neighbor are types of weak ties among which there is
little connection. For Granovetter, what is salient about this latter weak
sector is the fact that its members are in turn tied to other people who

FIGURE 9.1   Undirected Graph Demonstrating the Critical Role of a
Boundary Person in Transmitting Information Between
Two Dense Networks

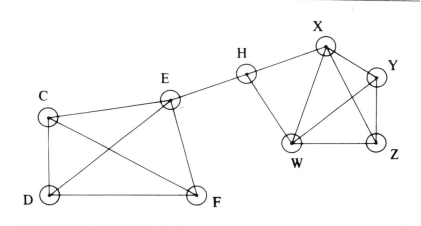

have no connection (except of an indirect sort) to our subject. Hence, people who are only weakly connected to the individual are most important "in that they are the channels through which ideas, influences, or information socially distant from ego may reach him" (Granovetter, 1973: 1371). It follows that the fewer indirect contacts people have, the more insulated they will be from events and information in the environment beyond their tight-knit, strong ties.

Granovetter put his hypothesis to work on a sample of white-collar "job changers," asking them to report on the frequency of contact they had maintained with those persons who were instrumental in supplying critical job information to them. Using this and supplementary interview data as the bases for measuring tie strength, he found that only 16.7 percent found jobs through contact with their strong ties, while 55.6 percent said they only maintained occasional contact with those who linked them to jobs, and 27.8 percent reported that they rarely saw those contacts who led them to jobs. Thus, there was good evidence to suggest that weak ties are critical sources of new information, while strong ties tend to recirculate old information.

The second study reinforces Granovetter's (1973) conclusion about the impact of network structure on the transmission of information to members. Here, however, the nature of the information examined provides a closer analogy to the situation which our consultees were grappling with. The study concerns the transmission of information about a preventive health service—family planning—to lower-class mothers. Liu and Duff (1972) found that mothers who participated in social networks composed of social intimates who were structurally close-knit were less likely to receive new information about family planning. However, they, too, found that in those cases where the information was transmitted, the weaker ties—to neighbors, for example—were responsible for introducing the information. The authors also found that family planning information was communicated more frequently to those lower-class mothers who lived in socioeconomically heterogeneous neighborhoods than to mothers residing in homogeneous milieus. This finding is consistent with the more general thesis we have been illustrating, a thesis which maintains that people are more likely to receive new information from the environment through the mediation of their second-order contacts, who function as bridges to more socially distant and diverse networks. Laumann (1973) arrives at the same conclusion on the basis of his study of urban social networks. He argues that "radial" networks—those which are more loose-knit, highly differentiated, and more heterogeneous in social composition—"are in some sense more flexible and consequently more adaptive to the demands of a modern industrial society that is undergoing continuous social change and in which many of its personnel are likely to be highly mobile both geographically and socially" (p. 115).

The preceding discussion and illustrations suggest that it would be of considerable value for our consultees to explore the extent to which the sole support mothers whom they seek to attract to their program are indeed embedded in close-knit social circles which are restricted to other sole support mothers. To the extent that their networks do not include members with contacts which branch outward to other, more demographically heterogeneous, networks, they may, indeed, be insulated from knowledge of the existence of the parent education programs mounted by the CC. While empirical social network data should be collected to test this hypothesis, our consultees were able to shed some light on this matter on the basis of their more general knowledge of the community situation of low-income mothers. In particular, two of their observations bear mention. First, most of the mothers were receiving welfare benefits and therefore had few contacts with persons outside the confines of their neighborhood.

They were not employed, since employment was a losing proposition, given welfare regulations which required them to return funds to the government once they surpassed a certain weekly salary; they were generally expected to be on call at home, should a social worker decide to make a home visit; and they did not tend to join clubs or organizations or attend church because of the social stigma attached to their status as welfare recipients. Second, the home environment to which they were closely bound was public housing, consisting largely of other low-income families, including a high density of sole support mothers. Thus, their neighborhoods were homogeneous in terms of the socioeconomic status of the residents, although, like the rest of metropolitan Toronto, the neighborhoods included a diversity of ethnic subgroups. From the point of view of our consultees, the ethnic diversity of these neighborhoods only served to reinforce the tendency of residents to cluster themselves in tight-knit and highly segmented networks; and even if some sole support mothers did maintain bridging ties to other ethnic networks, the latter showed an even lower rate of service utilization than did the sole support mothers. In support of these general observations, our consultees brought out the fact that a study (Marsden, 1975) conducted among 100 mothers in a public housing project only four miles from the CC had found that 90 percent had either no knowledge or very little information about the various family service programs operating in the local community.

Network Structure and Referral Functions

The study of the process whereby new knowledge is diffused among social circles has shown that even when people are reached directly through the use of mass media channels of information, they rarely act on this information without consulting members of their personal networks (Katz and Lazarsfeld, 1955; Rogers, 1962). People typically seek advice about the costs and benefits of acting on the new information, clarification about how the information bears on their own unique life circumstances, and feedback from their peers about the private and tentative decisions they have made which favor either action or inaction on the basis of the new information. Hence, when it comes to people's decisions about whether or not to enroll in a new social program or whether to adopt novel health behaviors, they turn to their family members and friends, using them as informal screening and referral agents.

John McKinlay's (1973) study of the patterns of use of prenatal services on the part of a sample of low-income women provides an excellent illustration of the ways in which lay consultants in contrasting network configurations affect levels of service use. Again, we chose to describe this study to our consultees because it involved a population of low-income women and the use of a preventive health program. In this study, the women were divided into a group of "utilizers" and "under-utilizers" based on the frequency and timing of their attendance at a maternity clinic. Controlling for social class, geographic proximity to the clinic, and education, McKinlay interviewed the 48 underutilizers and 39 utilizers about the frequency and locus of their contact with nonhousehold family members and friends. In addition, he collected data from them about the proximity and age of these two categories of network members. His goal was to first determine whether and how the social networks of the two groups differed structurally, and then to assess any differences in how the networks were activated for consultation about various personal and family health and welfare problems.

McKinlay found that the utilizers were much less involved with the kin sector of their network than were the underutilizers: they visited their relatives less frequently, in part because these kin tended to live farther away from their homes than the relatives of the underutilizers. In fact, group differences in the residential proximity of relatives and friends to the respondents and to one another were marked. While underutilizers lived close to both relatives and friends, the friends and relatives of the utilizers lived at some distance from one another. In general, these and other trends in the data suggested that there was an interlocking relationship between the kin and kith sectors of the underutilizers' networks, and that, in contrast, these sectors were unjoined among the utilizers. The utilizers tended to visit their friends more frequently than their relatives, and these friends tended to be workmates who were unconnected to the respondents' family ties.

The answers which respondents provided to questions about who they might consult about such problems as financial difficulties, obtaining housing, and concerns about pregnancy and childbirth revealed that the utilizers generally consulted fewer and a narrower range of network members than did underutilizers. Utilizers tended to rely primarily on friends and their husbands when they sought advice, but compared with underutilizers, they infrequently sought advice from anyone. On the other hand, underutilizers relied on a variety of proximal relatives and friends for informal consultation, a finding which McKinlay believes is consistent with the structural connectedness of the kin and friendship sectors of their networks. McKinlay (1973) casts his findings in the language of reference group theory:

> Respondents with proximate, close-knit and interlocking social networks will be likely to display greater conformity with their reference groups than will respondents with relatively inaccessible, loose-knit differentiated social networks, who may display conformity with or take a positive orientation to, a non-membership group, and employ it as a frame of reference [p. 288].

In the case of McKinlay's underutilizers, the dense and parochial networks in which they were embedded placed pressure on them not to use the maternity clinic's services. McKinlay also explains that another possible effect of involvement in an extensive network of lay consultants is to delay service utilization because the help seeker may be passed on from one lay consultant to another. One additional finding from McKinlay's (1973) study bears mention here because of its pertinence to the social situation of the sole support mothers whom our consultees were attempting to reach. The underutilizers in this study tended to live a "crisis existence," showing unstable marital ties to husbands who were chronically unemployed. In contrast, the utilizers and their spouses had stable employment and marriages. Hence, McKinlay argues that it may be easier for the utilizers to invest time in developing and maintaining a separate network of friends, while the more chronic stresses in the lives of the underutilizers make them at once more dependent on their ties to geographically close and interacting friends and relatives and less capable of turning attention to the work of establishing a separate peer network.

   Our consultees felt that the social situation of their local sole support mothers approximated that of McKinlay's underutilizers. Moreover, these mothers would be even more dependent on neighborhood-based peer ties alone because, as single parents, they would probably have a diminished kin component of the network, and as welfare recipients they would be largely home-bound. Our consultees speculated that the social networks of low-income sole support mothers would thus be characterized by a small number of proximate and close-knit ties which would be capable of exerting a good deal of pressure and expressing high agreement about whether or not attendance at parenting programs was advisable. We realized, however, that while small and cohesive networks of this sort had been found among McKinlay's (1973) underutilizers, such networks might function in the opposite way—enhancing utilization rather than diminishing it—in the face of a different sort of health or family welfare problem, and/or in the face of a service program which was organized along different lines. Bazelay and Viney (1974) found that network members are likely to hold different norms when it comes to engaging different services for different presenting problems. They interviewed a sample of 221 female residents of a subsidized housing community and found that in crises such as bereavement or marital breakdown the women would either rely on their own personal resources or seek help from close friends and relatives, while they tended to engage professional helpers for medical and financial crises. And even when norms favor the use of professional services, the manner in which these services are designed and delivered is likely to affect utilization rates. Some human services may be more threatening to the mother's self-esteem than others; some may suggest a greater element of social control than others; and some may appear to offer more immediate and tangible rewards than others. These considerations led us to the conclusion that we would have to assess social network norms while concurrently testing our hypotheses about the structural patterns of the networks.

We therefore drew the following research implications on the basis of our discussion of McKinlay's study. Data regarding the structure of the networks among sole support mothers would help to inform us about whether they were, indeed, involved in the sort of close-knit, homogeneous, and neighborhood-based networks which limit their access to novel information about social programs and which exert strong pressures regarding utilization when such information is introduced to members through mass media campaigns. In addition, data regarding the prevailing norms held by network members should be collected to tap two domains: (a) norms about the types of problems or health matters most appropriately addressed by professionally sponsored service programs as opposed to those which should be handled informally, through indigenous resources; and (b) norms about the elements or dimensions of service design which are most critical in affecting decisions about whether or not to use a given formal service. The importance of these latter norms was illustrated for us in the following extract from an interview conducted with the sister of one of McKinlay's (1973) underutilizers:

> I told my sister [the respondent] not to go to the clinic but to have her kids at home. At the hospital they only let the husband see the baby at first—it's a long time before we're [extended kin] allowed to see it. After all, we look after her till she's better [delivered], and she stays here with us. We've got as much right to see the baby as he

[respondent's husband] has. But they don't let you [McKinlay, 1972: 130].

This quotation revealed only one clash between the values held by an influential lay consultant and the manner in which the professional system had been organized to deliver this particular type of health service. We felt that there may be other elements of service design which are perceived by the lay system as antithetical to its own beliefs and which we ought to investigate more comprehensively among the mothers we wished to reach.

Networks as Support Systems

To this point, our discussion with our consultees had focused on studies which suggested that social networks which take certain structural forms tend to insulate people from novel information about social programs and that, in addition, they are capable of placing strong pressures on their members' utilization behavior, impeding utilization when norms are unfavorable and speeding utilization when there is consensus about the favorability of the service. However, as our consultees began to formulate hypotheses about the character of the networks which prevailed among the sole support mothers in their catchment area, it was clear that they were also beginning to formulate ideas about how these networks could be modified for the purpose of enlarging these mothers' rate of attendance at the agency's parent education programs. It might be possible, for example, to identify the opinion leaders in these networks and then to initially work closely with them, either for the purpose of training them in more competent child-rearing practices, training which they could then extend to members of their networks, or to simply convince them to act as informal referral agents who could channel their peers to the agency's programs. While these suggestions reflected growing appreciation on the part of our consultees of how social network analysis could inform their understanding of service utilization patterns, we began to realize that we had failed to give them another important perspective on the functions of people's networks of social ties. Specifically, we had thus far not alerted them to the possibility that among some neighborhood-based networks, low rates of service utilization might signify that members are enmeshed in a network of informal help capable of providing support and guidance for the parenting role. We therefore turned our attention to the task of reviewing studies which had focused on social networks as support systems, hoping that this literature would provide leads about the kinds of network structures which are best capable of providing support for the parenting role and those which are least capable of doing so.

As we uncovered the literature in this area, we found not one but several lines of research on the supportive functions of people's supportive ties. We found abundant research testifying to the health-protective effects of social support, but no agreement about what constitutes social support. On the one hand, the sociological and epidemiological literature we reviewed suggested that people who maintain a high level of social participation and who can therefore be characterized as socially integrated into the wider society are happier (Phillips, 1967), have lower rates of mortality (Berkman & Syme, 1979), and show fewer and less severe symptoms of psychiatric disequilibrium (Myers et al., 1975; Lin et al., 1979) than those who tend to be more socially isolated. However, because these studies were so macroscopic in nature, they shed little light on the sort of questions we were seeking to answer. These studies did not indicate whether health protection is predicated upon access to an optimal number of social ties or whether only certain configurations of social ties are implicated in maintaining people's physical and psychological well-being, and they revealed nothing about the resources which might be transmitted between people and which are capable of moderating the stress which might otherwise overwhelm them. In contrast to these molar approaches to operationalizing the support construct, we reviewed studies which claimed that access to a single intimate social tie was at the heart of social support. We read Lowenthal and Haven's (1968) study of social ties and adaptation among the elderly and found the counterpoint to the studies mentioned above. These researchers found that even when elderly persons had experienced a reduction in their level of social participation over a period of one year, access to an intimate social tie proved to be associated with a relatively high level of morale. These same findings were replicated by Conner, Powers, and Bultena (1979), who found that only certain social ties, not the sheer number of ties or frequency of interaction with others, were associated with a high level of life satisfaction among their elderly respondents. We were most impressed with Robert Weiss' (1974) formulation about the sorts of "provisions" which are necessary to maintain the mental health of people, because his ideas were, in part, grounded in his observations and interviews with single parents who attended Parents Without Partners. He found that while friendships among members of PWP seemed to make life more bearable and satisfied members' needs for social integration, they did not have the power to alleviate members' feelings of emotional isolation. Interviews he conducted with other people who had experienced a loss of other sorts of social ties (other than a marital tie) added to his understanding of the diverse provisions available through contrasting types of social bonds; and in his final scheme he lists six provisions of social relationships, adding that, ". . . individuals must maintain a number of different relationships to establish the conditions necessary for well being" (Weiss, 1974: 22). These include attachment, social integration, opportunities for nurturance, reassurance of worth, a sense of reliable alliance, and obtaining guidance.

Finally, we found only a single study which had examined social network variables in relation to support within a "normal" community sample of women. We found this study especially useful because it helped us to gain further insight into the reasons why dense and socially homogeneous social networks are less beneficial to people coping with life events and transitions than are more loose-knit, branching networks. Hirsch (1980) gathered social network data from 20 women who had recently been widowed and from 14 women who had recently returned to full-time university studies. He asked them to list up to 20 people with whom they maintained regular contact. In addition, during a two-week period they completed a "daily interaction rating form" on which they indicated how much time they had spent with each of these network members and the type of support (based on five categories previously determined) expressed in these interactions. Measures of overall support were determined, and measures of density of each woman's network were also calculated. Finally, each of the subject's relationships was rated in terms of its "dimensionality," which assesses the number of important activities shared with each network member. If, for example, a respondent engaged in at least two different kinds of activities or role relationships with another person, this tie could be described as multidimensional. Hirsch (1980) states that multidimensional relationships have greater social exchange value to the partners involved and that they represent stronger and more reliable ties.

In his results, Hirsch (1980) finds that the denser social networks were associated with poorer functioning on several measures of mental health. Specifically, women who participated in dense networks were found to have poorer mood and lower self-esteem scores than those with more loose-knit networks. In addition, the more dense their networks, the less support, in the forms of socializing, emotional support, reinforcement, and cognitive guidance, was provided. When Hirsch examined the density of his respondents' networks in terms of the extent of connectedness between the friendship and the family sectors, he found here too that the greater the density, the less support was provided. Finally, he found that access to multidimensional friendships was related to higher self-esteem and more satisfying socializing and tangible assistance.

Hirsch (1980) tries to explain why low-density networks with large numbers of multidimensional relationships are more adaptive for these respondents. Given the tasks facing these women—the need for both the widows and the women resuming university studies to enter and gain satisfaction from new activities outside their domestic lives—they were best assisted in developing new social identities through involvement in networks which branched into the wider social environment and through social ties which were not exclusively based upon their domestic sphere of activities. Hence, they did not have to relinquish existing social ties in order to move into these new spheres of activity, but only needed to emphasize those social relationships which were based on activities which were more closely related to their new involvements in the community. Hirsch characterizes the overall pattern of his findings as follows:

> The greater diversity of interest and segregation of different spheres of activity characterizing low density, multidimensional natural support systems can be seen to serve as an insurance policy. This policy may serve to protect individuals from having problematic changes in particular spheres of their lives become too encompassing, threatening and debilitating. The policy may provide rewarding alternative social identities and activities, facilitating a smoother reorganization of one's life, at less psychic cost [1980: 19].

In terms of the course of our consultation, Hirsch's explanation of the benefits which arise from participation in loose-knit networks and from relationships which are based on multiple fields of interaction led us to surmise that the social networks of our target population were probably not well suited to helping members effect new social identities which were not tied to their status as welfare recipients. If indeed we were correct in characterizing their networks as dense and composed of other sole support mothers with whom they shared a very narrow range of activities, then it is likely that their networks only reinforce the prevailing shared social identity and their current parenting practices. While their existing social contacts may provide them with certain basic supportive resources, Hirsch's (1980) study suggested to us that this field of social contacts is probably not structured in such a way or composed of the kinds of social relationships to qualify it as a support system capable of enhancing its members' social adaptation. We therefore hypothesized that low utilization of the CC's parenting programs could not be attributed to the existence of a competing natural support system which adequately tends to the family needs of sole support mothers. When we consider this hypothesis alongside our earlier speculations about the effect of tight-knit and socially homogeneous networks on the transmission of new information and on people's service utilization decisions, we gain the overall impression that these sorts of networks tend to be highly constraining for people. They are likely to lock people into monolithic standards for behavior, insulate them from news about novel resources in the environment, and discourage them from experimenting with foreign ideas about problem-solving.

Summary: A Research Framework for Assessing Network Influences on Service Utilization

No amount of tinkering with the elements of program design nor alteration in the site of program delivery will increase the rate of program utilization if the intended audience is subjected to the influence of a powerful reference group which fails to sanction the program's mission, fails to see the value of the program's resources, or defines the program as one which competes for the loyalty of the group's members. The professional community has paid too little attention to the social orbits in which their potential clients are embedded, preferring instead to concentrate on the technology reflected in the content of their social programs. And where attention has been paid to designing programs which suit the consumer, knowledge about the latter has been based on broad demographic descriptors such as income level, ethnicity, educational attainment, and geographic location. Granted that some agencies have gone the extra distance toward tailoring their programs to the needs of their catchment areas by, for example, examining indicators of social problems in the locale or by reviewing health statistics, they have nevertheless ignored the fact that these broad characterizations of people and their settings provide only equally broad guidelines for identifying the targets of intervention and the means of intervention. More important, these sources of information say nothing about the field of social forces which interpose themselves between the calculation of needs, the summary demographics, and the ultimate utilization of professional services.

Throughout this chapter, we have tried to show how concepts drawn from research on social networks can be fruitfully applied to the analysis of service underutilization, and we have grounded our discussion upon a specific case study of one agency's efforts to extend a preventive program to a low-income population of sole support mothers. Our goal was to provide the staff with leads about how these mothers' social worlds might be structured and about how these structures might influence their use of the agency's parent education services. Our more general purpose was to identify a subset of network variables which may influence rates of program utilization and which, therefore, should be included in future research on this topic. In order to identify these network variables, we found it useful to first consider three ways in which social networks may exercise control over people's use of services. As systems of communication, they may insulate people from information about the existence of social programs; as referral systems, they may condition people's attitudes toward specific social programs; and as support systems, they may meet people's needs for support and guidance directly. These three "network functions" are summarized in Figure 9.2. By reviewing studies which have examined these three network functions, we were able to specify a set of network properties which ought to be included in future research on program utilization. These properties have been organized into three categories and are listed in Figure 9.2 under the heading, "Network Characteristics." Considered together, the network characteristics and network functions outlined in Figure 9.2 constitute a research framework for the study of service utilization. This framework formed the basis for a grant proposal which our consultees have subsequently submitted.

In terms of the method of data collection, we recommended that our consultees first attempt to identify a set of key informants in the neighborhood, people who would be nominated by others as long-term residents who are knowledgeable about local social groupings. These informants could be approached to provide information about the range of social networks which they perceive in their locale and to nominate at least one person from each network. In short, we suggested that a snowball sample might be the most efficient way of beginning the research process since it would provide preliminary data about the feasibility of a full-scale network study. The basic purpose of this first stage, then, would be to determine the extent to which the neighborhood is characterized by social isolation of its residents, or by the existence (as we hypothesized) of small, tight-knit, and socially homogeneous networks. In the former case, a full-scale study of the variables included in Figure 9.2 should not be undertaken; agency staff should instead concentrate on community organization tactics which would be directed toward building networks and fostering social support among residents. The task of weaving a social

FIGURE 9.2   Research Framework for the Study of Network
Characteristics and Functions which Influence
Service Utilization

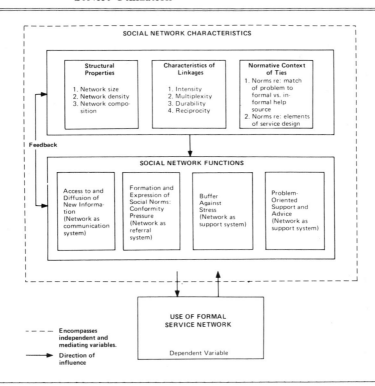

fabric into the community should take precedence over fostering greater
utilization of agency services. Indeed, it is likely that residents of such a
community would place a higher priority on gaining a sense of social
integration than they would on attending a program to improve their
parenting skills.

It is likely, however, that preliminary research would identify some
isolated persons and some intact social networks in the community. In
fact, throughout the course of our consultation our discussion of the
literature in relation to our consultee's knowledge of the community
situation of sole support mothers led us to hypothesize that we would
uncover the existence of small, dense, and socially homogeneous networks

in the locale. Those who are enmeshed in these networks should be approached and interviewed with a mind to collecting data about the variables outlined in Figure 9.2. Efforts should be made to gather information about the communication system of their networks, the extent to which they act as referral systems, and about the extent to which they serve socially supportive functions for their members. In particular, respondents should be questioned about their knowledge of social programs in the community, their use of network members as lay consultants regarding the decision to use these programs, and the extent to which their needs are met by the available support from these associates. These same respondents should be asked to provide data about the properties of their networks so that calculations of the density, size, composition, and internal segmentation can be made and related to network functions and to the utilization behavior of members. Respondents can also provide information about the prevailing norms regarding the occasions when they would be prompted to use professional help sources and their attitudes toward alternative elements of program design can be gauged.

The theme we have sounded throughout this chapter is that social network research has invaluable potential as a tool to analyze and improve the functional relationship between a community primary group and a formal service program. While it is clear that the conduct of such research poses new problems in the areas of field research and data analysis, and while the network processes under study are complex, we can only take advantage of a social network perspective on problems of service use if we employ a conceptual model and a framework for research which reflects rather than masks that complexity.

References

Albee, G.W., & Joffee, J.M. (Eds.). *Primary Prevention of Psychopathology.* Hanover, NH: University Press of New England, 1977.

Auerbach, J.B. *Parents Learn Through Discussion: Principles and Practices of Parent Group Discussion.* New York: John Wiley, 1968.

Bazelay, P., & Viney, L. Women coping with crisis: A preliminary community study. *Journal of Community Psychology,* 1974, *2,* 321-329.

Berkman, L.F., & Syme, S.L. Social networks, host resistance, and mortality: Nine-year follow-up study of Alameda County residents. *American Journal of Epidemiology,* 1979, *109,* 186-204.

Bloom, B.L. *Community Mental Health: A General Introduction.* Belmont, CA: Wadsworth, 1975.

Bott, E. *Family and Social Network.* London: Tavistock, 1971.

Brim, D. *Education for Child-Rearing.* New York: Free Press, 1965.

Bullough, B. Poverty, ethnic identity, and preventive health care. *Journal of Health and Social Behavior* 1972, *13*, 65-71.

Chilman, C. Helping low-income families through parent education. *Children*, 1963, *10*, 127-132.

Chilman, C. Programs for disadvantaged parents: Some major trends and related research. In B.M. Caldwell and H.N. Ricciuti (Eds.), *Review of Child Development Research. Volume 3.* Chicago: University of Chicago Press, 1973.

Conner, K.A., Powers, E.A., & Bultena, G.L. Social interaction and life satisfaction: An empirical assessment of late-life patterns. *Journal of Gerontology*, 1979, *34*, 116-121.

Craven, P., & Wellman, B. The network city. *Sociological Inquiry*, 1973, *3*, 57-88.

Freeburg, N., & Payne, D. Parental influence on cognitive development in early childhood. *Child Development*, 1967, *38*, 65-87.

Gershon, M., & Biller, H. *The Other Helpers: Paraprofessionals and Nonprofessionals in Mental Health.* Lexington, MA: D.C. Heath, 1977.

Gordon, I.S. *Parent Involvement in Compensatory Education.* Urbana: University of Illinois Press, 1970.

Granovetter, M. The strength of weak ties. *American Journal of Sociology*, 1973, *78*, 1360-1380.

Hereford, C. *Changing Parent Attitudes Through Group Discussion.* Austin: Hogg Foundation for Mental Health, University of Texas, 1963.

Hirsch, B.J. Natural support systems and coping with major life changes. *American Journal of Community Psychology*, 1980, *8*, 159-172.

Hunt, J. The psychological basis for using pre-school enrichment as an antidote for cultural deprivation. *Merrill-Palmer Quarterly*, 1964, *10*, 209-243.

Katz, E., & Lazarsfeld, P. *Personal Influence.* New York: Free Press, 1955.

Kelly, J.G., Snowden, L., & Munoz, R.F. Social and community interventions. *Annual Review of Psychology*, 1977, *28*, 323-361.

Kraft, I., & Chilman, C. *A Survey of Research: Helping Low-Income Families Through Parent Education.* Washington, DC: Department of Health, Education and Welfare, 1966.

Laumann, E.O. *Bonds of Pluralism.* New York: John Wiley, 1973.

Lin, N., Ensel, W.M., Simeone, R.S., & Kuo, W. Social support, stressful life events, and illness: A model and an empirical test. *Journal of Health and Social Behavior*, 1979, *20*, 108-119.

Liu, W.T., & Duff, R.W. The strength in weak ties. *Public Opinion Quarterly*, 1972, *36*, 361-366.

Lowenthal, M.F., & Haven, C. Interaction and adaptation: Intimacy as a critical variable. *American Sociological Review*, 1968, *33*, 20-30.

Marsden, L.R. *North York Family Formation Study.* North York, Ontario: North York Board of Education, 1975.

McKinlay, J. Some approaches and problems in the study of the use of services: An overview. *Journal of Health and Social Behavior*, 1972, *13*, 115-151.

McKinlay, J. Social networks, lay consultation, and helping behavior. *Social Forces*, 1973, *51*, 275-292.

Myers, J., Lindenthal, J., & Pepper, M. Life events, social integration and psychiatric symptomatology. *Journal of Health and Social Behavior*, 1975, *16*, 421-429.

Phillips, D.L. Mental health status, social participation and happiness. *Journal of Health and Social Behavior,* 1967, *8,* 285-291.

Pickarts, E., & Fargo, J. Parent education: Toward parental competence. *Family Coordinator,* 1970, *19,* 124-133.

Reissman, F. Issues in training the nonprofessional. *Poverty and Human Resources Abstracts,* 1967, *2,* 5-17.

Rogers, E. *Diffusion of Innovation.* New York: Free Press, 1962.

Rutter, M.L. Dimensions of parenthood: Some myths and suggestions. In *The Family in Society.* London: Her Majesty's Stationery Office, 1974.

Schofield, W. *Psychotherapy: The Purchase of Friendship.* Englewood Cliffs, NJ: Prentice-Hall, 1964.

Weiss, R. The provisions of social relationships. In Z. Rubin (Ed.), *Doing Unto Others.* Englewood Cliffs, NJ: Prentice-Hall, 1974.

Whitten, N.E., Jr., & Wolfe, A.W. Network analysis. In J.J. Honigmann (Ed.), *Handbook of Social and Cultural Anthropology.* Chicago: Rand McNally, 1974.

10

Prevention Policy
The Federal Perspective

Thomas F.A. Plaut
National Institute of Mental Health

Background—Recent Developments
in the Prevention Area

The concept of prevention in the mental health field is not new. Current interest in this field is an extension of work going back almost 20 years (Caplan, 1964). The public health concept of prevention is evidenced in the emphasis on consultation and education services in the Federally initiated community mental health centers program that had its start in the mid-1960s.[1] However, only in the last five or six years has there been a renewed interest in prevention at the national (and Federal) level(s). The impact of the "Lalonde Report" (Lalonde, 1974) in the United States has been substantial. This report, by the Canadian Minister of Health at that time, suggested that the long-range means to reduce morbidity and mortality from a broad range of health conditions was through modifications in persons' lifestyles. More recently, the Report of the U.S. Surgeon General (*Healthy People,* 1979) has emphasized the same general theme. In addition, the field of prevention has received increased attention as a means of reducing ever-escalating medical care spending. Some concern is being expressed that advocacy of prevention can be a cover for cutting public expenditures for medical care. In 1979 the U.S. Surgeon General convened a working meeting to develop national prevention goals for 1990 in a range of different areas. These include physical fitness and exercise, stress, drug and alcohol problems, communicable diseases, hypertension, accidents, industrial hazards, and neonatal mortality.

More narrowly within the mental health field, the publication of the Report from the President's Commission on Mental Health probably will be marked as a key step in the development of Federal prevention initiatives. One of the eight major recommendation chapters of the report is entitled "A Strategy for Prevention" (President's Commission on Mental Health, 1978a: 51-54). It should be noted that there was no such emphasis on prevention in the report of the only previous national mental health commission (Action for Mental Health, 1961). Specifically, the commission recommended that (1) NIMH established a Center for Prevention, (2) primary prevention be the major priority of this center, and (3) $10 million be provided for NIMH prevention activities with a 10-year goal of 10 percent of the total NIMH budget being devoted to activities directly related to prevention. Furthermore, the report of the Task Panel on Prevention (President's Commission on Mental Health, 1978c: Appendix) reviews and synthesizes much recent research and conceptual work. The establishment of an Office of Prevention in NIMH in the summer of 1979 was a direct outgrowth of the commission's work and the follow-up activities within the U.S. Department of Health and Human Services (Report of the HEW Task Force, 1977). In the fall of 1979 the Alcohol, Drug Abuse and Mental Health Administration (parent agency of NIMH) convened a national meeting on prevention that drew several hundred participants (*Proceedings,* in press). Even prior to the stimulus provided by the work of the President's Commission, NIMH had initiated some significant prevention activities under the leadership of Steve Goldston. These included the publication of *Primary Prevention: An Idea Whose Time Has Come* (Klein and Goldston, 1977) and the initiation of an NIMH Primary Prevention Series. In a legislative first in 1979, the U.S. Congress specified that $4 million of NIMH's research budget was to be earmarked for prevention activities. The President's budget request had also included funds for prevention services activities, but these were not acted on by Congress because of delay in passage of the necessary enabling legislation— the Administration's Mental Health Systems Act. This legislative proposal included a special section on prevention, and it is anticipated that final congressional action will retain some form of authority for limited Federal prevention services grants to States and/or communities. There does not appear to be any sentiment in Congress for the appropriation of more than these very limited demonstration (capacity building) funds.

In 1979 the NIMH Office of Prevention issued two special prevention research grant announcements. They invited applications to test the effectiveness of programs directed at assisting children who were in situations of "risk" or to undertake research directed at developing such interventive approaches. The two "risk" situations were marital disruption (separation/ divorce) and severely disturbed parents (mentally ill, alcoholic, or drug abusers). NIMH also stated that its plans were for support of smaller-scale research activities in 1980 in areas such as the following: promoting parental competence among teenage parents, surveying the nature of psychosocial services for children in pediatric wards, examining community-based services dealing with death and dying, surveying prevention-related training activities in the four mental health disciplines, and organizing small "state-of-the-art" research workshops in a number of areas that appear to have potential for the development of preventive interventions.[2]

General Policy Issues in
Mental Health Prevention

(I) *Is there an adequate knowledge base?* Within the mental health community—particularly among clinicians, academicians, and many Federal managers—the basic question revolves around adequacy of the current knowledge base for the undertaking of preventive efforts. Although early leaders in the prevention field were psychiatrists (Caplan, 1964; Lindemann, 1944), recently more public criticism of preventive activities has come from psychiatry (Eisenberg, 1977; Lamb and Zusman, 1979) than from psychology. Leading spokespersons for prevention have included psychologists such as Albee and Joffee (1977) and Cowen and Zax (1968). There have also been significant approaches to prevention that move away from traditional medical model single-factor etiological theories. Bloom (1979) emphasizes the potential utility of focusing on "precipitating" rather than "predisposing" factors and on events (crises) which appear to be associated with increased frequency of a variety of mental disorders rather than being predictive for increased rates of a single or specific illness. The work of the Jessors (1977) stresses the complex interaction of many factors in the development of social and psychological problems. Cassel (1976) has written persuasively about the role of general, environmental, stressful factors in accounting for differential rates of a number of medical disorders.

To some prevention advocates, it appears that a "double-standard" is being applied in relation to the adequacy of the knowledge base for action. That is, more evidence regarding effectiveness seems to be required before preventive programs are supported than is the case for treatment activities. In American society, generally there is greater public demand to "do something" when a person is ill or suffering than to undertake preventive efforts. Prevention is accepted in principle, but when hard resource allocation choices are made, the decision usually goes for treatment services. The White House Office on Science and Technology has recently estimated that no more than 15 percent of generally accepted medical technology (surgery, pharmacological treatments, and so on) have been fully evaluated and found to be effective.[3]

(II) *What are appropriate targets for prevention/promotion activities?* Prevention efforts have been directed at a number of different target groups or populations. The failure to clarify the matter has been the subject of considerable criticism from those opposed to prevention programs. Some have argued that the priority targets for preventive work should be the *major mental illnesses (schizophrenia and manic-depressive disorders).* However, there is little evidence regarding the effectiveness of programs geared specifically to reduce rates of these severe disorders. Some argue that the focus should be on reducing rates of *other clearly defined "mental conditions";* for example, those listed in the Diagnostic and Statistical Manual of the American Psychiatric Association (DSM-III). Klerman (in press) has suggested another target group: *persons suffering from moderate to severe anxiety or depression* (but not necessarily diagnosable as being ill in terms of standard psychiatric nosology). Eisenberg and Parron (1979) propose a focus on preventing *developmental attrition,* "a sequential and cumulative failure to attain levels of cognitive and affective development sufficient for personal and social competence." (p. 148). Finally, the *promotion of mental health* (improved coping, for example) has often been singled out as a goal of prevention programs. At a recent Federally sponsored workshop (Martin, 1979), a new concept of *primary promotion* was proposed. This was an explicit effort to move away from an "illness model" and from the focus on specific conditions. Instead, the emphasis is on developing "wellness" in whole populations, on promoting and reinforcing the strengths of community systems and attacking those that are viewed as "dysfunctional." There is no consensus on which of the above classes of potential targets for prevention/promotion programs is most important. Different assumptions underlie the various approaches and different strategies undoubtedly are called for. To the extent that there is agreement on the use of terms, greater clarity will occur in future discussions and dialogues.

(III) *Factors to consider in choosing objectives for prevention programs.* What elements should be considered in making choices among various prevention program alternatives? Below are listed a number of factors that could form the basis of such a decision-making process:

(A) *What is the social cost or burden of illness (Rice et al., 1976) involved in the particular problem or condition?* Factors that could be included are death, disability, days of work lost, impaired functioning, or extent of suffering consequent on the condition. Using single or multiple indices, it would be possible to rank possible target populations or illnesses.

(B) *What is the current knowledge base regarding causes (etiology) of the condition, and how persuasive is the evidence that interventions are effective?* Mention previously has been made that many critics of prevention programs point to the lack of research which would support the belief that programs will have the desired impact. In determining what preventive efforts to undertake, it is reasonable to take into account the likelihood that the planned intervention will have the anticipated effects.

(C) What is the feasibility of the proposed program? Reference here is to such factors as political acceptance of the program, nature of public attitudes, balance between risk and gain factors, and availability of funds to actually carry out the effort. For example, would allocation of funds generate such resentment from clinical service providers or certain subgroups in the community that the end results would be counterproductive?

(D) *How appropriate is it for the particular program or unit of government to take the lead in developing or organizing the activity?* Is it appropriate for a local community mental health program to spend significant staff time and other resources to persuade county commissioners to increase the availability of public housing, or to secure the ouster of a police chief who is felt to be racist? Ensuring improved prenatal care for teenage mothers may well have preventive implications from a mental health standpoint; however, is it the responsibility of a local mental health program to take the lead in a campaign to bring this about? Should mental health programs, including those of a preventive nature, rather focus on those activities and actions that are particularly within the areas' of expertise and specialized skills of mental health professionals?

(IV) *What are the boundaries of mental health prevention activities?* There is agreement that mental health prevention activities can be directed at bringing about change in individual or family behavior. Less clear, as was suggested above, is the extent to which there is support for mental health programs seeking to bring about broader societal changes. For example, there is considerable evidence that rates of mental disorders are related to social class and to other measures of economic deprivation. Should prevention programs then seek to bring about greater equity in the society generally; to bring about income redistribution; to reduce poverty, racism, or sexism?

In recent years, the interest in stress reduction and stress management has grown rapidly in the general health field (Holmes and Rahe, 1967; Monat and Lazarus, 1977; Dohrenwend and Dohrenwend, 1974). Helping (persuading?) people to modify their lifestyles has also become a key objective of a number of preventive health and health education programs (Farquahar et al., 1977). Other approaches, sometimes described as "holistic health" (Pelletier, 1977) emphasize not only stress management, but also diet, exercise, relaxation, and so on. Many of these efforts have as their objective not only the reduction of mental distress, but also the possible impact on physical health. This suggests opportunities for previously unexplored collaboration between mental health programs and medical care (and other health) programs.

Suggesting to people that they can take responsibility for their own health (physical and mental) is consistent with current trends for consumer activism and less dependence on medical and other professional specialists. However, there is some danger that emphasis on individual responsibility may lead to a disregard of societal and institutional factors that often have major effects on people. Ryan (1971) has pointed out the essentially conservative nature of this approach—that is, "blaming the victim."

Assisting in the development of mutual-aid, self-help groups (Caplan and Killilea, 1976; Silverman, 1978) have become accepted elements of some community mental health programs. It is interesting to note that the potential contribution of such groups has been more widely acknowledged within some aspects of the medical care field than is generally the case in mental health. Programs to modify attitudes and practices in certain social institutions—that is, schools, police, day care centers, and so on—are now often found in community mental health centers, usually as part of the consultation and education activities. While some such efforts are directed at early case-finding and referral, others emphasize the "humanization" of the particular institution or social setting.

One position on the controversy regarding the place of social action in mental health prevention programs has been articulated by Eisenberg and Parron (1979: 152):

> Some of the corrective measures are medical in form; all are societal in substance. Mental health professionals bear a special responsibility to bring to public attention the urgency of concerted social action. Surely, in an era of serious neglect by the Federal Government, at all levels we must become activists for social change on behalf of the neglected and disenfranchised.

(V) *Difficulties in the evaluation of prevention programs.* How will you know if the program "worked," if it had any effect at all? Questions of this sort are frequently addressed to prevention advocates. The problem of evaluation of prevention programs does indeed appear to be a particularly difficult one. There is little disagreement that such programs need to be evaluated. However, the unspecific nature of the proposed goals (objectives) often makes this a difficult, if not impossible, task. For example, improving persons' coping skills or providing "support-system" help to individuals grieving for a recently deceased spouse are not likely to lead to any specific set of outcomes that are easily measurable.

Evaluation of prevention programs involves all of the difficulties associated with the evaluation of psychotherapy—and probably some others in addition. In therapy evaluation, one can usually point to the presence of some specific symptoms or behaviors that one wishes to eliminate or modify. For most preventive efforts, there is much less clarity and specificity regarding the desired changes. Some of the effects of preventive programs on individuals are likely to be measurable only over very long periods of time. This is particularly the case for those activities directed at reducing rates of a major mental illness, since the "pre-morbid" phase of most such conditions is known to be a matter of months and, in most cases, requires years before clearly identifiable symptoms develop.

One way to overcome such difficulties is to identify "better" and "poorer" ways of dealing with specific tasks or situations and then determine whether the preventive efforts result in a shift in the desired direction. This does, however, leave unanswered whether there is any direct relationship between these ways of dealing with the situation and some subsequent, generally agreed-upon index or measure of mental health (or illness).

It has been argued that all prevention programs need to be evaluated. While this is a desirable goal, it is unrealistic to expect that most local prevention programs can undertake the type of evaluation that would add to current knowledge regarding the effectiveness of the program. Such basic evaluation studies might well be undertaken only on a selected basis in collaboration with groups of experienced evaluation researchers. Such a strategy need not involve total abandonment of efforts to assess the relative quality of different preventive efforts. It has been suggested (Woy, 1979) that all prevention programs be examined on a regular basis through some form of peer review. The use of such "collegial" review methods is now well established in the health field, such as Professional Standards Review Organizations (PSROs) and the local peer review committees of the various mental health disciplinary organizations. To the extent possible, specific evaluation criteria could be developed, but considerable weight would still be attached to the "judgments" made by the experts constituting these review groups.

Principles Underlying the
Current Federal Mental Health
Prevention Program

Although the NIMH prevention program was not formally established as a separate component until the fall of 1979, a number of key guiding principles can be identified. Four of these principles are discussed below.

(I) *Emphasis on knowledge development.* Accent is being placed on the development of new knowledge and the careful testing and evaluation of all services demonstration programs. This is in contrast to an approach that would emphasize wide-scale dissemination of essentially untested programs and substantial support of ongoing or proposed community-based service programs. A priority will be to interest qualified investigators to undertake research directly related to prevention. In this research-oriented approach to the development and testing of interventive models, a wide range of types of intervention and target populations will be studied.

(II) *Priority to primary prevention efforts, but some attention also to secondary prevention.* The bulk of available resources will be directed to the primary prevention area, but some funds will also be set aside for secondary prevention activities. Secondary prevention efforts would include studies of how to improve the early identification (case-finding) skills of various caregivers. These would include, but not be restricted to, nonpsychiatric physicians. On any given day, more identifiable psychiatric "casualties" are seen by persons in the general medical care delivery system than by workers in the specialty mental health care system (President's Commission on Mental Health, 1978b: 8). Promotion approaches in the mental health field will also be studied. These include, but are not restricted to, traditional health and public education.

(III) *Major effort to collaborate with and utilize other components within the Department of Health and Human Services.* The NIMH Office of Prevention is committed to working intensively with all other relevant components of the institute—research, services, training, and education. This approach also applies to cooperative efforts with other components of the Public Health Service and other units in the department, such as the

Office of Human Development Services and the Department of Education (formerly the Office of Education). In each case, existing programs of other units within the department will be examined to see what opportunities they present for mental health prevention/promotion activities. The newly developing area of behavioral medicine presents unusual opportunities for bridge-building with the mental health prevention field. An example of this is the interest in stress which cuts across NIMH and the "categorical" disease institutes within the National Institutes of Health (heart, cancer, and so on).

(IV) *Planned strategy to improve quality of work in the prevention area.* Central to the program philosophy is attracting highly competent workers throughout the United States to the research, training, and action (services) aspects of prevention work. The objective is to "legitimize" (and make attractive) this area for quality scientific and other professional endeavors. The goal, then, is to get prevention "on the agenda" of many groups, organizations, and institutions. A major method for achieving this objective is the building of linkages among previously unrelated individuals or groups: the establishment of networks among researchers, among training institutions, among services personnel, and among all three of these groups.

Conclusion

The prevention/promotion area remains in an early developmental stage. Many issues are unresolved due to lack of necessary data and disagreement on concepts and ideology. The continuing identification and analysis of these issues is essential if the area is to move ahead. To act as though there were no residual issues is to invite attacks by critics from a broad range of fronts—laboratory researchers, clinicians, and opponents of any efforts at planned social change. It is hoped that future years will see a larger proportion of mental health workers involved in some aspects of prevention and a larger proportion of the total national mental health dollar invested in this area.

Notes

1. This is not to imply that "consultation and education" is synonymous with "prevention." In the absence of a public health preventive orientation, consultation and education services would never have become part of the federal mental health legislation in the mid-1960s.

2. Principles underlying the current NIMH prevention program are outlined below.

3. Reported by G. Klerman at a meeting of the National Advisory Mental Health Council, December 1979.

References

Action for Mental Health. Report of the Joint Commission on Mental Illness and Health. New York: Basic Books, 1961.

Albee, G.W., & Joffe, J.M. (Eds.). *Primary Prevention of Psychopathology. Volume 1. The Issues.* Hanover, NH: University Press of New England, 1977.

American Psychiatric Association. *Diagnostic and Statistical Manual for Mental Disorders—III.* Washington, DC: Author, 1980.

Bloom, B.L. Prevention of mental disorders: Recent advances in theory and practice. *Community Mental Health Journal,* 1979, *15,* 179-191.

Caplan, G. *Principles of Preventive Psychiatry.* New York: Basic Books, 1964.

Caplan, G., & Killilea, M. (Eds.). *Support Systems and Mutual Help: Multi-Disciplinary Explorations.* New York: Grune and Stratton, 1976.

Cassel, J. The contributions of the social environment to host resistance. *American Journal of Epidemiology,* 1976, *104,* 107-123.

Cowen, E., & Zax, M. Early detection and prevention of emotional disorders: Conceptualization and programs. In J.W. Carter (Ed.), *Research Contributions from Psychology to Mental Health.* New York: Behavioral Publications, 1968, 46-59.

Dohrenwend, B., & Dohrenwend, B.P. (Eds.). *Stressful Life Events: Their Nature and Effects.* New York: John Wiley, 1974.

Eisenberg, L. The perils of prevention: A cautionary note. *New England Journal of Medicine,* 1977, *297,* 1230-1232.

Eisenberg, L., & Parron, D. Strategies for the prevention of mental disorders. In *Healthy People, the Surgeon General's Report on Health Promotion and Disease Prevention.* Background Papers, DHEW (PHS) Publication No. 79-55071A. Washington, DC: U.S. Government Printing Office, 1979, 135-155.

Farquhar, J., Maccoby, N., Wood, P.D., et al. Community education for cardiovascular disease. *The Lancet,* 1977, *1,* 1192-1195.

Healthy People, the Surgeon General's Report on Health Promotion and Disease Prevention. Background Papers, DHEW (PHS) Publication No. 70-55071. Washington, DC: U.S. Government Printing Office, 1979.

Holmes, T.H., & Rahe, R.H. The social readjustment scale. *Journal of Psychosomatic Research,* 1967, *11,* 213-218.

Jessor, R., & Jessor, S. *Problem Behavior and Psycho-Social Development: A Longitudinal Study of Youth.* New York: Academic Press, 1977.

Klein, D.C., & Goldston, S.E. (Eds.). *Primary Prevention: An Idea Whose Time Has Come.* DHEW (ADM) Publication No. 77-447. Washington, DC: U.S. Government Printing Office, 1977.

Klerman, G.L. Keynote address. *Proceedings, First Annual Conference on Prevention, The Alcohol, Drug Abuse and Mental Health Administration.* DHEW (ADM) Publication. Washington, DC: U.S. Government Printing Office, in press.

Lalonde, M. *A New Perspective on the Health of Canadians.* Ottawa: Government of Canada, 1974.

Lamb, H.R., & Zusman, J. Primary prevention in perspective. *American Journal of Psychiatry,* 1979, *136,* 12-16.

Lindemann, E. The symptomatology and management of acute grief. *American Journal of Psychiatry,* 1944, *101,* 141-152.

Martin, K.M. Reflections on the workshop on primary prevention and mental health. Office of Mental Health Programs, Indian Health Service, PHS, DHEW. Washington, DC: U.S. Government Printing Office, 1979. (unpublished)

Monat, A., & Lazarus, R.S. (Eds.). *Stress and Coping: An Anthology.* New York: Columbia University Press, 1977.

Pelletier, K.R. *Mind as Healer, Mind as Slayer: A Holistic Approach to Preventing Stress Disorders.* New York: Delacorte Press, 1977.

President's Commission on Mental Health. *Report to the President. Volume I.* Washington, DC: U.S. Government Printing Office, 1978. (a)

President's Commission on Mental Health. *Report to the President. Volume II.* Washington, DC: U.S. Government Printing Office, 1978. (b)

President's Commission on Mental Health. *Report to the President. Volume IV.* Washington, DC: U.S. Government Printing Office, 1978. (c)

Proceedings, First Annual Conference on Prevention, the Alcohol, Drug Abuse and Mental Health Administration. DHEW (ADM) Publication. Washington, DC: U.S. Government Printing Office, in press.

Preventing Disease/Promoting Health: Objectives for the Nation. Working Papers developed by the Department of Health, Education and Welfare at a public conference, Atlanta, Georgia, August, 1979.

Report of the DHEW Task Force on Implementation of the Report to the President from the President's Commission on Mental Health. DHEW (ADM) Publication No. 79-848. Washington, DC: U.S. Government Printing Office, 1977.

Rice, D.P., Feidman, J.J., & White, K.L. *The Current Burden of Illness in the U.S.* Occasional Papers of the Institute of Medicine. Washington, DC: National Academy of Sciences, 1976.

Ryan, W. *Blaming the Victim.* New York: Random House, 1971.

Silverman, P.R. *Mutual Help Groups: A Guide for Mental Health Workers.* DHEW (ADM) Publication No. 78-646. Washington, DC: U.S. Government Printing Office, 1978.

Woy, R. Personal communication, 1979.

11

Primary Prevention
Policy and Practice

Carolyn F. Swift

Southwest Community Mental Health Center,
Columbus, Ohio

Revolutions, in retrospect, are inevitable events. Prospectively, their success is less certain. Their coming may or may not be heralded with bloodshed or fanfare. The recent revolution in Iran erupted with little forewarning to western observers: The entrenched acceded to the besiegers in a relatively unanticipated and bloodless coup. Other revolutions are preceded by a series of escalating critical events punctuated with public declarations of dissent and culminating in the birth of a new order. The much-heralded and long-awaited prevention revolution in the mental health field appears to be of the latter variety.

The concept of prevention has been surfacing in the health field with increasing frequency and expanding authority over the last century. In 1850, a Report of the Sanitary Commisson of Massachusetts set forth the belief that

> a vast amount of unnecessarily impaired health, and physical debility exists among those not actually confined by sickness: —that these preventable evils require an enormous expenditure and loss of money, and impose upon the people unnumbered and immeasurable calamities, pecuniary, social, physical, mental, and moral, which might be avoided: —that means exist, within our reach, for their mitigation or removal: —and that measures for prevention will effect infinitely more than remedies for the cure of disease [quoted in Fielding, 1977].

Bloom (1971) reminds us that some 60 years ago Adolf Meyer advised communities to go beyond "mere mending" to prevent the systematic production of mental problems. A decade later Harry Stack Sullivan outlined the prevention-treatment dichotomy that is still debated today: "Either you believe that mental disorders are acts of God, predestined, inexorably fixed, arising from constitutional or some other irremediable substratums . . . or you believe that mental disorder is largely preventable and somewhat remediable by control of psycho-sociological factors" (quoted in Fielding, 1977).

A look at some of the prevention advocates emerging in the last few years compels the conclusion that primary prevention has joined the ranks of apple pie and motherhood as an American value. For example, the President's Commission on Mental Health has identified prevention as a "necessary ingredient of a systematic approach to promoting mental health" (1978: 51). The Surgeon General's Report on Health Promotion and Disease Prevention (1979) has cited prevention as the primary strategy through which further improvements in the health of the American people can be made:

> There are three overwhelming reasons why a new strong emphasis on prevention—at all levels of government and by all our citizens—is essential. . . . Prevention saves lives. . . . Prevention improves the quality of life. . . . Finally, it can save dollars in the long run. In an era of runaway health costs, preventive action for health is cost-effective" [1978: 9].

The Joint Commission on Accreditation of Hospitals has listed prevention as the foremost service goal of their balanced service system (1979: 9). Late in 1977, Dr. Gerald L. Klerman, as new Administrator of the Alcohol, Drug Abuse and Mental Health Administration (ADAMHA), established prevention as the fourth major agency priority. An ADAMHA Prevention Committee was established to develop a planning document to guide the agency's prevention efforts through 1982 (ADAMHA Prevention Policy Paper, 1979: A-4). In June 1979 the National Institute of Mental Health (NIMH) set up an Office on Prevention, with a first-year budget of $4 million for research projects. Finally, in a staff paper (1978), the Institute of Medicine called for a stronger federal prevention policy and organized a conference to formulate a national prevention strategy.

These are not fringe groups; rather, they represent the broad spectrum of the health field, including the conservative medical establishment. The call to arms for prevention by such a prestigious array of power blocs in the health system inevitably affects policy and practice in the field, which in turn shapes trends for prevention in the 1980s. The chain of historical events coupled with pronouncements from the health establishment and the prevention avant garde point to the decline of the unidimensional treatment model of health care in the United States. Prevention rebels are finding their ranks swollen with treatment professionals espousing prevention goals. This swell of support for prevention from all levels of the health care system has been interpreted as assuring success for prevention programs (Goldston, 1977; Klerman, 1979; Surgeon General's Report, 1979). Albee (in press), on the other hand, cites recent psychiatric literature opposing prevention efforts in mental health and warns that the chorus of support is a siren song that will not be backed up with adequate funds. Primary prevention is on its way to becoming a major buzzword of the eighties, a glamor stock soaring high on word-of-mouth tips of future promise. Whether it will be held for appreciation by committed investors or sold short by buyers looking for a quick buck is yet to be determined.

Development of Federal
Prevention Policy During the Seventies

Franks (in press) cites two legislative events as key in developing prevention policy at the national level over the last decade. First, the National Health Planning and Resources Development Act of 1974 (P.L. 93-641) included prevention in two of its priorities—disease prevention and public education about health care. Guidelines for state health plans and health systems plans in implementing P.L. 93-641 required plans for the prevention goals of health promotion, health protection, and prevention and detection services.

The second significant legislative event was the National Consumer Health Information and Health Promotion Act of 1976 (P.L. 94-317). Franks (in press) documents the influence of *Preventive Medicine, USA* (1976) on this legislation. This publication, produced with the combined efforts of the National Institutes of Health, John E. Fogarty International Center for Advanced Study in the Health Sciences, and the American College of Preventive Medicine, provided recommendations that shaped the legislative mandate to the secretary of Health, Education and Welfare. The secretary was charged with formulating national goals and supporting research and demonstration projects for health information and promotion as well as preventive health services and education in how to use health care, and also was charged with analyzing and recommending resources needed to accomplish these goals.

Against the background of this legislation and a series of prevention/ health-promotion conferences and reports from health groups, the President's Commission on Mental Health (1978) produced its recommendations on prevention. The commission's recommendations constitute the single most significant event in this century in their impact on the development and delivery of community mental health prevention programs. Their influence is currently being felt in pending legislation, the restructuring of the federal and state mental health bureaucracies, the creation of a new federal-state partnership in the delivery of community mental health services, and the eruption of research proposals and service programs targeted to prevention programs for children.

Of the six recommendations on prevention made by the commission, five are targeted to children—prenatal and early infant care for all women; periodic developmental child health assessments; comprehensive health and mental health care for all children; developmental day care programs; and family counseling and support as well as full evaluations whenever out-of-home placements for children are considered. The sixth recommendation was to establish a Prevention Center within the National Institute of Mental Health to coordinate federal prevention programs, to be funded at $10 million the first year and to receive 10 percent of the NIMH budget by 1988.

Four of the themes of the overall commission report have significance for prevention. First, the emphasis on prevention throughout the report ensures that prevention issues will be addressed within the legislative-regulatory system. Second, the transfer of power to the states for planning, funding, and implementing mental health programs creates problems for prevention programs, since few states have either a commitment to or expertise in prevention. The commission's directive to make mental health services available to unserved and underserved populations opens the door to flexible, innovative forms of mental health service delivery, including the possible separation of preventive from treatment services (see discussion of the Mental Health Systems Act below). Since many of the priority populations—children and youth, the aged, racial and ethnic minorities, the poor—are considered to be at high risk for the development of mental illness due to environmental hazards or discrimination, prevention programs are especially relevant for these groups. Finally, targeting children as the population group to be served can be expected to restrict the development of prevention programs for other populations.

The commission's recommendations were based on the report generated by the Task Panel on Prevention, which was chaired by George Albee. Table 11.1 charts the task panel's recommendations, their translation into the commission's recommendations, and the subsequent institutional response through the Mental Health Systems Act and the establishment of the NIMH Office on Prevention. As expected, there is a shrinkage process from the initial task panel's recommendations to their final (to date) impact on the system. The process begins with the commission's eclipsing of the task panel's recommendations. For example, both groups agree on the emphasis on children as the priority population. However, the task panel, in citing stress reduction, environments, and the strategy of increasing coping skills, gives examples of successful prevention programs in the schools. Clearly, schools are a common environment for children as well as a common source of stress. With the exception of Headstart programs, the commission does not pursue this direction. The task panel, while not emphasizing institutional stressors, recognizes the necessity to reduce stress due to racism, poverty, sexism, ageism, and urban blight. The commission does not deal with these issues in their recommendations on prevention.

Both the task panel and the commission recommend the structural change of the establishment of an NIMH Primary Prevention Center. This recommendation is not reflected in the Mental Health Systems Act. In June 1979 an "Office" on Prevention was established at NIMH under the direction of Tom Plaut. However, the office commands neither the clout nor the budget envisioned by the two study groups. Currently, the three major mental health constituency groups—the Mental Health Association, the National Council of Community Mental Health Centers, and the National Association of State Mental Health Program Directors—support amendment of the act to include the primary prevention center as recommended by the commission.

Community Mental Health Center
Commitment to Prevention

Since the locus of primary prevention activities in community mental health centers (CMHCs) is in consultation and education (C & E) units, a review of the resources and activities of these units gives some sense of the past CMHC commitment to prevention. C & E units were assigned the prevention role in the initial CMHC legislation in 1963.

TABLE 11.1   Official Recommendations of the President's Commission on Mental Health (1978) and the Institutional Response (1979)

Official Recommendations of the President's Commission on Mental Health		Institutional Response	
Task Panel on Prevention	PCMH Report (recommendations numbered as in Report)	MH Systems Act (Titles)	NIMH Implementation
I. *Emphasis* Priority for infant/children populations their environments stress reduction increase coping skills	Recommendations 1-5 are targeted to infants and children 1. prenatal/infant care 2. child health assessment and developmental review 3. comprehensive health and mh services for all children. 4. developmental day care 5. foster care	Children/youth are one of the priority pops. II. State prevention programs IV. CMHC prevention & C & E programs; "single service entity" programs	Office on Prevention Research initiatives: 5 out of 7 target children and their families; e.g., children whose parents are divorced, emotionally disturbed, etc.
Reduce stress of racism, poverty, sexism, ageism, urban blight.	Not addressed in prevention section	as above	Worshops on state of the art for prevention for priority populations.
II. *Structural* NIMH Primary Prevention Center	NIMH Primary Prevention Center	not addressed	NIMH Office on Prevention, June, 1979.
Prev. offices in state mental health authorities	Establish responsibility for prev. progs. in states (footnote to #6)	II. State Prevention program authority	Liaison with state MH authorities

TABLE 11.1 (Continued)

Official Recommendations of the President's
Commission on Mental Health

Task Panel on Prevention	PCMH Report (recommendations numbered as in Report)	Institutional Response	
		MH Systems Act (Titles)	NIMH Implementation
Prevention field stations		as above	not addressed
Prevention grants to local agencies (e.g., CMHCs)		IV. prevention and C & E grants	Management and accountability for prevention services, research and training programs
Prevention training and research	6. Prevention training and other appropriate activities	II. State prevention grants	
NIMH prev. center to coordinate federal prevention programs.	6. NIMH Prev. Center to coordinate federal prevention programs.	not addressed	Coordinates only NIMH prevention programs.
III. Funding: $12-$15 million now, $20-$25 million a year by 1985.	6. $10 million the first year, and 10% of NIMH budget by 1988.	II. $5 million in 1980 for state prev. prog.	$4 million research budget in 1980.
IV. Management and Review NIMH prev. prog. mandated 10 yrs. citizens' advisory committees	6. Projects NIMH budget for 10 years not addressed	II. 4-yr state programs IV. 8-yr CMHC C & E and prevention prog. IV., VI.	Office on Prevention is a permanent office within NIMH not addressed

Four of the five essential elements of service required of a comprehensive community mental health center focus on new methods of treatment and care. The fifth, consultation and education to community agencies and professionals, is concerned with the prevention of mental illness and the promotion of mental health [U.S. Department of Health, Education and Welfare, 1966].

While heralded as a bold new approach by President John Kennedy in his 1963 Presidential message, prevention activities were given neither the political clout nor the monetary resources to fulfill their mission. Snow and Newton (1976) trace the behind-the-scenes realities that ensured that the prevention mission envisioned by Kennedy could not be realized.

In the most recent five-year period for which data are available (1973-1977) an average of 4.1 percent of all CMHC staff hours in federally funded centers was devoted to C & E activities (NIMH Survey and Reports Branch, 1978). The figures show a decline of 33 percent over the period, from a high of 4.8 in 1973 to 3.2 percent in 1977. Consideration of artifacts of the reporting system in combination with reimbursement policies reveals the 4.1 figure to be a conservative estimate and the declining trend a possible illusion. As staffing grants and other federal funds have run out over the last five years, CMHCs have been resourceful in repackaging and labeling some C & E activities to ensure their reimbursability.

In the years of plenty—during the heyday of federal staffing grants— there was little concern about collecting fees for C & E offerings. The increasing numbers of CMHCs "graduating" from this support have found it necessary either to find funding for programs or cut them off. Clinical and C & E services provide alternative options in dealing with certain populations or problems in living. Families with problems in parenting, for example, may be routed to clinical treatment or enrolled in C & E classes in Parent Effectiveness Training. Abused wives may be assigned to therapy or to assertiveness training classes. Increasingly, clinical treatment plans are being written to include C & E classes as a necessary part of treatment, thus making the participation of diagnosed clients eligible for third-party reimbursement. Unfortunately, one of the unintended "side effects" of the practice of attempting to recover maximum fees for C & E classes is an increase in the number of participants who are given a clinical diagnosis and processed through the treatment system, as opposed to simply attending the class as students or members of the general public. Here the principle of the right to treatment in the least restrictive environment is violated by funding realities. When this practice is followed, staff time is prorated as clinical and the resultant fee is credited to clinical services within the center.

Case consultation has historically been a major activity of CMHC C & E units—with a focus on schools. By consulting with teachers around problem children, C & E professionals not only assist in resolving particular cases but increase the expertise of the teacher in dealing with other, similar cases in the future. Case consultation, then, has both clinical relevance for the case at hand and prevention relevance for future cases. By labeling such case consultation as a collateral clinical contact, CMHCs can recover third-party payment for the activity. Again, the staff time as well as the fee is credited to clinical services. The result of these reclassifications of C & E activities is a reduction in reported C & E staff time.

If this interpretation is correct, the data should reflect reduced hours devoted to C & E consultation and reduced hours devoted to children as a target population. In fact, C & E services to children have dropped almost 10 percent in the last three years (for which data are available), and case consultation has dropped 33 percent.

Concurrently, of course, "graduate" centers—those graduating from the eighth year of their staffing grants—are being forced to reduce services as federal funds disappear, and C & E services are being cut first precisely because of their economic vulnerability (Comptroller General, 1979; Weiner et al., 1979). Quite simply, they have not paid for themselves. A decline in C & E services over the last three years could be explained by this budgetary reality. In the absence of data showing an increase in collateral clinical contacts, or in clinical clients assigned to C & E classes, it is impossible to interpret definitively the decline in C & E staff hours. However, it is reasonable to assume both variables are operating: Traditional C & E activities are being reclassified into reimbursable clinical services, and C & E activities are being cut for economic reasons.

What proportion of C & E resources has been committed to prevention? Perlmutter (1976) estimates that half of all C & E activity in CMHCs can legitimately be classified as primary prevention. Focusing only on NIMH grant funds, using Perlmutter's estimate of half of all C & E activity as preventive and the NIMH figure 4.1 as the average percentage of CMHC C & E staff time, NIMH has spent roughly $128,299,900 on CMHC primary prevention activity since the CMHC program began in 1963. Table 11.2 shows the breakdown of C & E receipts from NIMH funding mechanisms by years. Since these grant programs have been in effect for varying

TABLE 11.2   Community Mental Health Center Receipts for
Consultation and Education Services from NIMH Grant
Mechanisms, 1965-1979

NIMH Grant Mechanism	Years Supplied	Total CMHC Dollars Expended	C & E Share (%)	Prevention Share (%)	Prevention Dollars
Staffing grants	1965-1978	$1,236,600,000	4.1	2.05	$25,350,300
Part F grants (for children)	1972-1979	154,800,000	75.0	50.0	77,400,000
C & E grants	1976-1979	28,500,000	100.0	50.0	14,250,000
Operations grants	1976-1978	551,200,000	4.1	2.05	11,299,600
Total Dollars Expended		1,971,100,000			128,299,900

NOTE: Data compiled from NIMH Survey and Reports Branch, 1978; Premo, 1980; Williamson, 1980.

periods, the years over which funding has been supplied range from 1965, when the first staffing grants were awarded, to 1979. C & E and operations grants were first awarded in 1976, and Part F grants in 1972. It should be noted that the data shown under "Total CMHC Dollars Expended" include only funds in which C & E services participated as recipients. Therefore, this figure should not be used as an estimate of total NIMH expenditures for CMHCs over this period—for example, no funds for construction grants are included in this estimate.

In Table 11.2 the prevention share of funding is figured as half of the C & E share (except for Part F grants). Assignment of the C & E share for staffing and operations grants is straightforward, based on the NIMH estimate of C & E staff time. The figure for Part F grants is more of a "guesstimate" based on my experience in the field. Some program recipients classify their programs as involving prevention but not C & E. I have estimated such programs as accounting for 12.5 percent of all Part F programs. Figuring C & E's share of Part F programs at 75 percent, and alloting half of this (37.5 percent) to prevention, the total prevention Part F share is figured at 50 percent. Based on my experience with this program, this 50 percent share for prevention is an underestimate.

In addition to NIMH mainstream funds, CMHC C & E units have aggressively sought and successfully won funds from a variety of other federal, state, and private sources for their centers and their communities: from the Law Enforcement Assistance Administration, the National Institute of Drug Abuse, the National Institute of Alcoholism and Alcohol Abuse, the Department of Labor (Comprehensive Employment Training Act funds) and more. Since income from federal grants, according to NIMH reporting procedures, is not reported as C & E income (it is reported in a separate category of "Other Government Funds"), attempts to document the sources and amounts of C & E income and prevention's share of that are analogous to attempts to photograph the Loch Ness monster. Afficinados suspect there's something out there, and with patience and sensitive equipment we may eventually document it. To date, however, we must content ourselves with speculation on the size of the mass below the surface, based on relatively infrequent sightings.

C & E and prevention services historically have not been expected to generate income. As a result, staff have not been trained to ask for fees and the community has not been prepared to pay them. This approach to C & E services is reflected in the language of the Mental Health Systems Act, which refers to grants for "non-revenue producing activities." Here C & E is lumped with evaluation, case finding, administration, and coordination. Clearly, if primary prevention services are to be delivered in CMHCs, funding mechanisms must be found at the local as well as the federal level.

A key strategy for C & E units in building community resources is to assist other community agencies in locating and applying for available funds, and to include CMHC C & E staff in the application as consultants or trainers. The total funds brought into the community through the efforts of C & E staff are not assessed by any monitoring system and therefore not credited to C & E's fund-raising track record. In sum, C & E's record in generating funds for prevention programs, as reflected in NIMH statistics, is an underestimate of the actual dollars brought into both CMHCs and communities.

ADAMHA Commitment to Prevention: 1979-1980

Within the Department of Health, Education and Welfare, the Alcohol, Drug Abuse and Mental Health Administration budget includes over $59 million for prevention for 1979 and 1980. Table 11.3 breaks these figures

TABLE 11.3 ADAMHA 1979-1980 Institute Prevention Budget Summaries by Major Categories (dollars in thousands)

Institute	Health Promotion		Health Protection		Capacity-Building		Disease Prevention		Totals	
	1979	1980	1979	1980	1979	1980	1979	1980	1979	1980
NIAAA	2422	1940	231	371	0	0	1661	8028	4314	10339
NIDA	2037	2309	600	1100	3740	3768	0	50	6377	7227
NIMH	8701	9668	0	0	1708	8380	0	2315	10409	20363
Totals	$13160	$13917	$831	$1471	$5448	$12148	$1661	$10393	$21100	$37929

SOURCE: ADAMHA Prevention Policy Paper (1979).

TABLE 11.4 NIMH 1979-80 Prevention Budget Summaries by Major Categories (dollars in thousands)

Program Category	Health Promotion		Health Protection		Capacity-Building		Disease Prevention		Totals	
	1979	1980	1979	1980	1979	1980	1979	1980	1979	1980
Research	3322	4557	0	0	0	500	0	2265	3322	7322
Community Programs	5068	4769	0	0	0	6000*	0	0	5068	10769
Program Support	311	342	0	0	0	0	0	0	311	342
Training	0	0	0	0	1708	1880	0	0	1708	1880
Totals	8701	9668	0	0	1708	8380	0	2265	10409	20313

*Dependent on passage of the Mental Health Systems Act.
SOURCE: ADAMHA Prevention Policy Paper (1979).

out by year, by institute, and by program focus—health promotion, health protection, capacity-building, and disease prevention. Table 11.4 shows an analysis of these funds for NIMH by the categories of research, community programs and program support, and training ($50,000 budgeted to a "cross-cutting initiative" in disease prevention has been omitted from Table 4). While these figures establish a benchmark for estimating commitment to prevention at the ADAMHA level of HEW, in fact, most federal preventive activities occur outside HEW. Unfortunately, there is little reliable budget information available on these other federal programs.

> At the Federal level of government alone, a conservative count of agencies with responsibilities or functions related to prevention shows 11 departments, 17 independent agencies, three quasi-official agencies, five permanent or temporary offices within the Executive Office of the President, and four agencies within the Legislative Branch. This count does not include Congressional Committees and Subcommittees with jurisdiction in health or prevention related areas . . . [Activities outside HEW] include food and nutrition programs administered by the Department of Agriculture, occupational health and safety programs administered by the Department of Labor, environmental control programs administered by the Environmental Protection Agency and other agencies, and most consumer product safety programs [Franks, in press].

There is obviously a need for an overall federal prevention policy and coordination of the many federal prevention programs. A review of the budgets for the various institutes shows that NIMH has the highest commitment to prevention for the two years in terms of dollars—almost twice that of either of the others—and that most of the funds are to be spent in health promotion and capacity-building. Out of a two-year commitment of some $30 million to prevention, only $2 million is targeted for disease prevention programs in NIMH. In distributing scarce dollars over the program categories of research, training, and community programs, NIMH has chosen to put minimal funds into training ($3.5 million) and to channel over half of their budget into community programs ($15.8 million). The major NIMH emphasis within communities, as reflected in the budget, is health promotion. These priorities may be appropriate. However, the question is raised as to how program priorities are set. One of the recommendations of the Task Panel on Prevention was that a Citizen's Advisory Committee be established to advise and assist the proposed Center on Prevention. Significantly, no active citizen's group now exists to provide the sort of input and monitoring that would ensure relevance of ADAMHA and/or NIMH prevention programs to community concerns.

Prevention Issues in the Eighties

This brief review of the increasing influence of prevention as an idea in the mental health field, the development of federal prevention policy, and the community mental health commitment to prevention—both in Washington and in the field—signals the readiness of the prevention revolution to declare its independence in the 1980s. A series of challenges must be successfully met before this revolution can become a reality. In addition to the obvious issue of funding, a number of other issues and events critical to the future prevention are emerging in the mental health field. They include:

- a reconceptualization of prevention,
- possible separation of prevention and treatment service delivery,
- decentralization of power from federal to state governments,
- prevention programs aimed at systems change,
- a growing constituency for prevention in community mental health,
- new careers in prevention, and
- an emphasis on evaluation and cost-effectiveness.

Reconceptualization of Prevention

The battle-weary primary-secondary-tertiary prevention terminology developed to serve the field of public health has achieved an awkward fit, at best, in the field of mental health. There are a number of reasons for this: secondary and tertiary prevention are both treatment; the end states targeted for prevention and their causes have not been identified for mental health with the precision characteristic of physical health prevention efforts; and there is a growing consensus to conceptualize health in positive rather than negative terms, and "prevention" is a negative term.

A first-generation refinement split the concept of prevention into health promotion and disease prevention. The ADAMHA Prevention Policy Paper (1979) further expands the concept to include health protection:

ADAMHA's prevention framework . . . makes use of a continuum of health-related behaviors and disorders. Primary prevention is emphasized and three approaches are described: health promotion/education; health protection; and disease prevention [p. 2] . . . .

Health promotion embodies an approach to fostering positive behaviors and general good health practices primarily through public education and information dissemination. Health promotion activities are designed to 1) encourage individual behavior change and 2) improve socioeconomic and physical environments. . . .

Health protection embodies an approach to fostering general health through direct public regulatory and control activities, particularly those related to environmental factors affecting health (e.g., water purification and chlorination). . . .

Disease prevention encompasses services to prevent the occurrence of specific disorders, using strategies derived from analysis of risk factors for such disorders. Although the term "disease prevention" usually refers, in the ADM field, to the prevention of identifiable ADM disorders such as depression or alcohol addiction, it may also refer to preventing certain "high-risk" behaviors such as drug abuse and drinking or their untoward health consequences (e.g., suicide, automobile accidents, or cirrhosis) [ADAMHA Prevention Policy Paper, 1979: 4-6].

Official ADAMHA prevention policy is to develop new knowledge rather than fund ongoing service programs. Within that effort to develop new knowledge, emphasis is placed on risk factor research, evaluation, joint projects among the institutes in ADAMHA, and cooperation with other agencies.

Since programs follow funding, the ADAMHA definitions and intervention mechanisms will shape the next few years of prevention activity in the field of community mental health. Social science departments and medical schools of universities, community mental health centers, and hospitals are the most likely recipients of ADAMHA prevention funding.

Possible Separation of
Prevention and Treatment Service Delivery

With the growing constituency for prevention from the various quarters of health and mental health, the issue of where prevention will be housed becomes increasingly pressing. The field of physical health clearly separates prevention and treatment. The public health clinic functions as the prevention arm of the medical care system, providing immunizations, well baby clinics, prenatal care, and programs designed to screen normal populations for a variety of health risks. Hospitals and the private practice model of health care serve the treatment function of physical health.

While the community mental health center would appear to be the logical site for the delivery of preventive mental health services, the predominance of the treatment model in this system threatens to block the effective development of prevention programs in centers (Snow & Newton, 1976). The current divisive scramble for dollars among the 12 mandated services will strengthen already strong treatment programs at the expense of prevention programs in C & E units (Comptroller General, 1979; Weiner, et al., 1979). The research funding projected by ADAMHA for prevention will increase prevention research programs in universities and hospitals, but will do little to augment prevention services in centers.

The forthcoming community mental health legislation will play the pivotal role in determining the future of prevention programs within centers and communities. The Carter administration's Mental Health Systems Act, developed within the context of the Report of the President's Commission on Mental Health (1978), has a number of features that will significantly affect mental health prevention programs, if passed in their original form. These features are discussed below.

Title II of the Act, the Prevention Title, would give state mental health authorities the power to determine prevention funding and programming. The implications of Title II are discussed in the next section.

The "single service entity" is a provision of the act that would fund a public or nonprofit private "entity" to provide only one of the comprehensive mental health services (Title IV, Section 402). Conceivably, such an "entity" could be set up to implement prevention programs through the provision of C & E services. One of the implications of this section is the possibility of separating the delivery of preventive from clinical services, paralleling the separation of prevention and treatment services in the field of physical health.

A feature of the act intended to reinforce the continued coexistence of the two services under one roof is the provision for grants for non-revenue-producing activities. Under this section (Title IV, Section 405) grants would be provided for community mental health services that do not generate funds to cover their programs. Since the total funds available for such grants for a catchment area are minimal ($1 per capita), however, and since there is no requirement for minimum funding of any of the so-called non-revenue-producing activities, C & E and prevention programs could be ignored, with available funds going to case management or evaluation. While this section was originally intended to support C & E and prevention programs within community mental health centers, in its watered-down final version it provides little guarantee that such programs will receive any funding at all. For this reason the National Council of Community Mental Health Centers has protested the inclusion of community mental health center prevention funding in this section, and has supported the eligibility of centers for prevention funding under the major prevention title of the act (Title IV).

Decentralization of Power
from Federal to State Governments

Commensurate with the commissions's efforts to develop a partnership between states and the federal government in the delivery of mental health services, Title II of the Act assigns to state mental health authorities the responsibility for planning and implementing prevention programs. Under this title, prevention funds for research, training, and demonstration programs would go to the states, which would have the option of contracting to other agencies—such as universities, hospitals, or community mental health centers—for prevention functions. Given the record of most state mental health authorities for committing the majority of their mental health resources to maintaining state institutions, putting the states in charge of prevention funding smacks of putting the fox in charge of the chicken coop.

John Wolfe, Executive Director of the National Council of Community Mental Health Centers (NCCMHC), gave the following testimony before Congress on the act:

> The new role of the states as projected in the Mental Health Systems Act needs careful review and revision. NCCMHC supports an increased participation of the states in the planning and delivery of community mental health services. There should be an equal Federal-State-local partnership which has not existed in the past. As proposed, however, the Systems Act will grant the states an undue amount of authority over community mental health centers. Since most states still struggle with the problems of deinstitutionalization, it is unwise to give them unlimited and unregulated authority over community mental health centers, especially in regard to federal funding and evaluation. . . .

> Naturally, the interest of the states is with their own institutions. State funding for state institutions has not corresponded to the decrease in patients entering state hospitals. Since there are only very limited amounts of Federal funds available for mental health

services, it does not make good management sense to have them pass through another level of bureaucracy before they reach the people for whom the money is intended. Nowhere will this be more tragic than in the area of prevention, where the states lack the requisite expertise and commitment [Wolfe, 1979].

The three major mental health constituency groups—the Mental Health Association, the National Council of Community Mental Health Centers (NCCMHC) and the National Association of State Mental Health Program Directors—have agreed on prevention language for the act, according to which funds would be allotted to both states and public and nonprofit private agencies including community mental health centers. Prevention programs under this proposed revision would include

> planning, training, and coordination; identifying populations at-risk of mental disabilities, providing educational support or related services for specified populations designed to lower incidence of mental disability or promote mental health. Such programs shall be responsive to national prevention priorities and shall contribute through evaluation and reporting to the improvement methods [Mental Health Association, 1979].

The legislation is still pending at this writing. However, the entry of state mental health authorities into the administration and review of mental health prevention programs is a likely future development. When that happens the funding of these programs will be subject to the pressures of state and local politics.

Prevention Programs Aimed at Systems Change[1]

Almost all clinical mental health interventions are directed toward changing the person, not the environment. Environmental change is effected primarily through C & E units implementing prevention programs in CMHCs. While the concept of adjustment includes the notion of person-environment fit, the paradigmatic approach in the history of community mental health has been to fit the person to the environment. If the combination turns out to be a mismatch, the implicit assumption is that the person is at fault; with appropriate counseling or greater effort the match could be made to work. In fact, environmental measures account for more variance in behavior than measures of personality, biographic, or demographic variables together.

There is increasing recognition that the prevention professional must go beyond interventions focused on strengthening the host to those involving systems change. Major prevention policymakers—such as the Task Panel on Prevention of the President's Commission on Mental Health, The Surgeon General, ADAMHA—and other professional groups—such as the American Psychological Association (Task Force for the Delivery of Psychological Services)—agree on the importance of developing strategies to reduce or eliminate noxious environmental stressors. Difficult ethical and political issues will inevitably accompany efforts to change the environment, whether these efforts be focused on chlorination of water, noise pollution, racism, or sexism. Despite the difficulties, systems change is one of the major prevention waves of the 1980s. Through the application of current knowledge about such stressors as noise, crowding, economic fluctuations, cultural and linguistic alienation, and social isolation, the community mental health professional can be instrumental in preventing negative outcomes and promoting healthy environments for persons who will otherwise remain outside the community mental health system.

A Growing Constituency for
Prevention in Community Mental Health

There is an increasing recognition of primary prevention as the mission of the community mental health movement. This is evidenced in the emerging constituency for primary prevention that can be traced full circle from consumers through the professional community, regulatory agencies, legislators, and political leaders and back to the consumers who elect them.

The first grass-roots constituency—consumers—is becoming increasingly vocal in its endorsement of prevention concepts. CMHC consumer boards across the country, charged with formulating mission statements for their centers, are identifying prevention as the mission or one of the major goals of center services. Health planning agencies, functioning through inter-locking consumer committees, task forces, and boards, are increasingly promoting health education as a prevention approach to resolving health problems at the community level. The Mental Health Association has a long record of support for the concept of primary prevention. The current President, Beverly Long, was an articulate advocate for prevention on the President's Commission on Mental Health.

One of the barriers to implementation of prevention goals has been the lack of an identified discipline claiming "ownership" of prevention.

Support has been scattered throughout a range of health professional and academic disciplines, with parallel organizational efforts taking place over the last decade.

Professionals from a second level of support form a prevention constituency. The National Association of Prevention Professionals (NAPP), founded by a core of persons from the field of substance abuse, is an organization that now includes a broad range of prevention advocates. Through the clout of its membership, NAPP provided the impetus and subscriber base to initiate the *Journal on Prevention,* due to begin publication in 1980. The journal's editorial board and projected subject areas reflect community mental health concerns.

The National Council of Community Mental Health Centers includes, as part of its administrative structure, a Council on Prevention comprised of six representatives from member centers across the country. The council is charged with examining critical issues, establishing task forces, developing position papers, and recommending policy designed to promote and enhance prevention and C & E activities in CMHCs. Concerned with the "second-class citizen" image of C & E often projected by the clinical camp, the council recommended to NIMH that the term "indirect" be discontinued in reference to C & E services. CMHC primary prevention programs are implemented through C & E services. Such services have conventionally been referred to as "indirect" compared with clinical services, which have conventionally been referred to as "direct." Since primary prevention as an intervention strategy occurs prior to the development of pathology and prior to the involvement of treatment professionals, the council views it as a reversal of the order of events to refer to such primary interventions as "indirect." NIMH administration has complied with the request and dropped the term "indirect" from the recent revision of draft guidelines for C & E services. The council has established task forces to develop environmental assessment methodologies as well as comprehensive guidelines for C & E services. In a recent review and comment on the revision of NIMH draft guidelines for C & E, the council recommended language clarifying the goals of C & E as preventive. Current activities include advocating for prevention programs and funding for community mental health centers in the Mental Health Systems Act, sponsoring national conferences on C & E and assisting C & E professionals in forming a national organization, and promoting cooperative relationships between CMHCs and self-help groups as a prevention strategy. The Council on Prevention and NAPP established formal liaison in 1979, and agreed to promote mutual prevention concerns on a variety of fronts.

A unique approach to educating CMHC leaders to prevention concepts was incorporated in a series of primary prevention conferences held throughout the country in 1978 and 1979. Co-sponsored by NCCMHC and NIMH, the conferences recruited as participants three-person CMHC teams made up of a center board member, the executive director, and the C & E director. Each of these three roles is critical in implementing prevention programs in CMHCs: board approval and support is necessary for the allocation of funds to prevention; the director's cooperation is crucial in administering resources to prevention programs; and the C & E director's expertise in and commitment to prevention determine the success of CMHC prevention programs. In addition to the innovation of participant teams, this series of conferences brought together prevention advocates from academia and CMHCs as faculty.

The American Psychological Association Task Force on Alternative Models for the Delivery of Psychological Services (1979), established in 1978, identified "a significant effort in primary prevention" as one of eight criteria used in evaluating alternative models. In assessing the role of CMHCs in delivering psychological services, the task force report cites the CMHC mandate to serve entire catchment areas as a strategy for reaching large populations with cost-effective psychological services. CMHCs are cited as serving a significant prevention function "by working to develop effective natural support systems, self-help groups, and through consultation with agencies, settings and community care-givers," as well as by intervening in natural or man-made disasters (1979: 15).

Regulatory agencies, in implementing their task of formulating guidelines and setting standards for the delivery of mental health services, have responded to pressure from consumer and professional groups by adopting prevention philosophy and goals. In revising the draft guidelines for C & E services in 1979, NIMH has elevated prevention to the status of the primary goal, with consultation and education as means to accomplish the goal. The NCCMHC Council on Prevention advocated for this emphasis in working with the NIMH Community Mental Health Services Branch to revise the draft guidelines.

In 1978 the NIMH Staff College pioneered the first comprehensive training program dealing with management issues in CMHC C & E services. Since then the week-long workshop has been conducted seven times across the country, training almost 250 C & E directors. The relationship between C & E and prevention is one of the major topics of the course.

The Staff College plans to add an advanced course on C & E in 1980 in response to requests from the field.

The legislative activity that serves as an end result of the constituency-building process and also as a catalyst for future development of prevention programs has been discussed earlier. Following the growth of prevention concepts through the political circuitry of groups representing consumers, professionals, regulatory agencies, and legislative/political bodies is an exercise in tracing political power. The growing prevention constituency at each of these levels reinforces the chant of prevention optimists: It's an idea whose time has come.

New Careers in Prevention

A necessary first step in planning prevention programs is an epidemiological analysis of mental health problems in the community. While CMHC evaluation units can provide some relevant needs assessment data, the continuous tracking of local and national incidence and prevalence trends for targeted dysfunctions (teenage pregnancy and alcoholism) requires a new position within CMHCs. The function of such a position is similar to what Parcell (in press) calls a "health engineer."

> Health engineers could examine workplace settings for general factors affecting the long-range health and well being of workers, as opposed to more immediate dangers leading to on-the-job accidents. They would assess employees' individual health problems involving overweight, smoking, substance abuse and misuse, and similar health factors. Such health assessments could draw on both a systematic analysis of health information about individuals participating in the program and on the application of epidemiological studies of health problems involving variables such as age, sex, ethnicity, socioeconomic status, and geographical location. Through needs assessments of this kind health engineers could help to develop prevention programs tailored to the needs of specific employed groups and promoted through methods appropriate to each group.

> Health engineers would have expertise in one or more of several different disciplines such as physical education, nutrition, health education, counseling, and stress management [in press: 145-146].

CMHC prevention units increasingly will include media specialists, epidemiologists, and educators whose disciplines do not fall into the traditional categories of psychiatry, psychology, and social work. They will require interdisciplinary training and cross-department, cross-agency teaming to deliver a broad range of prevention services to their communities. The increased ADAMHA budget promises programs. It does not promise people to staff them. A critical question for the eighties, then, is how to develop the person-power to deliver prevention programs.

Emphasis on Evaluation
and Cost Effectiveness

The level of evaluation of community mental health center services in general is primitive, and evaluation of C & E and prevention programs lags behind even this elementary norm. The difficulties in evaluating these services adequately are rooted in:

— lack of consensus about service categories;

— lack of evaluation expertise in C & E and prevention staff;

— the priority placed on clinical services, with the resulting pressure to assign scarce CMHC evaluation resources to clinical rather than C & E services;

— lack of widely accepted models for evaluation of C & E and prevention programs;

— lack of adequate management information systems for C & E and prevention services;

— the longitudinal thrust of many C & E and prevention programs (changes in staff and lack of funding make it difficult to monitor and evaluate programs over a number of years); and

— the myriad design and statistical problems resulting from implementing programs in a field setting rather than in a laboratory; events—political, economic, environmental—intervene unexpectedly, disrupting data collection and analysis.

The Task Panel on Prevention of the President's Commission on Mental Health cites a large body of research documenting the effectiveness of prevention programs. Most of this research has been conducted in university or hospital settings. The classic research methodologies used—for example, pre- and posttests and control groups—while appropriate for application to CMHC programs, are rarely used. Minimal evaluation standards for programs need to go beyond the current process measures and client satisfaction scales that constitute the bulk of evaluation in CMHCs today.

Ciarlo (1977; Ciarlo and Davis, 1977) and his associates have taken a bold approach to evaluating community mental health services. Their model projects a way to measure the impact of services on the community, on targeted populations, and on the individual client. The long-range goal of community mental health services is to promote mental health and prevent mental illness in the community To meet this goal, and to know it has been met, some estimate of the mental health of the community is needed to provide a norm against which comparisons can be made. After mental health services have been available in the community for a period of years, does the mental health of the community improve? Does the mental health of high-risk groups vary systematically from community norms? While Ciarlo and his associates have not used their model to address these questions, they have attempted the ambitious task of sampling the mental health of the Denver community through the use of the Denver Community Mental Health Questionnaire. A random sample of residents was assessed on eight mental health scales—alcohol abuse, drug abuse, antisocial behavior, somatic complaints, disorganized behavior/ thinking, emotional distress, maladaptive behavior, and personal and social handicap. The resulting scores were then standardized to arrive at community norms for each of the mental health scales.

Applications of this methodology to the clinical client are obvious. Consumers of clinical services are assessed on these scales at intake, at various intervals during treatment, and at termination to determine their deficits (if any) from community norms. The goal set for treatment is to raise the client to within one standard deviation of the Denver population norm on the relevant scales of functioning. When standard clinical treatment of target populations does not result in improvement—this appears to be the case, for example, with drug-abusing clients—changes in treatment are suggested. If there is still no improvement and treatment options have been exhausted, it is suggested that the least costly humane treatment be used.

The method also has value for assessing preventive interventions. The success of intervention with high-risk-(or other target) populations could be tracked by periodic comparisons of their mental health with that of the larger community. This measure would supplement other, more standard measures, such as the number of persons subsequently seeking clinical treatment.

This approach to evaluation of community mental health services projects a model for comparing the relative effectiveness and efficiency of clinical versus preventive services. By offering preventive services to one section of the catchment area and clinical services to another, demographically comparable area, costs of services as well as the level of mental health of the residents of the two areas could be tracked over time and conclusions drawn about the relative effectiveness of the two service models in meeting community mental health goals.

Built into this model is a plan to periodically retest the Denver community to note any shifts in the mental health scales in the general population. Thus, a set of measures of the mental health of the community over time is generated. Interpreting shifts in the general community's mental health is tricky, at best, since uncontrolled community events may be responsible for any shifts observed. A Three Mile Island or a Son of Sam could jar the norms independent of ongoing community mental health programs. In spite of the difficulties in control and interpretation, this program is a refreshing attempt to use evaluation to further the community mental health mission.

Are prevention programs cost effective? This is a survival issue. The era of the unlimited federal dollar has been replaced by the era of Proposition 13. Local, state, and federal legislators are accountable to taxpayers for their support of health programs, and in the face of inflation and reduced sources of funding, hard choices are being made among human service programs: those that can deliver the most effective service at the least cost will survive those whose effectiveness cannot be demonstrated. The NIMH Draft Guidelines for Program Evaluation (for P.L. 94-63) specify that in each CMHC's annual program evaluation the impact of C & E services in attaining center and program goals be addressed in

- explicit statements of the intended consequences of C & E services,
- attempts to measure such consequences,
- estimates of the cost of C & E services, and
- an assessment of the relative efficiency of "direct and indirect" services in achieving center goals.

Clearly, what is needed is an overall evaluation methodology for C & E and prevention services.

Wisconsin's Department of Health and Social Services (1978) has developed a series of comparative cost figures for prevention versus treatment of mental retardation, mental illness, and alcoholism. According to this report, if the cost for maintaining one mentally retarded person for one year in a Wisconsin state facility ($24,000) were invested in prevention programs instead, a long-range savings of over $2 million could be realized if only two cases of mental retardation were prevented.[2] The report projects that an initial investment of $5,000 to prevent mental illness through mutual support groups and school programs would result in a long-range savings of $50,000 if only one case of recurring mental illness were prevented.[3]

The sort of detailed comparative analysis projected by the Wisconsin report needs to be executed throughout the prevention community. The ADAMHA emphasis on evaluation and the restriction of prevention funds to research projects only (as in the Office on Prevention) signals the prevention community that the name of the game in the eighties is accountability.

Conclusions

This chapter has provided an overview of the growing influence of primary prevention in the mental health field, the development of federal prevention policy, and the interaction of community mental health policy and practice in translating prevention concepts into programs. The revolution is not yet. The question of whether the prevention revolution is destined to remain a guerrila action, engaging the mainstream in periodic skirmishes, or whether it will swell through popular support to rival or eclipse the treatment approach to health, is left to be decided in a future annual review.

Notes

1. Portions of this section first appeared in the *Community Mental Health Journal* in an article by the author entitled, "The NCCMHC Task Force on Environmental Assessment" (Volume 16, 1980).

2. An investment of $24,000 in prevention of developmental disabilities could buy the following services: (1) a lead poisoning screening program (including outreach personnel) for 414 children at a cost of $58 per child (the cost includes two blood tests per child, medical treatment, and environmental check for all positive tests found—positives run from 7 percent to 22 percent of all children screened); and

(2) a genetic consult, ultrasonic scanning, and amniocentesis and chromosome analysis for 80 "at risk" pregnant women at $300 per woman.

These programs/services would affect many people. If they prevent only two cases of mental retardation which require institutionalization, in one year a savings of $24,000 in treatment costs would be realized; in two years, a savings of $48,000; and in the long range (50-55 years) a savings of over $2 million would occur (Wisconsin's Department of Health and Social Services, 1978: 11).

3. This estimate calculates that case at ten episodes involving 28 days of hospitalization, nine outpatient visits, and supportive living services for a total cost of $5,000 per episode. This $5,000 investment in prevention would buy: (1) 48 paraprofessionals to each lead one 8 week/2 hours per week mutual support group for 10 people in crisis at a cost of $6.50 per hour (this figure does not include training, coordination, or materials); and (2) two paraprofessional child-aides for 15 hours per week at $3.00 per hour for one year. Each aide sees 8-10 normal school children with "school adaption problems" twice weekly. (This figure does not include training and consultation; Wisconsin's Department of Health and Social Services, 1978: 12).

References

ADAMHA Prevention Policy Paper. Office of the Administrator, Office of Program Planning and Coordination/Division of Prevention, ADAMHA, 1979.

Albee, G. Preventing prevention in the community mental health centers. In H. Resnik, C. Ashton and C. Palley (Eds.), *The Health Care System and Drug Abuse Prevention: Toward Cooperation and Health Promotion.* Pyramid, a Project of the Prevention Branch, Division of Resource Development. Washington, DC: National Institute of Drug Abuse, in press.

American Psychological Association Task Force on Alternative Models for the Delivery of Psychological Services. Final report and recommendations, October, 1979.

Bloom, B.L. Strategies for the prevention of mental disorders. In G. Rosenblum (Ed.), *Issues in Community Psychology and Preventive Mental Health.* New York: Behavioral Publications, 1971.

Ciarlo, J. Monitoring and analysis of program outcome data. In I. Davidoff, M. Guttentag, and J. Offutt (Eds.), *Evaluating Community Mental Health Services, Principles and Practice,* DHEW (ADM) Publication No. 77-465. Washington, DC: National Institute of Mental Health, 1977.

Ciarlo, J., and Davis, C. Outcomes for adult clients. In I. Davidoff, M. Guttentag, and J. Offutt (Eds.), *Evaluating Community Mental Health Services, Principles and Practice,* DHEW (ADM) Publication No. 77-465. Washington, DC: U.S. Government Printing Office, 1977.

Comptroller General. Legislative and administrative changes needed in community mental health centers program. *Comptroller General's Report to the Subcommittee on Oversight and Investigations, House Committee on Interstate and Foreign Commerce.* Washington, DC: U.S. Government Printing Office, 1979.

Fielding, J.E. Health promotion: Some notions in search of a constituency. *American Journal of Public Health,* 1977, *67,* 1082.

Franks, P. Health policy and health planning: A framework for federal, state and local prevention initiatives in the 1980s. In H. Resnik, Carolyne A., and C. Palley (Eds.), *The Health Care System and Drug Abuse Prevention: Toward Cooperation and Health Promotion.* Pyramid, a Project of the Prevention Branch, Division of Resource Development. Washington, DC: National Institute of Drug Abuse, in press.

Goldston, S.E. An overview of primary prevention programming. In D. Klein and S. Goldston (Eds.), *Primary Prevention: An Idea Whose Time Has Come.* DHEW (PHS) Publication No. 77-447. Washington, DC: U.S. Government Printing Office, 1977.

Institute of Medicine. Perspectives on health promotion and disease prevention in the United States: A staff paper. National Academy of Sciences, Washington, DC: January, 1978.

Joint Commission on Accreditation of Hospitals. *Principles for Accreditation of Community Mental Health Service Programs,* Chicago, Illinois, 1979.

Klerman, G.L. Prevention policies for alcohol, drug abuse and mental health (1). Presented at the ADAMHA Prevention Conference, Silver Spring, Maryland, September 12, 1979.

Mental Health Association. "Consensus Language" proposed as amendment to the "Mental Health Systems Act." National Council of Community Mental Health Centers, National Association of State Mental Health Program Directors, November 28, 1979.

NIMH Survey and Reports Branch. Provisional data on federally funded community mental health centers, 1976-1977. Washington, DC: Division of Biometry and Epidemiology, National Institute of Mental Health, May, 1978.

Parcell, C. New insurance industry approaches. In H. Resnik, C. Ashton, and C. Palley (Eds.), *The Health Care System and Drug Abuse Prevention: Toward Cooperation and Health Promotion.* Pyramid, a Project of the Prevention Branch, Division of Resource Development. Washington, DC: National Institute of Drug Abuse, in press.

Perlmutter, F. An instrument for differentiating programs in prevention—primary, secondary and tertiary. *American Journal of Orthopsychiatry,* 1976, *46,* 533-541.

Premo, F. Chief Operations Liaison, Program Analysis Section, Community Mental Health Services Support Branch, NIMH. Personal communication. December 19, 1979.

Report of the President's Commission on Mental Health. Volume I. Washington, DC: U.S. Government Printing Office, 1978.

Preventive Medicine, U.S.A. A task force report sponsored by the John E. Fogarty International Center for Advanced Study in the Health Sciences, National Institutes of Health and the American College of Preventive Medicine. New York: Prodist, 1976.

Snow, D.L., & Newton, P.M. Task, social structure, and social process in the community mental health center movement. *American Psychologist,* 1976, *31,* 582-594.

Surgeon General's Report on Health Promotion and Disease Prevention. *Healthy People.* DHEW (PHS) Publication No.. 79-55071. Washington, DC: U.S. Government Printing Office, 1979.

U.S. Department of Health, Education and Welfare. *Essential Services of the Community Mental Health Center: Consultation and Education.* DHEW Publication No. 1478. Washington, DC: U.S. Government Printing Office, 1966.

Weiner, J., Woy, R., Sharfstein, S., & Bass, R. Community mental health centers and the "seed money" concept: Effects of terminating federal funds. *Community Mental Health Journal,* 1979, *15,* 129-138.

Williamson, R. Program Analysis Section, Community Mental Health Services Support Branch, National Institute of Mental Health. Personal communication. January 15, 1980.

Wisconsin's Department of Health and Social Services. *A Community Guidebook, Planning for Prevention Programs.* Division of Community Services, 1978.

Wolfe, J. Testimony before the Senate Subcommittee on Health and Scientific Research. Washington, DC: National Council of Community Mental Health Centers, May 24, 1979.

12

Prevention Activities at the State Level

Betty Tableman
Michigan Department of Mental Health

This is a report on how one state negotiated the Okefenokee Swamp (Kessler & Albee, 1975). Michigan's foray into the prevention thicket started in 1975. In that year, two other states (Massachusetts and Ohio) assigned staff to the relatively uncharted area of prevention programming. Today, seven states are in the process of operationalizing prevention programs (California, Georgia, Michigan, North Carolina, Ohio, Rhode Island, and South Carolina), and a number of others are exploring possibilities. It may be useful to summarize the Michigan experience.

Background

Michigan's program has evolved within a context of internal sanction and outside support. Impetus from the inside came from a new mental health code which specified prevention as one of the services to be undertaken by community mental health boards. The director of the Department of Mental Health, who had a background in public health, assigned me to survey the field of prevention and to make recommendations (Tableman, 1975). After a six-month literature search, several psychosocial prevention strategies were identified and recommendations for establishing a prevention unit were made. Shortly afterward, I was appointed as the director of the state's first prevention office.

Support from within the department was matched by support from the outside. For example, the Mental Health Association in Michigan, a respected advocate for mental health, along with a number of mental health professionals provided encouragement and support during the early stages of the state prevention program.

Another group that has played a key role in developing the prevention program is our Advisory Committee. The Advisory Committee is a small but knowledgeable group composed of the following: community mental health directors from each of the department's administrative regions, representatives from the Department's Citizen Council and other relevant organizations (the board association, the directors associations, the organization of mental health professionals, the mental health association), at-large representatives from several universities, and staff from the state Education and Substance Abuse agencies.

The Advisory Committee serves as a support system to our prevention staff, advises on policy issues, and brings matters of concern to the attention of the department's director. To avoid conflict of interest, the Advisory Committee does not serve as a grants review committee, although it has functioned as a hearing board and has advised me regarding termination and redirection of funded projects.

Functions and Goals

Since it was established in 1975, I have administered the State Prevention Program with assistance from an experienced professional and a full-time secretary. At the outset, we were assigned responsibility for supervising a Genetics Screening Laboratory which is part of the Michigan Department of Mental Health. The laboratory, under the direction of a geneticist, screens developmentally disabled youngsters for chromosomal and metabolic defects. Although the Genetics Laboratory has been significant, our primary function has been to develop demonstration projects (see Figure 12.1). During the last four years the budget for pilot prevention projects has steadily increased from $400,000 in 1976-1979 to $900,000 in 1979-1980.

In addition to developing prevention projects, the state prevention program was recently given responsibility for monitoring consultation and education (C & E) services. A required service in all federally funded community mental health centers, C & E services include a range of "indirect services" not defined as prevention within our current conceptual framework.

Because our conception of prevention serves as a guide for our pilot projects, it is important to articulate our perspective on the subject. First, we have tried to draw a sharp distinction between primary prevention and treatment and rehabilitation. We reason, for example, that if the objective for prevention is to reduce the incidence of emotional, cognitive, and

FIGURE 12.1   Functions Assigned to Prevention Staff

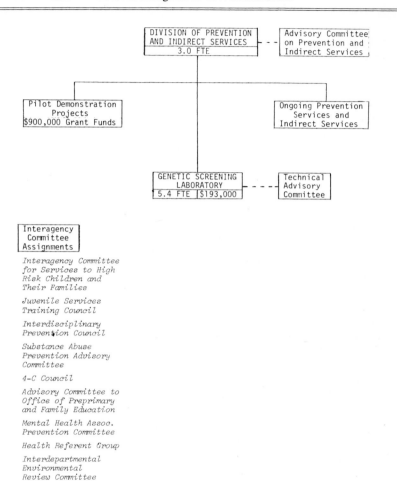

behavioral disorder, then case-finding—which is designed to bring people into treatment as clients—is not an appropriate function for prevention services. Similarly, crisis intervention, despite its historical links to prevention, is essentially a response to clinical emergencies and thus is part of treatment services. Avoiding reinstitutionalization, sometimes referred to as tertiary prevention, is a rehabilitation, not a prevention function.

From our perspective, prevention programming is based on the premise that adaptive and maladaptive behaviors are learned. The outcome for any individual is perceived as the consequence of the interaction between the constitutional vulnerability of that individual and the social and physical environmental accommodation to that vulnerability. Individuals negotiate transitions and crises in terms of their coping capabilities and the social supports available to them. Our programming is essentially attempting to maximize coping capabilities and support systems in high-risk populations (see Figure 12.2). We look for populations defined in terms of a common demographic or experiential variable which has been shown to be correlated with high rates of deviant behavior. This approach assumes a body of information derived from clinical and epidemiological studies.

Populations at risk are essentially children or adults in situations which have the potential for generating stress and deficits in physical and/or emotional resources over an extended period of time. The population at risk, therefore, is not a population subjected to a single critical event, but a population which is likely to be experiencing continuing stress and deprivation (Birch, 1974).

The child whose parents are divorcing, the child with a psychotic parent, the premature infant, the widow deprived of a primary support system, the unemployed wage earner confronted with role loss and income loss—all are confronting events which are not self-contained but can have continuing impact.

The crucial issue in prevention programming is not methodology, however important that may be, but the definition and recruitment of high-risk populations. How one defines and accesses the population to be served will in effect determine whether efforts are targeted or diffuse, whether those reached are actually at risk or merely willing participants. Generally, too little attention is paid to identifying the relevant characteristics of the population at risk and to implementing a systematic recruitment process. Wherever possible, we have attempted to access high risk populations by *systematically connecting with an ongoing service stream*—the maternity unit for newborns in at-risk situations, the circuit court for children of divorce, the mental health case management function for children of disordered adults. Our objective, once we get beyond the pilot demonstration phase, is to situate the prevention service so that it becomes an integral part of an ongoing service process.

In summary, I believe that progress in developing prevention programming is contingent on identifying clearly articulated and generally accepted content. We need to get beyond the stage where prevention is defined

FIGURE 12.2   Variables Affecting Adaptive/Maladaptive Behavior and
Prevention Domains

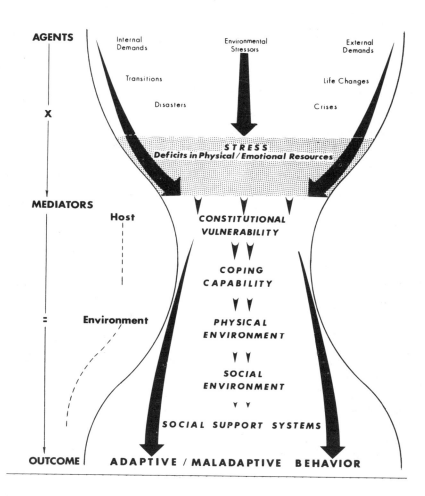

by a laundry list, where each practitioner can infuse into the umbrella
term "prevention" his or her idiosyncratic meaning, where advocates can
talk past each other because each is concerned with a different facet of the
problem.

In the Michigan program I am beginning to conceptualize prevention
programming as concerned with (1) biomedical approaches, (2) children at

risk, (3) adults at risk, and (4) problem-solving and general capability approaches. Whether this is the most useful categorization or whether a more finite categorization is needed (for example, school-based programming, infant programming) I do not know; I do know that legislatures and administrators can relate better to the specificity of "infant programming" than to the generality of "prevention."

Pilot Demonstration Projects

Pilot demonstration projects are being seen in Michigan as the route to implementing the statutory expectation that all community mental health boards will undertake prevention services. (While one-fifth of all boards in Michigan have prevention services developed prior to 1975, it is expected that many of the preexisting services will be redirected as models emerge from the projects). The process as outlined in Figure 12.3 assumes the development and evaluation of a pilot project, the development and evaluation of a replication project, and eventually a decision to encourage dissemination statewide as a base service or as a local option. Integral to the whole process is a clear understanding of how the project works and documentation through a replication manual and sometimes videotape. Although we are in our fourth year of funding, we are just entering the replication phase of the cycle for some projects. The sequence of service development and evaluation is a longer one than we had anticipated.

At the beginning of Michigan's program, we made a conscious decision to spread funds as widely as possible in community-based projects. Since our mission was perceived as translation of existing knowledge into community settings, we did not seek university-based research proposals. With one exception, our service projects have been contracts with community mental health boards. This decision enabled us to diversify our efforts so that we are currently trying out some seven different types of programming. It has spread involvement in prevention programming to more than one-third of Michigan's boards. It has given us a real sense of what is required to operationalize our conceptualizations.

We have learned a great deal about the mechanics of pilot demonstrations: (1) A high level of staff capability and sophistication is required to undertake pilot demonstrations. (2) Service-oriented staff are not invested in the collection of evaluation data. (3) Projects require a start-up phase before an evaluation design is implemented. (4) There is a high and seemingly inevitable attrition from control groups. (5) In pilot demonstrations we are not only exploring service methodologies, we are also exploring service delivery issues and outcome evaluation issues.

FIGURE 12.3   Process for Development of Prevention Service Models

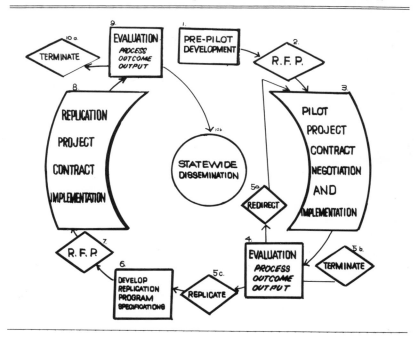

Our work is based primarily on continuing literature searches which point toward characteristics of risk populations and useful methodologies. I find research studies and specialized materials on infancy, adolescence, competence-building, high-risk studies, and aging more useful than general materials on prevention. One of the unrecognized aspects of prevention programming is the wide range of subject areas with which a small staff must become conversant.

While we are open to suggestions from the field, we operate primarily through written specifications outlining the general characteristics of the model we want to develop. We talk at length with applicants about what they propose to do and select that agency which seems to have a competent administrative setting and the firmest sense of what we are trying to accomplish. A period of intensive negotiation develops the contractual agreement.

To date we have initiated 20 service projects: 15 are still continuing. In three instances, we have underwritten projects with the objective of gaining the cooperation of other departments: a school-based infant stimulation project, a psychiatric nurse in a high-risk pregnancy clinic (our grant was to the Department of Public Health), and a mental health-substance abuse project to implement affective education in elementary schools. In these situations we are anticipating a time-limited involvement of the Department of Mental Health.

Descriptions of Specific Projects

Stress Management Training

This project was developed by a coordinator in a rural county who was funded initially to undertake a needs assessment, to be followed by service development. Interested in stress management, she worked with a staff member from the Cooperative Extension Service to formulate a training package, drawing on available materials on stress and life planning, relaxation, and communication skills. With departmental consultation, the effort was directed toward women receiving aid for their dependent children.

Designed as a prevention initiative, the intervention package can also be used with client populations, and, we believe, with that group of distressed women, nonpsychotic and not in crisis, who come to mental health agencies. Recruitment of the trainee is undertaken by social services caseworkers and is followed by personal contact from the prevention coordinator. Transportation to the ten weekly sessions is arranged and paid for by Social Services, and a carpool enhances the opportunity for participants to discuss the sessions and to establish social connections. The sessions are a combination of explicit teaching using visual aids and personal examples and group therapy. Two women from Mental Health and the Cooperative Extension Service share the leadership role. The experience has an electric effect on the participants, who are isolated and stressed women. Better communication with family members, a sense of control over their lives, establishment of friendships, participation in community activities, and movement off AFDC seem to be the consequences of this group experience. Pretests and posttests six months after the completion of training showed significant changes in several measures designed to assess anxiety, stress, and depression.

This project is being replicated in a large urban setting as a collaborative effort with the State Department of Social Services.

Children of Disordered Adults

This project developed out of the literature indicating that 50 percent of the children of severely disordered adults were likely themselves to exhibit some degree of deviancy (Anthony, 1974). The department's client data sheet was revised to include the number and ages of children of clients. Recruitment is undertaken through a systematic review by mental health center case managers and therapists of children attached to adult clients receiving inpatient, aftercare, and outpatient services. Service is initiated on an outreach basis through home visits. Interventions have included interpretation of the parent's behavior to the child, and interpretation of the child's needs to the parent; an effort to provide exposure to a stable adult for the child; advocacy with the schools; and recreational experiences and other opportunities for group and individual counseling. Unanticipated were the use of parent training and remedial reading.

An interesting side benefit of these projects has been the information provided to the adult's therapist as a result of the home visit. We are currently trying to understand the component parts of the intervention, to determine how problem-solving training can be incorporated into the intervention, to establish the linkage between these projects and infant mental health services (since approximately one-third of the children attached to adult clients will be infants and toddlers), and to pilot a rural model which combines various categories of prevention services for children.

Services to Children of Divorcing Parents

Just getting underway, this project seeks to enroll parents and their children at the time of filing for divorce through a collaborative arrangement with the circuit court which will send letters to parents and lawyers and provide names to the project. Families will be assigned randomly to three interventions: a pamphlet describing the impact of divorce on children and providing information about resources; a single educational presentation providing the same information and a ten-week parent's group, children's group, and adolescent group. Because 34 percent of the children in families filing for divorce are age five or less, an infant specialist will be added to this project. The first setback to this project came when it was discovered that only 10 percent of parents were living at the addresses provided by the circuit court. Each new project has its own set of surprises and lessons to be learned.

Infant Mental Health Services

The Michigan program has had a heavy investment in infant services concerned with the interaction between caregiver and infant as the basis for sound affective and cognitive growth. Because this programming is relevant to such community concerns as preventing child abuse and neglect and providing support for teenage parents, it has generated widespread interest and support.

Infant mental health projects nicely illustrate the building of linkages with other existing service. The effort in these projects has been to establish a means of systematically reviewing and gaining access to new-born children. Thus, three of the five projects have training hospital nurses to assess situational factors and observe mother-infant interaction in the hospital in order to identify those newborns who are in circumstances which place them at risk for attachment disorders. This screening strategy is still in the process of validation. A fourth project has a hospital-based infant specialist using clinical assessments. A fifth project is serving a caseload of pregnant adolescents receiving care in a hospital clinic.

Project services are carried out through weekly (or initially more frequent) home visits. Support, developmental guidance, and therapeutic interventions are designed to facilitate attachment, parental responsiveness, and the psychosocial development of the infant.

Evaluation results from the Bayley Scales of Infant Development at one year have been inconclusive, consistent with the experience in other infant projects around the country. Since there is some indication that this measure of infant behavior is not necessarily predictive of later psychopathology before age two and a half, the evaluation approach will be broadened to assess parent-infant interaction and to include a range of short-term and long-term outcome measures.

Other Areas of Programming

Other areas of programming are listed in Table 12.1. In addition, we propose this year to develop and evaluate a bereavement services project. In addition to the pilot projects, there have been a number of support projects. We have developed a training package for infant mental health specialists in collaboration with the Child Development Project, University of Michigan, as well as several films. We are putting together some materials on needs assessment and on community mental health response to plant closings. We also have a project assessing the feasibility of developing prevention services as an adjunct to a family planning clinic.

Unresolved Issues

Two issues remain unresolved in the Michigan program: reasonable approaches to evaluation and the process of transfer from project funding

TABLE 12.1   Summary of Michigan's Pilot Demonstration Projects

Population	Recruitment	Methodology
1. Infants in situations which place them at risk	a. Situational and observational screener in the maternity unit. b. Referral from 2. and 3. c. Referral from professionals.	Home visits; developmental guidance; support; psychotherapeutic intervention.
2. Children of disordered adults	Referral from inpatient services; access through mental health center's case management function; outpatient services.	Home visits. Interpretation to parents and to children; advocacy with group and individual recreation and discussion; parent education; remedial reading.
3. Children of divorcing parents	Recruitment through circuit court at the time of filing.	a. Pamphlet b. Single session presentation c. 8 session groups for (1) parents (2) elementary age children (3) adolescents
4. AFDC Women—Stress management training	Recruitment through social services; intake and service interviews.	Outreach to recruit; transportation; ten session training in problem solving, life planning, communication and relaxation techniques.

TABLE 12.1   Summary of Michigan's Pilot Demonstration Projects (Cont)

Population	Recruitment	Methodology
5. Low income families—parent training	Referral from other agencies; Headstart projects; neighborhood centers.	Outreach to recruit and to see if learning is applied; 10-session training in communication, play, discipline, behavioral management techniques, etc.
6. Elementary school children— Affective education	Teachers in participating schools.	Teachers are trained in process and in use of cumulative curriculum K-6.
7. Teenage parents and their infants	a. Referral from physicians, schools, public health, etc. b. Collaborative agreement with alternative school program.	Volunteer friend assigned to each girl. Counseling, infant stimulation.
8. Unemployed	Never adequately developed; project was terminated for this reason.	Azrin's Job Find Club
9. Selected pregnant women	High-risk pregnancy clinic.	Support, interpretation, advocacy.
10. Children at risk in rural county (combined model)	a. See 2 and 3 above. b. School referral. c. Mental health center referral.	a. See 2 and 3 above. b. Volunteer friend.

to the ongoing budget. Since positive evaluation results are the criteria for the continuance and ultimate acceptance of pilot demonstration projects, evaluation issues have become a central and crucial concern. We have underestimated the complexity of obtaining evaluation data for community-based prevention projects.

To begin with, we have encountered difficulties in establishing control groups when the service population is obtained by referral, nonadherence to random assignment in the face of pressures to provide service, and problems of tracking elusive control subjects over time in order to obtain outcome data. We are finding it essential to allocate a greater share of resources to this effort.

Even more basic is the issue of what will be evaluated and what measures will be used and the context for evaluation. Prevention projects are being held to a high level of outcome accountability which is realistic only if the means exist to document outcome accurately. Reliance on available standardized outcome measures is reasonable for those areas in which measurements have been well articulated (for example, children's behavior and affect). It is not so reasonable where existing standardized measures do not adequately tap the relevant dimensions and where measures to document clinical judgments are still being formulated. In the infant projects, for example, assessing impact requires some measure of psychosocial adjustment, and such measures are still in the process of development and standardization. We are learning that at this stage of development, a broad-brush approach to outcome evaluation using a range of reports and data is necessary for a rounded and fair assessment of prevention projects. We will be making wider use of outside consultants in putting together outcome hypotheses and measures.

Finally, we want to give a more significant role to *process evaluation.* In the infant projects, for example, we are currently using an on-site assessment by consultants expert in infant programming. In this way we can get a more complete picture of how the projects are operating, whether the quality of the work is acceptable, and whether the caseload is an appropriate one. Projects may have to go through a developmental sequence in which evaluation assesses the positive aspects, acknowledges the weaknesses, and formulates the next stage (Price, 1978). Table 12.2 outlines the natural history of two of our projects and shows how this developmental approach and assessment of basic program viability leads to later phases of program development.

The second major issue we have to confront is transfering prevention services from project funding to the ongoing budget. As projects move from pilot demonstration to replication with satisfactory evaluations,

TABLE 12.2 Natural History of Two Prevention Projects

Consideration	Washtenaw Job Find Club	Kalamazoo Infant Intervention
Process evaluation by outside experts	No	Yes
Methodology implemented?	Azrin's methodology implemented and documented.	Home visit intervention implemented. Staff can describe sequence, process, content.
Recruitment of target population?	*By self referral through newspaper publicity, ads; referral from counselors, personnel offices. Systematic process with (a) MESC, (b) CETA, (c) Schools not implemented.	By hospital screener. Low rate of service refusal and withdrawal.
Appropriateness of served population?	*Primarily female.	Assessed as appropriate.
Control group?	Noncomparable. Recruited from MESC lines.	Random assignment of screener referrals.
Data obtained?	Yes	*High attrition of control subjects.
Outcome data:	(a) Job finding results corroborate Azrin study. *(b) Zung depression scale shows no significant change.	*(a) Bayley Scales of Infant Development at one year show no significant difference between intervened and control. (b) Medical records search shows less accidents, injuries, negative comments for served group.

TABLE 12.2 (Continued)

Consideration	Washtenaw Job Find Club	Kalamazoo Infant Intervention
Should other measures have been used?	Not considered.	Yes
Appropriate area for mental health operation?	(a) General thrust may be more appropriate for an agency concerned with employment. (b) Appropriate as supplemental service for client populations.	Yes
Options?	†(a) Terminate. Turn over to agency concerned with employment. (b) Define target population more precisely. Redesign referral process. Redesign evaluation.	(a) Terminate †(b) Redesign evaluation. Tighten implementation of evaluation. Validate screener. Document intervention.

*Concerns
†Decision selected

251

there must be a structured way to accomplish this transition. Project applicants have always been apprehensive about what might happen once project funds are terminated. If boards which have had prevention projects are asked to choose between the prevention project and other existing services—in essence, a cut in funding—it is unlikely that prevention services can be selected in competition with departmental priorities and pressures related to deinstitutionalization.

This is a knotty and as yet unresolved problem. It would appear that prevention services will need some kind of specific protected allocation. Perhaps funding for prevention services will be the reward for those boards which have their base program under control. We are currently examining ways to maintain and disseminate successful projects.

In any case, prevention activities in Michigan have developed rapidly over the past five years. The next five years will almost surely see still other states begin programs at the state level. It is hoped that the Michigan experience can offer some beginning maps as these states explore their own uncharted territory.

References

Albee, G.W. Primary prevention. *Canada's Mental Health,* 1979, *27,* 5-9.

Anthony, E.J. A risk vulnerability intervention model for children of psychotic parents. In A. Koupernik and C. Koupernik (Eds.), *The Child in His Family: Children at Psychiatric Risk.* New York: John Wiley, 1974, 99-121.

Birch, H.G. Methodological issues in the longitudinal study of malnutrition. In D.F. Ricks, A. Thomas, and M. Roff (Eds.), *Life History Research in Psychopathology. Volume 3.* Minneapolis: University of Minnesota Press, 1974.

Cowen, E.L. Baby steps toward primary prevention. *American Journal of Community Psychology,* 1977, *5,* 1-22.

Kessler, M., & Albee, G.W. Primary prevention. *Annual Review of Psychology,* 1975, *26.*

Price, R.H. Evaluation research in primary prevention: Lifting ourselves by our bootstraps. Presented at the Primary Prevention Conference sponsored by the Community Mental Health Institute, National Council of Community Mental Health Centers, Denver, Colorado, June 11, 1978.

Tableman, B. *Report to Donald C. Smith, M.D. on the Development of a Prevention System.* Lansing: Michigan Department of Mental Health, 1975.

13

Implementing Prevention Programs

A Community Mental Health Center Director's Point of View

Saul Cooper

Washtenaw County Community Mental Health Center

Prevention is a many-splendored concept which surfaces periodically in the field of mental health. Its ascendency seems to have a varied causality. In some instances we find prevention surfacing when questions of efficacy and success in clinical programs are raised. At other times the popularity of prevention seems to be related to increased community concerns about highly specific populations or types of pathology. In some ways, community mental health ideology and services over the last 20 years have continuously highlighted prevention as a cornerstone of comprehensive services. The federal mandate for consultation and education was meant to assure prevention programming. No matter the cause, prevention programs whose time has come not once, but many times, are once again in the ascendency.

Definitional Issues

Aside from periodicity, we seem plagued with rather severe definitional problems. This may well reflect the state of the art; on the other hand, it may be that prevention in mental health centers is being defined by idiosyncratic practices. True change in program emphasis and direction is rare. We prefer to continue doing the same things; and relabeling is a much preferred behavior of choice.

We read a great deal about "new wine in old bottles" and "old wine in new bottles." Mental health historians in the future will no doubt speculate either about our hidden alcoholic tendencies or our preoccupation with manufacturing bottles. Let us hope that we can move away from the bar long enough to agree on some simple explicit definitions in the field of prevention. An inordinate amount of recent literature has wrestled with specifying prevention as primary prevention, which would appear to represent the purist point of view. Others in the field, especially those with continuing and intense clinical commitments, consider prevention as having primary, secondary, and tertiary aspects: Therefore, all mental health services are preventive in nature. Between the purist and the diehard clinician the field seems to be settling, at least in this cycle, as defining prevention activities somewhere between primary and secondary prevention. (This chapter will not attempt to present an extensive description of the similarities and differences between primary, secondary, and tertiary prevention. For this purpose, we would refer you to any basic public health text where the terms are dealt with in detail.) Presently, it would appear that while primary prevention has been popularly embraced by most academicians and reluctantly worshipped by most clinicians, in practice, we find that most prevention programs appear to represent mostly tertiary and secondary programming rather than primary.

A number of factors present in the mental health delivery system impinge on prevention programming. With the reduction of institutional beds, and with the tightened criteria for commitment, most mental health centers are faced with large numbers of so-called "after-care" clients. Services for these clients, many with long, chronic histories, place a heavy drain on resources. Resource allocation to more disturbed populations becomes inevitable as departments of mental health set "deinstitutionalization" as their highest priority. Unless the "magic pill" appears, primary prevention programs, at present, would seem to have very little to offer in dealing with this particular population group. Such clinical pressures represent considerable barriers to prevention programming.

Lack of specificity typifies most prevention programs in mental health settings. Any program which expects serious consideration must at the very least specify the target of the intervention, then must specify the intervention itself, and, finally, it must specify the outcome of the intervention. All too frequently we find programs geared to intermediary targets rather than to final targets—for example, programs geared to change teachers' attitudes in order to impact on the behavior of students. In such programs outcome measures which reflect changes in teacher attitudes obviously do not speak to the outcome intended for the target population: namely, students.

The target of a given intervention and the ultimate beneficiary of the intervention must be clearly specified. Under such program conditions one must be concerned with intermediate outcome as well as final outcome. Mental health centers with active consultation programs are reasonably successful in accessing caregivers; however, the beneficiaries of prevention programs have not been historically perceived as recipients of services unless they have defined themselves as a case.

Targeting a population infers a risk state for that population. Does our research allow us to define degrees of risk? More important, do we understand the etiological linkages between populations at risk and antecedent conditions? Clearly, basic research knowledge must be given a high priority if prevention programming is to hold much promise. Old questions of stigma and confidentiality must also be attended to if prevention programs are to succeed.

Along with definitional issues we find ourselves also constrained by a marked lack of systematic attempts at documenting prevention efforts. In order for practitioners to benefit from their own procedures and programs, as well as to learn from other practitioners, it becomes vital for prevention programs to have sufficient documentation systems. For such systems to be developed, one must, of course, first grapple with the definitional problems and then further develop a data-gathering process which can be carefully reviewed at whatever frequency might be necessary for effective management decision-making.

Our procedures for documentation in clinical practice have yet to be standardized in spite of more than 20 years of effort. How does one "count" two therapists with three family members in 50-minute interviews? Counting seems to be related to funding definitions. Sometimes we count therapist time, sometimes client time, and sometimes both. If we have a computerized management information system, we are likely to count everything in all possible combinations and then hope that the funding source will pick out what they deem relevant and fund us accordingly.

Documentation is clearly a necessary early step in developing credibility for prevention programs. Since both effort and efficiency measures are being increasingly required in mental health programs, we can likely assume that no prevention program can hope to survive which does not pay serious attention to definitional issues around effort and efficiency as part of a documentation system.

Domain Issues

Significant federal funding for prevention in recent years has come from the National Institute for Drug Abuse, the National Institute for

Alcohol Abuse and Alcoholism, and most recently from the National Institute of Mental Health. With three institutes supporting some degree of prevention programming, workers in the field of mental health are faced with an interesting set of domain issues.

Prevention programming in the schools, for example, seems to be largely a function of who gets there first. Programs designed to prevent drug abuse, alcohol abuse, or mental illness can hardly be distinguished in terms of their content. Does improving the self-concept of adolescents affect drug abuse reduction more or less than alcohol abuse reduction, or mental illness reduction? One might almost be led to conclude that the problem being prevented is determined much more by the source of funding than any other single variable.

Efficiency and effectiveness are endangered when various human service programs function under separate administrative units at the county or regional level. Prevention programs in the future must reflect collaboration across administrative and jurisdictional lines.

Is the Council on Aging in a given community the appropriate locus for prevention programs for the aged? Does the mental health center take on a leadership role? What about senior citizens' councils? Human service agencies have a long history of independent programming and independent funding. Prevention programs should not be doomed to repeat the same mistakes. Collaborative planning, funding, and programming at federal, state and local levels must be accomplished if we are to succeed in primary prevention.

Management Issues

Most clinical administrators are continually faced with developing a delicate program balance between the demands for services as reflected in clients' applications and the needs for services as reflected in a variety of needs assessments approaches. On the face of it, needs versus demands can never be totally balanced, and when typical administrators find themselves in the normative situation of having insufficient resources to meet already identified demands, they are most reluctant to look at other needs which may exist in the community. This needs-versus-demands issue is especially critical for those agencies interested in implementing prevention programs. It is almost as if clinical demands which are readily visible and which reflect the communities' press on the agency must be balanced against long-term prevention promises. In such a formula, clinical demands will almost always win.

One is faced with the wishful fantasy of a moratorium on clients presenting themselves to the agency, or the sudden influx of new and uncommitted funding which can be diverted to prevention programming. In addition, one finds a syndrome fairly frequently evidenced in mental health centers where administration espouses a commitment to prevention "when we get caught up on our clinical work." This fantasy allows one to play on both sides of the fence and promises very little prevention programming implementation in the forseeable future.

One starting point for administrators might well be a thorough assessment of their existing consultation and education programs. If one holds the level of resources constant, can the services be redirected toward prevention programming? Why do we continue to do what we are doing? How about a "sunset law" for both clinical and consultation services? A biannual review might help the center director in terminating certain community services in order to implement some modest prevention programming.

Constituency Issues

Complex community collaboration is at best a high-risk activity. It requires a considerable investment in time and energy and as such should be entered into only after much thoughtful consideration. However, if one chooses to begin prevention programming, then agency collaboration may well be a keystone. Such agency collaboration is surely necessary, but not sufficient. The nurturing of a nonprofessional constituency will immeasurably enhance prevention programs.

Service clubs (such as Kiwanis, Rotary, and Junior League) and church groups are particularly fruitful sources for constituency-building. Service delivery in a project framework is the typical approach to community activities by these organizations. If such organizations are given visible sponsorship and collaborative credit, they can often serve as the community base for preventive programs.

Any serious consideration of implementing prevention programs requires a focus on the politics of prevention at the local level. One must design a strategy which involves identifying relevant constituencies which might be interested in supporting prevention programs and use these constituencies to build both short-term and long-term commitments to the particular program being planned. Since most communities support and encourage mental health programs primarily as a response to social deviancy, and since most communities would prefer to deal with social deviancy by exclusion rather than by a treatment intervention, it becomes a high-risk strategy for mental health practitioners to promise that their particular prevention programs will effectively cope with problems that the community identifies. Further, one will ultimately run into the problem of etiological discrepancies. When the community chooses to feel that certain problems have distinct causes, they tend to respond unkindly to the mental health professional who designs a program that infers obviously different causes.

The politics of prevention, like the politics of mental health in general, have been largely overlooked by center directors. One sometimes wonders what there is in the training of center directors that makes them so uncomfortable with the political process.

Fiscal Support Issues

The history of fiscal support for mental health programs represents a major impediment for prevention programming. We find that fees and third-party reimbursements have always been required as a major income source. Most of the services delivered at a mental health center can ultimately generate some fee income. However, prevention programs, while ultimately fundable, rarely will attract sufficient fiscal support in the early demonstration stages. Federal operations grants which have included consultation and education have served as the fiscal support for many prevention programs; yet, as operations grants reach the end of their eight-year funding cycle, prevention, along with consultation and education, becomes a highly jeopardized activity, and both are frequently the first to disappear under the fiscal crunch. The movement of federal legislation toward an ongoing "capitation" process for funding consultation and education represents a hopeful sign for the future.

Here, again, one might seriously consider the development of a local constituency such as a service club which can be helpful fiscally in a way that is independent of the ongoing funding pattern of the mental health center. The role of the Junior League in the Primary Prevention Task Force of Erie, Pennsylvania, represents one such example.

Given the state of prevention technology and the fairly limited research base, one must be careful not to overpromise results in order to gain fiscal support. For example, assuring county commissioners that your prevention program will reduce juvenile delinquency and therefore free up funds presently being spent in the legal-judicial system is at best foolhardy. Even if you could guarantee such results, remember that funds could not be made available until your results are demonstrated. How, then, does the county support the original program of services for delinquents while simultaneously supporting the new prevention program. Two programs funded by one budget is not sound mathematics and certainly is not sound politics.

Organizational Issues

Most mental health administrators deal rather lightly with the basic question of who does prevention programming. If such services do exist in the agency, they frequently are seen automatically and without much thought as part of the consultation and education unit of the center. Such an organizational decision has a number of both positive and negative ramifications which need to be briefly explored. Consider, for example, the fact that the C & E unit is frequently made up of the least-senior personnel in the agency and is also frequently the smallest and least-funded organizational unit of the agency. At best, the C & E program will represent a very small and frequently insignificant part of the mental health center. At worst, it can be seen as irrelevant and existing only because of a federal mandate. Locating a prevention program within a C & E unit, therefore, reflects certain organizational messages which must be carefully considered.

If one could for the moment assume no organizational constraints, then a prevention program might be placed ideally within the director's office and have attached to it administrative support, as well as linkages to the major clinical components of the agency. While this ideal rarely will be achieved, it reflects the importance of legitimizing the program both for the agency staff and for the agency board by its very organizational location within the mental health center.

One further organizational note: In those agencies where consultation and education have been accepted early to maintain a forward-looking stance in the mental health field, we frequently find prevention simply being added to the consultation and education unit, thus a new set of letters C, E & P, has sprung up. Truth in labeling should demand that the center director require a change in programming to go along with the label change.

One finds that prevention programs, as practiced uniquely within C & E units, reflects the values of the director and the training and experience of the C & E coordinator. We seem doomed to repeat an old set of behaviors. In the absence of research findings we fall back on our personal experience in identifying necessary prevention programs. Professionals with a child guidance background will predictably evolve child-focused prevention programs with some clinically defined intervention procedure. In those agencies where programs are primarily educational in nature, one finds prevention programs geared in that direction. In effect, one must be cautious about provincialism wherever it occurs. Provincialism in a consultation and education unit is not by its nature any better or more appropriate than provincialism in a clinical unit.

If prevention programs are to succeed in mental health centers, the administration must carefully assess both internal and external consequences. Good programming requires both administrative support and resource commitment. Who determines the allocation of resources? Mental health center boards may respond quite positively to the concept of prevention; but professionals have the responsibility of specifying the potential short-term and long-term implications of prevention programs.

Both mental health boards and center directors have infinitely less difficulty in setting priorities when resources are expanding. However, the allocation of priorities when resources are shrinking poses an entirely different picture. Planning under these conditions requires a pro-active stance and considerable planning skills, both of which appear to be in short supply among boards and directors.

Research and Design Issues

Perhaps one of the most striking differences between prevention programming in public settings as opposed to prevention programming in academic settings has to do with the pragmatics of research and design. There are many special issues which concern practitioners in prevention programming. For example, can they legitimately set up control groups when required in a research framework, especially when their service delivery system in a public setting requires that they offer and deliver services to all who seek help? Further, how does one deal with short-term and long-term follow-up requirements of certain design approaches? Can the practitioner plan and design the prevention program with sufficient dollar support and therefore staff resources to put into practice a long-term follow-up which may not occur for six, twelve, or even 18 months after the actual intervention has taken place?

A more serious problem involves the potential case-finding aspects of the prevention program. Does the clinician or the prevention practitioner in the mental health center have a moral obligation to deliver services to those individuals defined as requiring intervention when first identified through a prevention program? Can one maintain individuals in a control group as they evidence further pathology and obviously also require intervention? Will the community allow prevention programming with long-term follow-up in the obvious face of people with problems not being treated?

If an outcome carries with it the implications that there will be a change in the base rate of some particular pathology for a special population group, will the local agencies responsible for collecting such information maintain a consistent position in data-gathering even if there is an implication that the rate of pathology might somehow be related to the quality and amount of service they deliver?

The problems faced by a prevention practitioner may be infinitely greater than those faced by the clinician, since over the years clinicians have rarely been put to the test of accountability in any clear-cut fashion. For the prevention practitioner to set out to prevent a particular problem in a particular population group really "puts the chips on the line" and in so doing allows for a degree of visible and public accountability which heretofore has not been faced by the mental health practitioner. The consequence of this situation is obvious. Successful prevention programming would add immeasurably to the credibility and perhaps even further fiscal support of mental health programs. On the other hand, the failure of prevention programming will be publicly visible and therefore will represent a much more serious threat to future funding for mental health services. The siren song of prevention, like other siren songs, needs to be approached by center directors with great curiosity, much enthusiasm, and considerable caution.

14

Strategies and Skills
for Promoting Mental Health

Richard F. Ketterer
Barbara C. Bader
Center for Human Services Research,
Ann Arbor, Michigan

Marc R. Levy
Six Area Coalition Community Mental Health Center,
Lincoln Park, Michigan

Despite the attention recently given to prevention in mental health, relatively little is known about prevention strategies or about the knowledge and skills required by prevention practitioners. In part, this problem exists because the field of prevention is still in a formative stage. First, few studies have defined the nature and range of prevention services, identifying the strategies and techniques used in service delivery. Second, opportunities for training and skill development in prevention have been limited, making it difficult for prevention practitioners to develop requisite skills. Third, the concept of prevention has different meanings for different people.

Since one's definition of prevention has implications for practice strategies and skills, we will first define our perspective on this important and emerging field, presenting a mental health promotion paradigm as an alternative to the traditional public health model of prevention. We will then discuss five major health promotion strategies and identify the knowledge and skills required in implementing them.

Mental Health Promotion
versus Disease-Prevention

The concept of prevention in mental health is generally traced to the field of public health, where prevention is divided into primary, secondary, and tertiary spheres. Primary and secondary prevention are designed to reduce the prevalence of disease or disorder: primary prevention by lowering the rate or incidence of new cases of disease and secondary prevention by reducing their duration through early case findings and effective treatment. Tertiary prevention is designed to reduce the severity of chronic disorders and is frequently labeled rehabilitation.

A premise underlying the public health framework of prevention is that disorders can be prevented by identifying and then eliminating the specific factors causing the disorders. Unfortunately, as Bloom (1979) has recently observed, this premise has proved considerably more useful in preventing a range of communicable diseases (such as cholera, malaria, and polio) and nutritional diseases (for example, beriberi, scurvy, and rickets) than in preventing mental and behavioral disorders such as depression and substance abuse.

Emerging as an alternative to the traditional public health perspective is a paradigm which defines mental and behavioral disorders as a consequence of multiple precipitating events, rather than as a result of a specific precondition. Bloom (1979) states: "It is a paradigm that does not begin with the assumption that every specific disorder has a single or even a multiple necessary precondition. Rather, this paradigm assumes that we are all variously vulnerable to stressful life events" (p. 183). Cassel (1976) makes a similar point when he asserts doubt that "any given psychosocial process or stressor will be etiologically specific for any disease" (p. 109). Rather, such psychosocial stressors are believed to increase susceptibility to disease without leading to a specific universally predictable disorder.

While stressful life events and conditions such as poverty and natural disasters cannot be shown to have specific adverse outcomes, they are believed to have pervasive though nonspecific adverse effects. Accordingly, Bloom (1979), Ryan (1971), and other advocates of an alternative approach argue that we need to shift attention away from prevention and toward mental health promotion. Promoting mental health means enhancing the competencies and well-being of individuals, groups, and communities through the application of multiple person-centered and system change efforts. Whereas traditional clinical interventions are aimed at changing psychological or psychosocial factors in an identified patient or client system, mental health promotion strategies are aimed at (1) improving the well-being and strengths of normal and at-risk populations through competence-training strategies; and (2) modifying social policies, social systems, and environmental factors which impede the mental health and well-being of groups in the community.

While funding for mental health promotion services has been sorely lacking (President's Commission on Mental Health, 1978), health promotion efforts in mental health have nonetheless been apparent. For example, consultation and education (C & E) staff in community mental health centers (CMHCs) have been offering prevention and health promotion services for almost two decades despite enormous barriers facing them (Ketterer & Bader, 1977; Ketterer, 1979). Similarly, affective education specialists, substance abuse prevention staff, community psychologists, and other nonclinically oriented mental health personnel have been struggling for years to provide health-promoting services in the mental health field. But what service strategies have health promotion professionals developed? Equally important, what knowledge and skills are required to effectively implement such strategies?

Toward a Typology of
Mental Health Promotion Strategies

A review of relevant literature suggests five major strategies employed by mental health promotion (MHP) professionals. These include (1) *consultation to natural support systems;* (2) *caregiver consultation;* (3) *organizational consultation;* (4) *community network/coalition-building;* and (5) *mental health education.*

Consultation to Natural Support Systems

A first strategy for promoting mental health is facilitating the development of natural support systems in the community. In recent years it has become apparent that social supports serve as a buffer protecting individuals from the effects of external stressors (Caplan, 1974; Cassel, 1973; Bloom, 1979). Citing results of numerous studies which examine the impact of social supports on health and mental health outcomes, Cassel (1973) concludes that the strength of social supports provided by an individual's primary group plays an important role in preventing mental and physical disorders.

Providing consultative services to natural support systems is illustrated by Collins and Pancoast (1976), who developed collaborative ties with natural neighbors, indigenous helpers who provide support to individuals and groups at risk. Their strategy involved (1) identifying high-risk neighborhoods, (2) conducting a preliminary assessment of the area using ethnographic techniques, (3) identifying natural neighbors and establishing a consultative relationship with them, and (4) assisting the natural helpers in carrying out their helping roles by providing ongoing consultation and support.

In a somewhat different vein, Silverman (1969) has attempted to facilitate the development of widow-to-widow programs which provide support to women who have lost their husbands, and Budman (1975) has developed psychoeducational groups which are started within an agency context but are later transported into the community. Like natural support groups, psychoeducational groups are aimed at providing a buffer to individuals facing developmental or accidental life crises.

In addition to creating natural support systems, Gottlieb and Schroter (1978) suggest that health promotion workers can play a role in facilitating communication and contact among natural helpers. They state:

> Once those persons who play a pivotal role in local natural delivery systems are identified, they can be convened by the professional both for the purpose of sharing knowledge of efficacious helping strategies and, more important, for the purpose of passing this knowledge on to other programs which are not currently enmeshed in natural helping networks [Gottlieb & Schroter, 1978: 619].

Caregiver Consultation

Just as it is important to develop and strengthen natural support systems, it is also crucial to improve the capacity of caregivers in the community, a goal that can be achieved through several consultative strategies. For example, client-centered case consultation is designed to assist mental health professionals in providing more effective services to their clients. Here, emphasis is placed on assisting consultees to provide more effective services to specific clients, not on improving their general skill level. In contrast, consultee-centered case consultation (Caplan, 1970), often referred to as caregiver consultation, is directed toward improving the overall effectiveness of the consultee, with secondary attention given to resolving specific client problems. The goal of caregiver consultation is to improve the knowledge and skills of the consultee in order that he or she will be able to provide more effective services in the future (Altrocchi et al., 1965; Berlin, 1964; Caplan, 1964).

Although originally designed for mental health professionals, caregiver consultation programs have gradually broadened to include other professionals such as clergy, police, and teachers as well as nonprofessionals such as bartenders, beauticians, and taxi drivers (Canter & Paulson, 1974; Hulme, 1974; Mann, 1971; Taynor et al., 1976). This type of consultation is important, since caregivers serve as gatekeepers to a wide range of community groups. By improving caregiver effectiveness, health promotion workers address the mental health needs of a much broader population.

Organizational Consultation

A third strategy for promoting mental health is to create more responsive human service organizations through organizational consultation and other system change interventions. System change efforts are based on the premise that key human service organizations—such as schools, churches, welfare programs, and law enforcement—profoundly influence the attitudes and behaviors of diverse community groups. Cowen (1977: 7) observes:

> Several things must happen for primary prevention to reap full benefit from a social environment approach. First, we must better understand how to assess social environments, their key impact dimensions, and how they vary on these. We must also establish clearer linkages between environmental qualities and people's personal development and behavior, both generally and in terms of specific person-environment matches. We assume that social systems are not neutral in their effects on people. They either contribute to or impair development. Charting the whys and wherefores of these relations will provide information that can be harnessed to engineer health-promoting environments.

Organizational change is typically carried out through process and program consultation. Process consultation is aimed at improving communication patterns and interpersonal processes within human service systems. Schein (1969) states that the goal of the process consultant is to "help the organization to solve its own problems by making it *aware* of organizational processes, of consequences of these processes, and of the mechanisms by which they can be changed" (p. 135).

Broader than process consultation, program consultation provides technical assistance on a range of problems of human service systems. MacLennan, Quinn, and Shroeder (1975) define program consultation in the following manner:

> Program consultation deals with problems concerned with the planning, development, management, evaluation, and coordination of services directly or indirectly affecting the mental health of the community. Participants in such consultations are generally administrators and planning staff. Initiative for seeking consultation may be

taken by agencies, departments, associations, institutions in the community, or by the community mental health center. Such consultation may result in the development of new services or policies, in the recommitment or redeployment of manpower, and in the addition of new functions to an agency. It may assist in the creation of mechanisms for more effective continuous coordination of services and exchange of information, in the provision of training or the development of research and evaluation. Activities may include working with individuals and groups on the development of plans and proposals, ex-officio participation on committees, or advising on the writing of technical materials [MacLennan et al., 1975: 6].

Program consultants must have extensive knowledge about the nature, methods, and goals of the program, which they use when providing advice on administrative and management issues. Where administrative issues are concerned, consultants typically establish working relationships with top administrators in the client system. The task, then, is to help administrators develop appropriate strategies for dealing with the management issues facing them, including problems of organizational and program design, decision-making procedures, performance review, board relations, program evaluation, job design, and personnel policies and practices.

Community Network/Coalition-Building

A fourth strategy for promoting mental health is to develop community networks to foster interagency coordination and to increase community involvement in and control of mental health resources. Iscoe (1974) contends that there is a close relationship between the development of community resources/power and key attributes such as self-esteem and sense of autonomy. Writing about the creation of competent communities, Iscoe points out that resources are needed so that "members of the community may make reasoned decisions about issues confronting them, leading to the most competent coping with these problems. . . . The concept of the competent community parallels the concept of positive mental health" (1974: 608-609).

The value of network-building can be illustrated through an example of collaboration between a community mental health center and a local community group. A minister and his volunteer youth leader approached the CMHC's consultation and education (C & E) unit to request assistance in generating community support for children's issues. Planning sessions were held with these individuals, and a collaborative strategy was developed which involved the C & E unit and appropriate community leaders. Contacts were made with churches, civic groups, and organizations serving children and families in the community, and individuals were encouraged to attend an organizational meeting around the theme "year of the child." A core group composed of representatives of local churches, civic groups, city government, mental health agencies, and schools became involved. This group met several times, setting program goals for the year and mobilizing for action. It organized an educational series focused on mental health topics, family issues, and substance abuse; sponsored a walk for children; created a "year of the child" float for a parade; and organized a community picnic. The schools, civic clubs, and mental health centers agreed to work cooperatively on several projects; the churches and the local parks and recreation department opened their facilities to community groups and activities; and, in general, the community became much more involved in children's issues.

The mental health staff involved in the initial planning for this community organization effort worked with only two community leaders. The "year of the child" theme allowed participating members and organizations to work on their own special interests while cooperating with others on projects having broad community appeal. Organizing and promoting community cooperation made it easier to reach the constituency being served, and community support for health promotion efforts appeared to increase.

Other examples of coalition-building are more directly political in nature. For instance, a rape or domestic violence network might go beyond simply bringing together professional caregivers and community residents, and might advocate on behalf of a client or service priority. Such a network might, for example, testify before city council in order to obtain funding for special services, or might lobby for support from civic and elected leaders. This work is increasingly becoming critical to the development and survival of specific programs.

Mental Health Education

A final strategy for promoting mental health is mental health education. The National Committee for Mental Health Education (1977: 2) defines mental health education as

a distinct group of interventions designed to assist people in acquiring knowledge, skills, and attitudes that directly contribute to their mental health and to their effect on the mental health of others. Such interventions enable people to cope with and act on their environment and seek to create environments which are more supportive of human life. Mental health education is applicable to a wide variety of purposes and target groups, and has unique potential for preventing emotional disability and for promoting growth in people and community groups.

What are the major purposes and target groups for mental health education efforts?

First, mental health education seeks to inform the general public about mental health problems and about available treatment and health-promoting resources. Research indicates that local residents often have minimal knowledge about mental health services offered in their community. For example, Goldman found (Heinemann et al., 1974) that only four percent of the community residents he surveyed knew that the local community mental health center existed. In another study, Heinemann and his associates (1974) found that only 15 percent of area residents surveyed were aware of the existence of the local CMHC. In light of the above findings, an important task of health promotion specialists is to increase the community's awareness of available health promotion and treatment services. In addition to promoting public knowledge about available resources, mental health educators also strive to provide general information to the community that promotes mental health, individual growth, and a more enriched life.

Second, mental health education attempts to develop important competencies within normal and at-risk groups. Such efforts, often referred to as competence training, are designed to improve the capacity of normal and at-risk populations to cope with predictable life transitions and to more effectively manage stressful situations. The premise underlying this approach is that disorders can be avoided by strengthening an individual's or group's capacity to handle environmental stress or life crises.

To illustrate educational efforts of this type, Shure and his colleagues (1971) developed a problem-solving curriculum for four-year-old Head Start children. The curriculum taught listening, attending, and problem-solving skills using games and dialogues presented for 20 minutes daily over a 10-week period. Evaluation results showed that children in the program improved on a number of criterion measures, including problem-solving skills, concern for others, ability to take initiative, and increased autonomy. Reviewing this literature, Cowen (1977) concluded that "implanting problem-solving skills apparently established a competence beachhead that radiated positively to a cluster of variables that we think of as 'good mental health' " (p. 13).

Zax and Specter (1974) and Bloom (1971) describe examples of intervention strategies aimed at teaching college students skills to overcome the stresses of college life, often viewed as a time of developmental crisis. Additional research is emerging which suggests the benefits of intervention at the time of situational crises, such as the birth of a child, the death of a spouse, or retirement. Education is viewed as an important means of developing skills to more effectively deal with such situations.

Third, mental health education attempts to increase the knowledge and skills of clients/patients and their significant others. These efforts are designed to assist clients in becoming more knowledgeable consumers of mental health services and to aid families and others involved with clients to play a more effective role in enhancing outcomes of therapeutic interventions. Educational programs are also designed to ease client transitions back into community life and to increase a community's acceptance of formerly institutionalized individuals returning to the community. Although research evaluating the effects of educational efforts in this area has been limited, Douglas, Westley, and Chaffee (1970) report success in improving attitudes toward the mentally retarded through the use of an extensive multimedia campaign. Evaluation results showed that improved attitudes toward the mentally retarded correlated with an increase in the amount of information about the mentally retarded provided through the media campaign.

A fourth goal of mental health education is to provide important information to people in the community who are in key positions to affect the lives of others. Formal and informal caregivers—from clergy, physicians, and school teachers to beauticians, bartenders, and employers—are recipients of educational efforts designed to increase their knowledge and ability to provide care and support, to recognize mental health problems, and to make appropriate referrals.

A final goal of mental health education is to influence public policies which affect the mental health and well-being of individuals and groups in the community. Keeping policymakers informed about mental health issues and sensitive to the effects of service programs on human lives, and developing position papers on key policy issues, are among the strategies available to health promotion professionals who wish to influence the public policy process.

The goal of influencing public policy has recently been identified as an explicit aim in a position paper issued by the National Committee for Mental Health Education (1977):

> A primary outcome of educational efforts in the public policy arena should be a greater understanding of and sensitivity to the mental health impact of all public policies by elected and non-elected policy-makers. Further, educational efforts in the area should seek to support and advance public policies which build upon and promote mental health [1977: 5].

Practice Skills

In a recent study of consultation and education programs in four CMHCs (Ketterer & Bader, 1977), C & E staff were asked to list the skills needed to deliver mental health promotion services. They identified 13 different skills ranging from interpersonal to consultation and research skills. Further analysis of these findings along with a review of the literature suggest that mental health promotion skills can be clustered into four discrete areas: consultation, education, organization, and action research. While few professionals are expected to become equally competent in all areas, it is important to identify the skills associated with each area.

Consultant Skills

Mental health promotion (MHP) specialists provide a range of consultative services from case and caregiver consultation to organizational and other system change interventions. Consultation services, as mentioned earlier, are generally aimed at improving caregiver systems, which in turn are expected to enhance the mental health and well-being of a much wider target population.

When functioning as consultants, MHP professionals must manage a complex set of tasks, including entry into the client system, implementation of change strategies, evaluation of the results, and, when possible, provision of follow-up services to the client. Recognizing the complexity of these tasks and the skills required to provide them, Lippitt and Lippitt (1978: 94) have humorously observed:

> Any list of the professional capabilities of a consultant is extensive—something like a combination of the Boy Scouts' laws, requirements

for admission to heaven, and the essential elements for securing tenure at an Ivy League college.

Insight into the knowledge and skills needed to function effectively as a consultant can be gleaned from a list of competencies generated through a recent survey of consultants (Lippitt & Lippitt, 1978). Results of the survey suggest the importance of the following consultant competencies: (1) thorough grounding in the behavioral sciences; (2) knowledge of administrative philosophies, policies, practices, and stages of growth of organizations and larger social systems; (3) understanding of human personality and attitude formation, and knowledge of how to design the change process; (4) communication, teaching, and counseling skills; (5) ability to form relationships based on trust with people from widely varying backgrounds and to work with groups and teams in planning and implementing change; (6) ability to diagnose problems with a client, to locate sources of help, power, and influence, and to understand the client's values and culture; (7) skill in designing surveys, interviewing, and other data-collection methods, as well as ability to use a variety of intervention methods effectively; (8) good problem-solving abilities; and (9) competence, integrity, maturity, willingness to take risks, openmindedness, honesty, and possession of a humanistic value system.

The above list suggests that consultants must simultaneously use both technical and interpersonal skills. Consultants must have excellent diagnostic, conceptual, and problem-solving abilities. They must be actively goal-directed: defining areas for consultation, suggesting ideas and alternatives to clients, referring clients to appropriate resources, and specifying desired outcomes. They must be knowledgeable about specific programs and how similar programs have resolved problems in the past. They must possess good communication skills, both orally and in writing, and must be able to both coolly assess difficult situations and "think on their feet." Moreover, because agency attitudes and needs have recently been shown to be the most critical determinants of consultation outcome (Larsen et al., 1976), consultants must develop the capacity to assess and influence an agency's readiness for consultation.[1] Finally, consultants must be able to do all of the above in a tactful, friendly, yet professional manner, generating trust, remaining flexible and tolerant of ambiguity, showing a good sense of timing, and being able to handle both frustration and criticism.

In summary, health promotion professionals working as consultants must acquire an extensive repertoire of skills. The effective consultant, then, is something of a "renaissance person" who possesses both technical and interpersonal competencies, and who is able to learn not only from formal training but from practical experience as well.

Educational Skills

Mental health professionals provide diverse educational and training services ranging from competence training for persons at risk to media campaigns designed to inform citizens about health promotion services. In their roles as educators, MHP professionals must possess a number of skills. Like consultants, educators must be able to communicate effectively, both orally and in writing. They must know how to plan and design training programs and be able to utilize a variety of educational and training techniques, such as role-playing, simulations, and problem-solving exercises. They must be able to use the media—radio, television, and newspapers. They must be able to work effectively with diverse groups, assessing their needs for information and developing educational programs to meet those needs. They must be competent in using multiple information dissemination strategies (such as pamphlets, leaflets, posters, bumper stickers, billboards, public service announcements, mailings, speakers, workshops and colloquia, and retreats) as well as in assessing the effectiveness of such efforts.

In addition to these skills, educators must be able to tailor their strategies to specific populations, while at the same time effectively overcoming resistances to change within each target group. They must be able to perform formal and informal needs assessments, to set clear objectives for educational efforts, to develop instructional materials, and to disseminate information that addresses identified needs. In addition to developing and using existing resources, they must identify and train natural helpers who can participate in the education/change process. They must do all of the above competently and efficiently, while at the same time dealing with "performance demands" and the necessity of communicating a great deal of information in limited time. In sum, the educator/trainer must be both a content and process expert who is skilled in designing learning environments and who has the energy and capacity to deliver in high-demand situations.

Organizer Skills

Health promotion professionals function as organizers when they attempt to develop networks and coalitions to address identifiable community needs. As with other health promotion roles, the organizer role requires diverse knowledge and skills. Commenting on this point, Zald (1967) notes that community organization "is an amalgam of many disciplines. Practitioners draw on a range of disciplines, from small group and psychodynamic theory to economics and political science" (p. 31). An analysis of the organizer role suggests that two broad competencies are required: linking/outreach and group skills.

Linking/outreach skills are required when organizers move away from the "home agency" and into the community. Organizers must have the ability to establish trust and a close working relationship with an ever-expanding network of individuals and groups brought together to achieve a common goal. Building trust in turn implies acting in a consistent and reliable manner with these frequently diverse constituencies. Organizers must also possess the ability to identify appropriate resources and to make them available to different client or consumer groups. To accomplish this, organizers must be able to access a range of resources (experts, sources for funds, and so on) as well as be knowledgeable about how to put such resources in the hands of appropriate client groups. Finally, effective organizers must have good political skills which enable them to build coalitions and to employ strategies designed to shift the balance of power in the community.

While linking/outreach skills are essential in working with diverse community groups, group and interpersonal skills are required to mobilize individuals into functioning groups. Key to this task are group facilitation and problem-solving skills. Facilitation skills enable the organizer to keep a group functioning effectively, achieving a balance between accomplishing group tasks and maintaining healthy interpersonal relationships among group members. Problem-solving skills, on the other hand, are required as the organizer assists groups in creatively and effectively moving through the stages of problem identification, proposal and review of alternative solutions, selection of a plan of action, implementation of the plan, and evaluation of the overall problem-solving effort. The organizer must assist the group in moving through the problem-solving steps while at the same time maintaining open communication among members and seeking advice from the outside where necessary. Finally, the organizer must use both group facilitation and problem-solving skills in promoting the emergence of leadership within the group, so that future group activities will draw more heavily on the capacities of group members.

Action Research Skills

A final role of MHP professionals is that of action researcher. While health promotion research has been associated traditionally with university-based social scientists, in recent years a growing number of community practitioners have recognized the need to incorporate research methods into overall intervention activities (Ketterer, 1979; French & Bell, 1973; Lippitt & Lippitt, 1978). Community consultants, for example, use action research techniques as a means of diagnosing and changing complex social systems. Similarly, educators and organizers alike are using research strategies to help them document community needs and to assess the effectiveness of intervention efforts (Blakely, 1979).

Health promotion professionals working as action researchers must have a basic understanding of the action research process, a problem-solving cycle in which data are used to analyze and solve problems being examined. This cycle consists of four major phases: (1) defining the problem; (2) collecting data; (3) analyzing and interpreting results, including key practice implications; and (4) feeding back findings to relevant client groups. The above tasks require that the MHP specialist possess several important skills, among them good analytic abilities. In the present context, analytic ability refers to the capacity to think systematically about an issue or problem, examining it fully before taking action. Having analytic skills also implies the ability to conceptualize from one's experience, a skill that enables the researcher to make sense out of complex and sometimes contradictory observations.

Along with analytic skills, action researchers must be knowledgeable about a number of data-collection methods. First, they must be able to identify and interpret existing documents, such as agency statistical reports, census data, annual reports, directories, and planning studies. These data are often invaluable in assessing community needs as well as in defining the parameters of health promotion projects.

In addition to using the above quantitative sources, action researchers should be familiar with qualitative methods developed by anthropologists and other social scientists (Patton, 1978; Parlett & Hamilton, 1976; Britan, 1978). Commenting on the value of qualitative methods, Barton and Lazarsfeld (1969: 182) state:

> Research which has neither statistical weight nor experimental design, research based on qualitative descriptions of a small number of cases, can nonetheless play the important role of suggesting possible relationships, causes, effects, and even dynamic processes.

One of the most useful qualitative methods is the key informant technique. This method consists of identifying and then conducting in-depth interviews with persons knowledgeable about a particular issue or problem in the community. Another useful method is the group conference approach, best illustrated by Delbecq's (Delbecq, et al., 1975) nominal group technique (NGT). The NGT entails a series of problem-solving steps starting with structured brainstorming and moving sequentially through priority-setting and, finally, consensus-building. Like key informant interviews, the NGT is especially valuable during the early phases of research, or where relatively little is known about a particular problem or issue. Finally, action researchers can employ observational techniques which put them in direct contact with the people and events they are studying (McCall & Simmons, 1969).

Besides collecting and analyzing data, action researchers must be familiar with data feedback and research utilization techniques and must be skilled in tailoring research findings to different target groups. Equally important, they must be able to tease out practice implications from multiple sources of data. It is not enough simply to present findings; efforts must be made to link findings to future action strategies. Finally, action researchers must be comfortable moving between researcher and change agent roles, including those of consultant, educator, and organizer. This, in turn, means either acquiring research and change agent skills or working in interdisciplinary teams in which these skills are represented.

A Note on Combining Practice Skills

Health promotion interventions often require professionals to function in multiple roles. Consider the example of a professional asked by the director of a community crisis center to consult about low morale among paraprofessional staff. Before devising a specific intervention strategy, the professional decides to conduct preliminary research to discover the underlying cause of the problem. Interviews are conducted with staff as well as with selected members of the center's citizen board. The results reveal that the major source of staff dissatisfaction is the lack of opportunities for staff development and training. Believing that this problem can be addressed, the MHP professional assists the agency in designing an appropriate in-service training program. Once the program is defined, he also serves as one of the trainers who will deliver the educational package.

In the above example, the MHP professional employs not only consultant skills but research and educational skills as well. In addition, to be effective, the professional combines knowledge about community crisis centers with generic intervention skills which are applied to the specific situation. In short, MHP professionals function in multiple roles, utilizing both generic intervention skills and knowledge about the unique culture and norms of the client system.

Implications

Given the complex and changing nature of the mental health promotion field, there is a need to establish directions for the future. What are some initiatives that can be taken by MHP professionals interested in the development of this emerging field?

Increased Understanding of
Health Promotion Services

One of the most important steps is to increase our understanding of mental health promotion services. What are the goals of different MHP services? What intervention methods are used to achieve health promotion goals? Who are the primary and secondary targets of health promotion efforts? What are the costs-benefits of person-centered versus system-centered interventions? These and other crucial questions need to be addressed in the coming years.

Generating knowledge about MHP services can be achieved through several research and development strategies. First, MHP professionals can develop procedures for monitoring ongoing mental health promotion services. In recent years, a number of consultation and education (C & E) programs have developed C & E information systems which provide valuable data for program planning and decision-making. Unfortunately, few programs have instituted comprehensive monitoring systems. What is needed is a plan for pilot testing and refining exemplary information systems and then disseminating them to other mental health promotion programs (Bader & Ellsworth, 1977).

Developing knowledge about MHP services can also be fostered by outside researchers who initiate applied research and evaluation activities. For example, Ketterer and Bader's study of C & E programs resulted in a typology of C & E services, as well as the identification of key program and service dimensions (Ketterer & Bader, 1977; Ketterer, 1979). Future efforts need to be directed toward evaluating the effects of specific MHP interventions. Commenting on the need for outcome evaluation in mental health consultation, Mannino and Shore (1975) write:

> We see a need for more studies in-depth that could attempt to delineate process variables and relate these to outcome variables. Also, we continue to see the need for multivariate studies which assess different levels of change in relationship to other factors, such as how the consultees' views and expectations of consultation affect outcome, or how experienced consultants and inexperienced consultants have different effects. In the final analysis, the more we can delimit the population studied, specify the activities performed, and use multi-level outcome variables, the more meaningful, and therefore more valuable, should be the results [Mannino & Shore, 1975: 19].

In sum, we need to initiate monitoring, evaluation, and other applied research efforts if we are to substantially increase our understanding of MHP services.

Staff Development and Training

In addition to research, efforts need to be made in the area of staff development and training. Although university-based doctoral programs in prevention and health promotion are developing (Iscoe et al., 1977), too few students are graduating from these programs to meet even the present demand for such qualified professionals. Interestingly, the lack of formal training programs has prompted MHP professionals to develop their own in-service and interagency training consortia. Unfortunately, lack of knowledge and resources have often hampered in-service training efforts, while interagency consortia are frequently plagued by problems of coordination and inadequate funds.

Recognizing these problems, the National Institute of Mental Health's Staff College has recently sponsored a series of five-day training workshops for C & E professionals working in community mental health. While this is a step in the right direction, it is not enough to meet the training needs of either C & E staff or MHP professionals working in other settings.

One idea we think has merit is the development of regional health promotion training centers similar to the evaluation resource center established by the National Institute of Mental Health. The goals of such resource centers would be to retrieve, package, and disseminate health promotion training centers similar to the evaluation resource center for packaging and disseminating training methods has already been developed (Rothman, 1974; Guba, 1968; Havelock, 1969) and needs only to be tailored to the mental health promotion field.

Interdisciplinary Teaming

Given the lack of adequate training and the complexity of health promotion efforts, many MHP interventions are beyond the knowledge base and skills of specific individuals. This problem can be addressed by establishing interdisciplinary teams that possess the range of necessary skills. Interdisciplinary teaming will often require MHP professionals to reach beyond traditional organizational boundaries to establish collaborative ties with other professionals. For example, in one community in Michigan a rape prevention project brought together prevention and health promotion professionals from dozens of different agencies and groups. Similarly, though at another level, a state mental health association we are involved with is sponsoring a series of health promotion conferences that are mobilizing the resources not only of diverse citizen groups, but also of interdisciplinary professional groups, such as C & E staff, public health educators, and community psychologists. These and similar efforts are needed to break down old barriers and to open the way for more viable and innovative ways of exchanging limited resources.

Constituency-Building

A final strategy is to develop greater institutional and public support for health promotion activities. The President's Commission on Mental Health (1978: 54-55) addresses this point directly:

> At present our efforts to prevent mental illness or to promote mental health are unstructured, unfocused, and uncoordinated. They command few dollars, limited personnel, and little interest at levels where resources are sufficient to achieve results. If we are to change this state of affairs, the prevention of mental illness and the promotion of mental health must become a visible part of national policy. To create visibility, there should be identifiable organizational components within Federal agencies that have direct responsibilities for mental health or whose programs affect mental health concerns. These components should be responsible for establishing priorities, developing programs, and advocating appropriate resources for the prevention of mental health and emotional disorders.

Despite the promise implied by the above statements, it remains unclear to what extent the recommendations of the President's Commission will be implemented. Consequently, it is important that political support for health promotion efforts be developed in order to influence the policy process.

At the present time, support for health promotion services derives from three major sources: (1) health promotion practitioners, (2) a small number of state and federal policymakers committed to health promotion goals, and (3) university-based community psychologists who have been advocating for prevention and health promotion for more than a decade. These groups have begun to establish local, state, and regional networks designed to support a health promotion perspective. The next step is to create a national network of health promotion personnel and, in the future, to expand it to include recipients of mental health promotion efforts. This strategy, we believe, will increase public support for mental health promotion services while heightening public awareness of the need to incorporate health promotion concepts and practices into everyday life.

Note

1. Readiness for consultation refers to an agency's definition of the problem, its recognition of the need for consultation, and the clarity of its expectations for the consultant.

References

Altrocchi, J., Spielberger, C., & Eisdorfer, C. Mental health consultation with groups. *Community Mental Health Journal*, 1965, *1*, 127-134.

Bader, B.C., & Ellsworth, S.L. Developing an information system for consultation and education services in community mental health centers. Presented in a symposium entitled "Developing and Documenting Consultation and Education Services in Community Mental Health Centers" at the 85th Annual Convention of the American Psychological Association, San Francisco, August 28, 1977.

Barton, A.H., & Lazarsfeld, P.F. Some functions of qualitative analysis in social research. In G.J. McCall and J.L. Simmons (Eds.), *Issues in Participant Observation*. Reading, MA: Addison-Wesley, 1969.

Berlin, I.N. Learning mental health consultation: History and problems. *Mental Hygiene*, 1964, *48*, 257-266.

Blakely, E.J. *Community Development Research: Concepts, Issues and Strategies*. New York: Human Sciences Press, 1979.

Bloom, B.L. A university freshman preventative intervention program: Report of a pilot project. *Journal of Consulting and Clinical Psychology*, 1971, *37*, 235-242.

Bloom, B.L. *Community Mental Health: A General Introduction*. Monterey, CA: Brooks/Cole, 1975.

Bloom, B.L. Prevention of mental disorders: Recent advances in theory and practice. *Community Mental Health Journal*, 1979, *15*, 179-191.

Britan, G.M. The place of anthropology in program evaluation. *Anthropological Quarterly*, 1978, *51*, 119-128.

Budman, S.H. A strategy for preventive mental health intervention. *Professional Psychology*, 1975, *6*, 394-398.

Canter, L., & Paulson, T. A college credit model of in-school consultation: A functional behavioral training program. *Community Mental Health Journal*, 1974, *10*, 268-275.

Caplan, G. *Principles of Preventive Psychiatry*. New York: Basic Books, 1964.

Caplan, G. *The Theory and Practice of Mental Health Consultation*. New York: Basic Books, 1970.

Caplan, G. *Support Systems and Community Mental Health*. New York: Behavioral Publications, 1974.

Cassel, J. The relation of the urban environment to health: Implications for prevention. *Mount Sinai Journal of Medicine*, 1973 *40*, 539-550.

Cassel, J. The contribution of the social environment to host resistance. *American Journal of Epidemiology*, 1976, *104*, 107-123.

Collins, A.H., & Pancoast, O.L. *Natural Helping Network*. New York: National Association of Social Workers, 1976.

Cowen, E.L. Baby-steps toward primary prevention. *American Journal of Community Psychology*, 1977, *5*, 1-22.

Delbecq, A.L., Van de Ven, A.H., & Gustafson, D.H. *Group Techniques for Program Planning*. Glenview, IL: Scott, Foresman, 1975.

Douglas, P., Westley, B., & Chaffee, S. An information campaign that changed attitudes. *Journalism Quarterly*, 1970, *47*, 479-492.

Egbert, L.D., Battit, G.E., Welch, C.E., & Bartlet, M.K. Reduction of post-operative pain by encouragement and instruction of patients. *New England Journal of Medicine*, 1964, *270*, 825-827.

French, W.L., & Bell, C.H. *Organization Development*. Englewood Cliffs, NJ: Prentice-Hall, 1973.

Gottlieb, B.H., & Schroter, C. Collaboration and resource exchange between professionals and natural support systems. *Professional Psychology*, 1978, *9*, 614-622.

Guba, E.G. Development, diffusion and evolution. In T.L. Eidell and J.M. Kitchel (Eds.), *Knowledge Production and Utilization*. Eugene: University Council for Educational Administration, Center for the Advanced Study of Education Administration, University of Oregon, 1968.

Havelock, R.G. *Planning for Innovation Through Dissemination and Utilization*. Ann Arbor: Institute for Social Research, University of Michigan, 1969.

Heinemann, S., Perlmutter, F., & Yudin, L. The community mental health center and community awareness. *Community Mental Health Journal*, 1974, *10*, 221-227.

Hulme, T. Mental health consulting with religious leaders. *Journal of Religion and Health*, 1974, *29*, 607-613.

Iscoe, I. Community psychology and the competent community. *American Psychologist*, 1974, *29*, 607-613.

Iscoe, I., Bloom, B., & Spielberger, C. (Eds.). *Community Psychology in Transition*. Washington, DC: Hemisphere, 1977.

Ketterer, R.F., & Bader, B.C. *Issues in the Development of Consultation and*

Education Services. Final report submitted to the Michigan Department of Mental Health, December, 1977.

Ketterer, R.F. *Developing Practice-Relevant Research about Consultation and Education Services in Community Mental Health Centers.* Doctoral dissertation, University of Michigan, 1979. (unpublished)

Larsen, J.K., Norris, E.L., & Kroll, J. *Consultation and Its Outcome: Community Mental Health Centers.* Palo Alto, CA: American Institutes for Research, 1976.

Lippitt, G., & Lippitt, R. *The Consulting Process in Action.* La Jolla, CA: University Associates, 1978.

McCall, G.J., & Simmons, J.L. (Eds.). *Issues in Participant Observation.* Reading, MA: Addison-Wesley, 1969.

MacLennan, B.W., Quinn, R.D., & Shroeder, D. The scope of community mental health consultation. In F.V. Mannino, B.W. MacLennan, and M.F. Shore (Eds.), *The Practice of Mental Health Consultation.* Washington, DC: Mental Health Study Center, Division of Mental Health Service Programs NIMH, 1975, 3-24.

Mann, P.A. Establishing a mental health consultation program with a police department. *Community Mental Health Journal,* 1971, *7*, 118-126.

Mannino, F.V., & Shore, M.F. The effects of consultation: A review of empirical studies. *American Journal of Community Psychology,* 1975, *3*, 1-21.

Meyer, M.L., & Gerrard, M. Graduate training in community psychology. *American Journal of Community Psychology,* 1977, *5*, 155-164.

National Committee for Mental Health Education. *Mental Health Education—A Concept Paper.* March, 1977. (mimeo)

Parlett, M., & Hamilton, D. Evaluation as illumination: A new approach to the study of innovating programs. In G.V. Glass (Ed.), *Evaluation Studies Volume 1. Annual Review* Beverly Hills, CA: Sage 1976.

Patton, M.Q. *Utilization-Focused Evaluation.* Beverly Hills, CA: Sage, 1978.

President's Commission on Mental Health, Volume I. Washington, DC: U.S. Government Printing Office, 1978.

Rothman, J. *Planning and Organizing for Social Change: Action Principles from Social Science Research.* New York: Columbia University Press, 1974.

Ryan, W. *Blaming the Victim.* New York: Random House, 1971..

Schein, E.H. *Process Consultation: Its Role in Organization Development.* Reading, MA: Addison-Wesley, 1969.

Shure, M.B., Spivak, G., & Jaeger, M. Problem-solving, thinking and adjustment among disadvantaged pre-school children. *Child Development,* 1971, *42*, 1791-1803.

Silverman, P.R. The widow-to-widow program. *Mental Hygiene,* 1969, *53*, 333-337.

Taynor, J., Perry, J., & Fredericks, P. A brief program to upgrade the skills of community caregivers. *Community Mental Health Journal,* 1976, *12*, 13-19.

Zald, M. Sociology and community organization practice. In M. Zald (Ed.), *Organizing for Community Welfare.* Chicago: Quadrangle Books, 1967.

Zax, M., & Specter, G.A. *An Introduction to Community Psychology.* New York: John Wiley, 1974.

15

Research and Evaluation in Primary Prevention
Issues and Guidelines

Kenneth Heller
Indiana University
Richard H. Price
University of Michigan
Kenneth J. Sher
Indiana University

The desirability and potential utility of primary prevention as a mental health goal has become increasingly accepted both by the public and by mental health professionals (*Task Panel Report on Prevention,* 1978). Prevention was highlighted in the 1978 report from the President's Commission on Mental Health and "should by all rights be the glamour stock on the mental health market" (Herbert, 1979). Yet, there have been so few adequately evaluated prevention projects reported that doubts about the viability of prevention at both conceptual and practical levels have begun to surface (APA Monitor, 1979; Lamb & Zusman, 1979). Now we may be faced with the possible untimely eclipse of a concept of great promise before data have been collected to evaluate potential utility or effectiveness.

The aim of this chapter is to help rectify this problem by reviewing both conceptual and methodological difficulties associated with primary prevention research and then providing a framework that would be useful in stimulating prevention research and more systematically evaluating prevention demonstration projects. In the discussion that follows, we will use the term "research" in its most general sense. Clearly, prevention in mental health requires an extremely broad array of inquiry methods. At one extreme, basic research generating new knowledge of the etiology and epidemiology of various psychological disorders is needed. However, the results of such research may have only remote implications for decisions about actual prevention program implementation. At the other extreme, evaluation of whether a particular program has met its goals may play an important role in the decision to continue that program in the future; but may contribute little to our understanding of the disorder or the processes by which it was prevented from occurring, without further research to test the generality of program effects or to pinpoint the most crucial program ingredients. At this point in the beginning stages of the development of a prevention knowledge base and technology, both basic research and program evaluation studies are needed.

There is no doubt that research in primary prevention is a complex undertaking with conceptual ambiguities and methodological difficulties which impede the systematic collection of evidence. However, these impediments should not become an excuse for inaction. In attempting to learn about prevention, more is to be gained by taking action than by doing nothing. Even ineffective programs can lead to useful information if they are conducted in such a way that their results can be reliably assessed and reasons for lack of success can be determined (Heller & Monahan, 1977). Thus, our critique of prevention concepts and methods will be undertaken in a constructive spirit; and we expect that the proposed framework for designing and evaluating prevention programs that flows from this critique will serve as a spur to future prevention research.

Political Impediments to Primary Prevention Research

The current controversy surrounding the viability of primary prevention is, in part, a function of competing political and professional interest groups. There is now a fairly extensive network of public and private providers of direct mental health services, some of whom believe that resources devoted to prevention programs will jeopardize their livelihood by diverting funds from treatment. They see the gains in funding mental health services over the last two decades threatened by the rhetoric of prevention advocates who champion their position by pointing to the inefficiencies and low social utility of psychotherapeutic services. Untrained in prevention, many worry about their place in a future mental health system that downplays what they do best—direct ameliorative help to distressed individuals.

A second source of political opposition to prevention comes from fiscal and political conservatives, who, in advocating a general governmental cutback in social services, are opposed to any new programs. They are concerned with what they see as the grandiosity of prevention proposals that are not keyed to specific circumscribed disorders. They see community-wide prevention proposals with a population focus as increasing the risk of government interference and regulation in the lives of ordinary citizens. They worry about the potential waste and cost of community-wide programs, since many individuals who would receive such services might potentially manage quite well without them.

Our goal in raising these issues is not to enter the debate on their substance—for example, whether prevention programs are or are not more costly, potentially wasteful, more likely to lead to excessive government regulation, or are a realistic threat to the livelihood of practicing clinicians. We believe that the best way to resolve these issues is to collect evidence from prevention demonstration projects that would facilitate rational decision-making. Some of the negative consequences anticipated by the opponents of prevention *could* occur, but withholding funding for demonstration projects because political and professional lobbying has convinced policymakers that they *will* occur ultimately is a disservice to all. Obviously, political lobbying and professional and organizational self-interests always will affect the fate of social innovations. The issue is whether political decisions will be made without evidence—whether prevention will be discarded before serious efforts to implement and evaluate the concept and its limits are attempted.

An example of the importance of evidence as a prerequisite for policy-making can be seen in some of the recent controversy surrounding the possibilities for prevention-oriented programs for the schizophrenic disorders. Eisenberg (Note 1) raises the possibility that to the extent that the schizophrenic disorders involve inherited predispositions, effective community-based treatment, by restoring patients to the community and increasing the likelihood of marriage and procreation, adds schizophrenia-related genes to the transmissible gene pool. The same criticism, of course, would apply to prevention programs that prevented the appearance of schizophrenic behavior but did not reduce genetic predisposition. While this argument may sound plausible, and indeed was used over 100 years ago to justify extended custodial care for mental patients and other "undesirables" (Caplan, 1969), the issue really cannot be decided without evidence. Equally plausible is the possibility that "schizophrenic genes," if not expressed, may actually lead to greater adaptability. For example, the association between creativity and schizophrenia in the same bloodlines has been noted (Heston, 1970). Furthermore, there are some genetic disorders in which a partial genetic loading actually contributes to greater immunity to other disorders (for example, a nondominant genetic loading for sickle cell anemia contributes to lowered susceptibility for malaria). The point is that there is absolutely no evidence that "schizophrenic genes" in the gene pool contribute to a weakening of the genetic stock, or that effective prevention programs would lead to a perceptible increase in the genetic loading for schizophrenia in the general population. Unfounded fears such as these, based upon untested speculation, should not determine prevention policy

The ultimate justification for prevention research is that some social good has been accomplished. For this reason, it is our strong conviction that prevention proponents will lose the political battle for funding without good data which is capable of documenting the effectiveness and social utility of prevention programs. We are not naively suggesting that political decisions are made on the basis of evidence alone. However, we do believe that data can and should be part of policy deliberations. If policy is made for political reasons despite contrary evidence, at least policymakers and their constituents should be aware that this is what has occurred.

To say that good research is needed will appear simply as a pious platitude if at the same time we do not address the impediments that have made research in this field so difficult. Nor would we be reacting constructively if we could not suggest how some of the complexities in the field could be resolved. Thus, we now turn to a discussion of some of the major conceptual and methodological constraints on research in primary prevention.

Conceptual Issues in
Primary Prevention Research

Despite the apparent simplicity and appeal of prevention, anyone who has seriously contemplated the design of a specific prevention project immediately is struck by the difficulties in implementation. The reality is that current prevention concepts do not provide an adequate conceptual base from which prevention research can be derived. There are a number of reasons for the current conceptual inadequacy.

Prevention definitions are goal statements that do not specify how prevention goals can be operationalized. The basic, widely accepted definition of primary prevention seems straightforward and easy to understand—reducing the incidence of disorder in populations. Most often definitions of primary prevention appear juxtaposed with those of secondary and tertiary prevention. Thus, Caplan (1964: 16-17) states that prevention involves programs for reducing

> (1) the incidence of mental disorders of all types in a community (primary prevention), (2) the duration of a significant number of those disorders which do occur (secondary prevention), and (3) the impairment which may result from those disorders (tertiary prevention)

Bolman (1969), in essential agreement with the above, adds some simplifying language to the definition:

> Primary prevention attempts to prevent a disorder from occurring. Secondary prevention attempts to identify and treat at the earliest possible moment so as to reduce the length and severity of disorder. Tertiary prevention attempts to reduce to a minimum the degree of handicap or impairment that results from a disorder that has already occurred. From the standpoint of the community, these distinctions are equivalent to reducing incidence, prevalence and extent of disability respectively [1969: 208].

Notice that neither of the definitions above specifies operations by which the goals of reduced incidence, prevalence, or lowered disability are to be achieved. While the goal of preventing psychological disorder implies a noble, socially useful undertaking that many could agree should have high social utility, it is astounding that the rhetoric of prevention advocates has not dealt with the core problem of specifying operations by which prevention goals might be realized.

Undoubtedly, there are a number of valid reasons why the specification of prevention operations rarely has been addressed systematically. The field of prevention is new and a great deal of effort was required initially to accomplish a conceptual reorientation. As Cowen (1973) has pointed out, the dominant view in the mental health fields involved an unquestioned acceptance of psychotherapy as the only way of helping people in distress. For many years conceptual alternatives were never seriously considered, "and without a change in how one looks at a problem a change in how one deals with that problem will not occur" (Heller & Monahan, 1977: 115).

A second impediment to specifying prevention operations is that knowledge about the etiology of mental disorders still is in such a rudimentary state that the design of prevention programs keyed to etiological factors is haunted by uncertainty and potential lack of precision. Historically, the primary advances in prevention occurred in those areas of public health in which diseases of bacterial or viral origin could be dealt with directly. In psychological disorders, single etiological factors responsible for the appearance of symptomatology are not likely to be found. Most psychological disorders appear to have multifactorial causation, and methodological limitations make it extremely difficult to find causal relationships between alleged etiological factors and eventual disorder. Prevention programing cannot depend upon the eventual discovery of a "magic bullet" (vaccine, vitamin, or drug) that will dramatically alter the incidence of disorder. The public health analogies to mental disorder are closer to those encountered in heart conditions and cancers than they are to disorders such as poliomyelitis or vitamin deficiency. Thus, the etiology of mental disorder needs to be conceptualized in multifactorial terms.

The importance of adopting multifactorial causation models in conceptualizing prevention activities. Price (1974) suggests that those concerned with mental disorder view etiology in terms of "multifactoral causation" or "risk factors" instead of simple causation. Following this orientation, Heller and Monahan suggest that

> the best analogy from physical medicine might be how we currently view the risk factors associated with the likelihood of heart disorders. We know that the risk factors associated with the appearance of heart attacks include genetic and constitutional factors, e.g., the extent to which there is a history of heart attacks in the family, age of onset, weight, and cholesterol level; but also includes life-style variables such as diet, amount of smoking and exercise, pace of life, and type of reaction to stress. There is no *one* "cause" of heart disorders but anyone demonstrating a large number of the above risk factors is statistically more vulnerable to the appearance of heart disorder than is an individual with a low risk loading. Similarly an individual can reduce the likelihood of a heart attack by reducing as many of the risk factors as possible—e.g., cut down on smoking, increase exercise, control diet, etc. [Heller & Monahan, 1977: 121].

What is particularly interesting about the heart disorder example is that over the last decade, the incidence of heart disorder in the general population has indeed gone down. While the reasons for reduced incidence are not completely clear, it does appear that large numbers of people have adopted lifestyle changes that have addressed a number of risk factors simultaneously. This example suggests a point that will be amplified in greater detail later. In order to discover the elements that should be included in a prevention package, research in prevention must tease apart the separate effects of individual risk factors (for example, the individual effects of weight loss, smoking, and alcohol consumption on the incidence of heart attacks). However, in order to maximize the likelihood of showing *population-wide* reduction in incidence, prevention programs probably will need to address a group of contributing risk factors simultaneously.

The cancer example in medicine also presents some interesting analogies to mental disorders. The exact causes of cancer are not known, but a number of risk factors have been identified in epidemiological and laboratory research with animals. The relative contribution of risk factors such as noxious environmental agents and personal predisposition also are unknown. It does appear that while not all individuals exposed to cancer-inducing conditions succumb, environmental contaminants do increase risk so that, given sufficient exposure, relatively immune individuals also would succumb. What is particularly intriguing about the cancer analogy is that appearance of disorder apparently often is delayed about 20 years after exposure. Thus, the best time to measure vulnerability is considerably delayed also.

In a similar manner, the risk period for many psychological disorders probably occurs not in childhood, when exposure to risk may be greatest, but in adulthood, when reaction patterns learned earlier become habitualized and entrenched. However, what complicates discovery of exact risk factors for the development of psychological difficulties is that a single discrete exposure to noxious environmental events probably does not cause irrevocable later symptomatology. As Barbara Dohrenwend (1978) has suggested, competent functioning is influenced by patterns of stressful events interacting with personal predispositional factors moderated by protective relationships with significant others. Thus, the risk factors associated with psychological disorder will be much more difficult to tease apart.

Still, there are advantages to conceptualizing prevention activities in terms of a multiple risk factor orientation. This view implies that intervention to reduce the incidence of dysfunctional behavior can occur at a number of levels. Prevention efforts might be oriented toward reducing the impact of environmental stress at community, organizational, or familial levels; or intervention programs might be aimed at strengthening the capacity of vulnerable populations to deal with that stress. The issue becomes one of empirical benefit. What types of interventions produce the best results at the least financial, societal, and psychic cost (Heller & Monahan, 1977: 121-122)?

The distinction between proximal programmatic objectives and distal prevention goals. The most popular way of thinking about prevention is in terms of "end-states" (Cowen, 1973) to be prevented. Yet, as we have already noted, global end-state goals cannot be dealt with in research without a clearer objective statement of the target behaviors to be reduced and a specification of the operations by which such goals are to be achieved. Furthermore, while reducing adverse end-states may be a distal goal of social interest, most prevention programs will have difficulty demonstrating an impact on such goals. To the extent that disorder develops over time in response to multiple interactive risk factors, other variables not accounted for in any specific prevention program also will influence the ultimate community-wide incidence of disorder.

If any single component prevention program by itself is unlikely to influence incidence rates, how can researchers hope to demonstrate effectiveness in this field? Basically, we must recognize that prevention research is faced with two separate problems. The first is to determine the effects on behavior of specific intervention programs. The second is to link proximal objectives such as effective behavior change (if the program was successful) with the ultimate reduction in rates for the end-state goals in question. For example, if the distal goal involves a reduction in delinquency rates, a first step would be to determine the risk factors that are most likely to contribute to high delinquency. Several could be specified, among which might be included poor school performance, troubled family relationships, parental alcoholism, antisocial behavior patterns among peers, few employment opportunities, and so on. Choosing one risk factor for example, school performance, a researcher might develop a program to improve poor school work through a tutorial reading program. However, is it likely that tutorial reading by itself will reduce delinquency rates? Probably not, and it would be misleading to expect that improved school performance alone would influence the distal goal of delinquency prevention. However, the research on whether school performance can be improved by a tutorial reading program should be done. When the data are in on how separate risk factors can be modified, we would be in a better position to mount intervention programs that combine a number of interventions which would be likely to impact on the distal goal. Thus, the steps we are advocating in the design of prevention programs involve collecting data on the effectiveness of specific intervention programs in modifying specific risk factors, and, as a separate question, determining what *combination* of interventions is most effective in producing an impact on ultimate prevention goals.

Competency enhancement as a prevention goal. Recently, many clinical and community psychologists have adopted a competency orientation; that is, they have begun to conceptualize their task as helping individuals develop psychosocial strengths (Albee & Joffee, 1977; Bloom, 1979; Kent & Rolf, 1979). In theory, competency enhancement is a legitimate prevention activity, for as Bloom (1965) points out, the prevention of disease can occur either by immunizing or strengthening the "host" (for example, immunizing an individual against smallpox) or by modification of the environment. Prevention activities from a competency enhancement view mean that programs could focus on building adaptive strengths with the assumption that a strengthened individual will be able to deal better with a variety of stresses that might eventually lead to disability. Thus, training children in social problem-solving skills has become a popular area in prevention research (Allen et al., 1976; Gesten et al., 1979; Shure, 1979; Shure & Spivack, 1979).

The issue is whether the basic assumption of this research is correct— whether individuals whose competencies are increased are less vulnerable to later disability. This empirical question will have to be addressed since we are skeptical of society's interest in funding "enhancement" programs that are not in some way related to distal goals of disorder prevention. While increased competency is a worthwhile objective in its own right, research still must be done to determine whether individuals so "immunized" are less vulnerable to disorder. We suspect that society will demand that such a link be demonstrated for the future continued funding of competency-based research.

Environment and person-centered interventions: risk situations and populations at risk. The concept of a population or a group at risk is well accepted in the prevention literature. A risk group can be defined as any group which, based on epidemiological evidence, shows a higher probability of developing psychological distress or disorder compared with the general population. Thus, children of emotionally disturbed or alcoholic parents, the unemployed, those entering retirement, or those who have been recently widowed all have been found to be at higher risk for psychological disorder than the general population.

Price (1980) suggests that as a conceptual aid in initiating prevention research, it may be useful to adopt a situation orientation to risk groups. People are members of risk groups not only because of individual characteristics they may possess but because they may be faced with situations that place high demands on adaptive capacity. In each of the examples above, altering some characteristic of the risk situation or event is at least as likely to reduce risk as is person-centered intervention whose purpose is to strengthen the coping capacity of the affected individual. For example, cooperative housing for the elderly can mitigate some of the isolation resulting from conjugal bereavement; alternative employment possibilities for the retired can prevent many of the consequences resulting from mandatory retirement; providing alternative adult parent figures as with Big Brothers and Big Sisters can partially compensate for the inconsistent parenting offered by disturbed or absent parents. Price (1979) argues that the advantages of a situational orientation to risk groups are both conceptual and practical. Attributions of causality (person or situation) strongly condition how we view the affected groups and how we intervene. Furthermore, the situational approach to prevention has a greater likelihood of leading to a focus on "movable" variables, those that can be more easily manipulated for the purposes of intervention.

Price (1979) proposes that researchers can utilize environmental data to design programs to increase adjustment in three ways: by means of setting *selection,* setting *change,* and setting *creation.* Settings can be selected, changed, or created in order to better "fit" individual needs and goals with setting characteristics. For example, helping individuals find recreation, leisure time, self-help groups, or educational institutions that best meet their needs qualify as setting selection interventions. Setting change might be accomplished by consultation and organization development, while setting creation occurs when groups develop alternative structures (for example, alternative schools) to meet their needs. Since much of the prevention literature is change-oriented, the possibilities of maximizing adjustive coping through setting selection often are overlooked. Most of us engage in setting selection naturally, on our own. That settings can be purposely selected as an intervention strategy comes as a surprise because we tend not to select settings in any conscious or systematic way. Setting selection strategies require careful attention to person and setting *assessment* in order to have some basis for matching. As Price (1979) notes, there is some reason for optimism about setting selection because the appropriate assessment tools are now coming into place.

The purpose of this section is to note that prevention research can be undertaken meaningfully from either a person- or environment-centered focus. We have emphasized the potential of conceptualizing prevention in terms of assessing and modifying risk situations because we believe that this perspective has still unrealized potential. Ultimately, an interactionist view that conceptualizes the development of disorder in terms of an interaction between persons and setting factors may prove to be of greatest value in reaching distal prevention goals. As a practical matter, we will probably achieve greater progress by first pinning down "main effects" (Nisbett, 1977) in prevention research. Thus, from the point of view of reaching proximal programmatic objectives, there are advantages to studying the separate effects of prevention programs aimed at either risk groups or risk situations.

Considerations in the choice of evaluation criteria: distinguishing between the preventive potential, effectiveness, cost, and popularity of intervention programs. Typically, in evaluating prevention programs the immediate concern is for effectiveness—Did the intervention "work" as anticipated in meeting the stated objectives? However, effectiveness is just one of several criteria by which prevention programs should be evaluated. Equally important in a full evaluation are *preventive potential* and *cost*; and distinguishing these from program *popularity*. *Preventive potential* refers to the extent to which the intervention contributes to the reduction in incidence of a prevention goal of high priority, one that is likely to have a fairly large mental health impact. For example, a program to improve the social skills of primary grade children might have greater priority than a similar program for mature adults; or a program oriented toward constructive recreational outlets for preteenagers in a high-crime neighborhood might have greater preventive potential than a similar program for adjudicated delinquents with chronic offense records. Of course, what might be considered a socially worthy project of high priority is subject to value judgments. In the examples just given, early intervention (that is, with children and high-risk preteenagers) is considered more socially valuable than later intervention. Other priorities for prevention activities might include problems that are important because of their frequency in the general population (such as family disruption associated with divorce) or problems that produce extensive social disruption (for example, widespread drug use). The point is that judgments of prevention potential can and should be made independent of other evaluation criteria. And, since they may be made covertly in the process of allocating research funds, such judgments should become more open. Procedures for rational decision-making outlined by Edwards, Guttentag, and Snapper (1975) and by Hammond and Adelman (1976) can be used in the process of determining prevention priorities.

Cost includes not only the financial expense associated with the program but also the extent to which it is labor-intensive. Programs which utilize high staff-client ratios or involve individual one-to-one relationships are extremely costly, particularly when the provider of service is a highly trained professional. For example, intensive individual psychotherapy programs are more costly to operate than similar programs staffed by paraprofessional counselors. Least costly of all might be group programs conducted by indigenous peer counselors. Another cost involves the negative side-effects that may accrue from program adoption. For example, without adequate staff preparation and training, programs to mainstream emotionally disturbed or retarded youngsters are likely to increase stress in schools and raise the probability that such children will be stigmatized by other children. If research indicates that all are equally effective in terms of distal prevention goals (such as delinquency prevention), cost becomes a major criterion in deciding which should be implemented.

All of the above can be distinguished from the public and professional popularity of a program. *Popular* programs typically are those which are concordant with the social values of the groups in question. Thus, a "prevention" program which deals harshly with first-offense drug users might receive wide endorsement from the public but yet show little preventive potential or effectiveness and, in the long run, might be quite costly to implement. Programs can be popular with professionals as well, advocated for reasons of social value concordance rather than because of other evaluation criteria such as cost or effectiveness. The current interest in child abuse prevention is an example of a professionally popular program with little data on preventive potential, effectiveness, or cost.

Distinguishing among these evaluation outcomes is important in the design and eventual adoption and dissemination of prevention demonstration projects. For example, if there is a choice, labor-intensive interventions should be avoided despite the fact that the one-to-one therapy tradition in the mental health fields will probably lead program designers to think first of interventions of this sort. Similarly, programs that clash with popular public values are least likely to be adopted regardless of effectiveness demonstrated. Most program designers know this to be the case and would claim that they never intentionally design an unpopular program. A problem occurs when public and professional popularity are confused. There are numerous instances of programs designed primarily in concordance with professional values, which, when mounted with outside grant funds, are never adopted in local communities beyond the demonstration grant period—primarily because of discordance with local customs and mores.

Methodological Impediments to
Research in Primary Prevention

There is no dispute that research in applied settings is a difficult undertaking. In an important methodological critique, Cowen (1978) points to a number of specific hazards associated with community research and notes that many of these hazards are not easily surmountable. Cowen's conclusions about the realities of community research are worth repeating:

> Communities are many things. One thing they are not is an ideal laboratory for antiseptic psychological studies. Their extraordinary complexity, omnipresent flux, action-service orientation, and susceptibility to day-to-day pressures present real and formidable barriers to "Mr. Clean" program evaluation studies. These factors place major constraints on the design of studies, the types of criteria that can be used, and the rigor of sophistication of the control that can be exercised. Although some of those problems can be reduced through judicious planning, others, quite beyond the experimenter's control, cannot. This is one reason why theory, logic, and the actual development and implementation of new community programs have outpaced the field's supporting research base. . . .

> Much can be done to strengthen community program evaluation technology and to design studies that reduce sources of confound or error. Weaknesses in specific measures or in classes of criteria typically used in community program outcome research dictate that greater emphasis be placed on converging sources of evidence. But we must still expect that community realities will remain to militate against ideal research studies. The vulnerability of findings from any single community evaluation study points to the importance both of replication and of tolerance for a slow accretive process, in which small pieces in a puzzle gradually cumulate toward weight-of evidence conclusions about major new programming approaches [Cowen, 1978: 803-804]

There are several useful sources that discuss difficulties in initiating and evaluating research in applied settings (Attkisson et al., 1978; Bennett & Lumsdaine, 1975; Campbell, 1969; Riecken et al., 1974), including some particularly helpful in overcoming impediments to meaningful community research (Bloom, 1968; Cook & Campbell, 1979; Muñoz et al., 1979; Price & Politser, 1980; Price, Note 2). At this point, we would like to summarize some key methodological points to be found in these sources which have particular relevance to research in primary prevention. Then we will note additional problems unique to primary prevention research. In noting these difficulties, our point is not to encourage despair about the possibilities of obtaining useful information about prevention, but to emphasize that progress in this field will be made in small steps by the slow accumulation of knowledge from studies none of which may be perfect. We agree with Goldstein, Heller, and Sechrest (1966) that "weak research is not worthless research" and that "a series of individually faulty research studies with no consistent methodological weakness may add up to a fairly convincing conclusion" (Goldstein et al., 1966: 18). This statement is not to be taken as an apology for poor research that is not as good as it could be, but is a realistic statement of what researchers and the potential consumers of their research might expect. For us, recognition of this reality implies *more* research, not less, so that the accumulation of needed evidence will occur.

Common Problems Faced by Research in Applied Settings

Specification of Target Behaviors

The target of intervention attempts needs precise definition. It is not sufficient to expect "better mental health" or "improved adjustment" to result from an intervention. These concepts are themselves so global and undifferentiated that their use might lead to reports of ineffective intervention when in fact specific effects might have been demonstrated. Future work in prevention should carefully spell out the specific effects expected from preventive interventions and then develop precise, specific measures of these targeted behaviors (Heller & Monahan, 1977: 141-142).

Specification of the Intervention

Parallel to the need for precision in measuring outcome is the need to more clearly define the intervention itself. If multiple-component interventions are used, each should be clearly defined and the outcome expected from each should be specified.

Without specification of target behaviors or interventions we will be unable to answer the questions: Did change occur as a result of the intervention? And, if so, what factors produced the change?

Representative Designs and
Generalization of Prevention Effects

Brunswik (1947) and Hammond (1954) have emphasized the importance of sampling from a universe of experimental conditions in order to reach conclusions that transcend a particular setting.

> Brunswik's main argument was that in order to generalize beyond a study's specific circumstances, one need not only have an adequate subject N, which most experiments do, but also experimental conditions that represent, statistically, the universe of circumstances to which the experimenter hopes to generalize [Cowen, 1978: 795].

The danger is in overgeneralizing from the results of a particular study, no matter how significant they may appear. For example, a social competency prevention program administered in one school to a sample of 200 third and fourth graders provides evidence about social competency in that one school, but not necessarily in other schools elsewhere. For purposes of generalization, the N of the study is *one,* not 200. Obviously, what this point highlights is the importance of replication. Because of the time-consuming nature of prevention studies, replication of one study at a time may be an inefficient way to proceed. A team of investigators working on the same problem using the same methodology but at different sites in the long run may be more effective. Such a coordinated effort probably would require an active research center for primary prevention at the national level.

Next, we turn to a consideration of methodological problems unique to research in primary prevention.

Problems Associated with
the Prevention of Low Base Rate Disorders

A special problem arises in prevention research in that the end-state disorders to be prevented often occur at extremely low rates in the general population. For example, problem drinking is estimated to occur in 10 percent of the general population; more severe alcoholism in three percent of the population; and schizophrenic disorders in one percent of the population. There are several problems for the researcher in working with such low base rate phenomena. (1) Finding sufficient cases to constitute a risk group can be difficult. For example, even assuming 100 percent concordance between risk markers and the eventual appearance of disorder, one would have to screen 1000 individuals in the general population to find ten who might be schizophrenia-prone and possible subjects for a prevention study. (2) If a community-wide methodology is employed, most individuals who would receive an intervention designed to prevent a low base rate disorder from appearing would probably never need it. Again, using the schizophrenia example, in a community-wide intervention study, 99 persons would needlessly receive an intervention that would be appropriate for only one in 100 individuals. (3) Regardless of the methodology used, even powerful interventions for low base rate disorders will have difficulty demonstrating statistical significance unless extremely large numbers of subjects are used.

This last point is illustrated in Table 15.1, which shows the sample size needed to find a statistically significant difference between two observed proportions. In this example, it will be assumed that the intervention group was found to have half as many cases of disorder after intervention as the control group (an apparently very effective intervention). However, as can be seen in the table, the sample size needed to detect a significant difference even for an effective intervention increases dramatically as the base rate of the disorder decreases.

There are no ideal solutions to the above dilemmas. One possibility is to accept less stringent criteria for statistical significance recognizing that, at least in the initial stages of research in which intervention programs are being refined, trends in the data will be worthy of follow-up. A second possiblity is to concentrate on problems of higher frequency in the general population. This is Cowen's (1973) point when he suggests that researchers become less concerned with rooted dysfunction. He argues that concentration on those with profound but infrequent disorders at the expense of the many who are less severely disturbed basically is less democratic. He argues that we should not automatically accept the proposition put forth by some (Joint Commission on Mental Illness and Health, 1961; Zusman & Lamb, 1977) that the severe mental disorders are the number-one priority for the mental health professions.

A third strategy involves sharpening the risk group methodology by collecting epidemiological data on risk situations and populations at risk so that intervention is provided to the most vulnerable groups. For example, Farberow (1974) reports that the total suicide rate for the United States in 1968 was 10.7 per 100,000 persons. When only white males are considered, this rate jumps to 16.9; and if we further restrict our population to white males over 55 years of age, the rate approaches 40 per 100,000. However, while it makes sense to target the intervention at the most

TABLE 15.1   Minimum Sample Sizes Needed to Demonstrate a Significant (.05) Difference Between Experimental and Control Groups*

If the proportion of problem cases in the control group after program completion was:	. . . and the proportion of the problem cases in the experimental group after program completion was:	. . . then minimum N needed per group would be:
.50	.25	22
.20	.10	69
.10	.05	151
.01	.005	1611

*For an intervention that reduced the incidence of problem behavior by 50 percent.

vulnerable groups, in this example, the group composed of older, white males still would be expected to yield only a small number of suicide casualties, making evaluation of suicide prevention difficult. Another example of a higher base rate problem can be provided. In 1970, the divorce rate in the United States was 1400 per 100,000 married men and women (National Center for Health Statistics, 1978). When only married men and women under 30 are considered, the divorce rate doubles to approximately 3000 per 100,000. Thus, it would make sense to target divorce prevention programs at younger married couples. Base rates would be high enough in many communities to permit meaningful statistical analyses of results.

The Need for Long-Term Follow-Up: Implications for Research Policy

While lengthy follow-up to test for deterioration effects is to be recommended in any intervention study, it is particularly crucial in prevention studies. Since primary prevention deals with groups before disorder has become manifest, the effectiveness of the intervention cannot be fully assessed until the groups in question have passed through their period of greatest risk. For example, the period of greatest risk for alcoholism and schizophrenic disorders extends from early to middle adulthood. Assuming preventive intervention occurred during childhood or the early teens, one would have to wait for decades to determine whether the interventions had been successful. The possiblity of having to wait for a period that might take up the productive lifetime of the researcher in order to determine whether a particular intervention was effective should give pause to any investigator.

The need for long-term follow-up also points to why prevention research requires a long-term policy committment at the federal level. Now that policymakers may be accepting the logic of prevention, they must recognize that it is often not realistic to expect immediate results. Federal agencies collecting prevention data need to be buffered from political forces that push for quick answers and which force investigators to overpromise in order to receive funding. Without an appreciation of how long it will take to produce definitive data on the reduction in incidence of many distal prevention goals there will be inevitable disillusionment with prevention as a realistic enterprise.

Fisher and Jones (1978) have illustrated the above point by describing an impediment to long-term risk research associated with current funding practices. They state:

> Since longitudinal programs must compete for funds with non-longitudinal programs, and since relatively short-term programs produce findings and publications rapidly, longitudinal projects are faced with a disadvantage in terms of repeatedly demonstrating productivity. To justify their existence in this competitive framework, investigators in longitudinal research often invest heavily in data analysis for grant renewals and yearly reports even though the analyses are on partial samples and are of little practical or theoretical use [Fisher & Jones, 1978: 228-229].

We are not suggesting that prevention researchers be given a "blank check" to do what they wish for 20-40 years without public accountability. For many prevention goals, the period of greatest risk occurs early. School phobia, delinquency, and problem-solving competency in children are examples of prevention targets that can be assessed more immediately. Furthermore, useful data can be collected even though decisions about the ultimate achievement of distal prevention goals are deferred. Data on proximal programmatic objectives can be assessed; and age-adjusted incidence figures can be collected to determine whether an intervention is "on track." For example, an alcoholism prevention program might be able to demonstrate a reduction in teenage drinking even though figures for the overall reduction in alcoholism in the general population had not yet been collected. Of course, the early incidence figures by themselves would not be sufficient. It is possible that a program might delay onset but not reduce ultimate incidence of a disorder. Still, a program that delayed onset would be socially useful by increasing the number of years of problem-free, productive living.

The need for lengthy follow-up has implications not only for funding policies and how long we should wait to expect meaningful results, but for organizational issues within the prevention project. Fisher and Jones (1978) note that the long-term time commitment and procedural difficulties of carrying out longitudinal research can lead to investigator "burnout," and that project responsibility by only one or two principal investigators may not be the best model for lengthy prospective studies. To complicate matters further, when project length is long, as should be expected in prevention research, turnover of key staff members becomes more likely. One way of possibly protecting against these potential difficulties is to distribute the responsibility for carrying out prevention research among several persons to maximize the likelihood for project continuity.

Guidelines for the Development and Evaluation of Prevention Programs

Basically, there are three components in a prevention program that need specification:

(1) *The prevention target*—consisting of the populations at risk and/or risk situations that are expected to lead to vulnerability;

(2) *the program or intervention*—consisting of person and/or environmentally oriented procedures to reduce vulnerability; and

(3) *the expected outcome*—consisting of proximal programmatic objectives and distal end-state goals.

A survey of existing prevention programs might reveal that not all have clearly specified each of the above components. Some might be clear about what was to be prevented—that is, the end state—but quite unclear about who precisely was to be reached and how prevention was to be accomplished. Other programs might be relatively clear about who was at risk, but much less clear about what they were at risk for and how prevention efforts should have proceeded. Still others might be clear about the prevention program to be undertaken but relatively less specific about precisely what was to be prevented and who was to be reached in the process of doing so (Price, Note 2).

In the initial stages of program development, lack of specificity about one or more components should not be of great concern. Indeed, we should recognize that effective primary prevention often involves a two-stage process. Program development is the first stage, and only when the details have been carefully worked out are we ready for the second stage—a full-fledged test of the effectiveness of program activities. Program designers cannot do both simultaneously, despite pressure from sponsors for quick results.

Although a program may start with a clear focus on only one of the components of a prevention program, eventually all will need to be considered. Hence, we now move to a discussion of the components of prevention programs emphasizing the questions that should be asked and information that should be collected for each. Table 15.2 presents these points in a summary format.

The Prevention Target

What specific risk situation or population at risk will be studied?

What is the evidence for the risk potential of the particular situation or the evidence for the suspected vulnerability for the group at risk?

In conceptualizing the prevention target, the point of entry is to define the risk group as specifically as possible. The place to begin is with the prior literature concerning the nature of the environmental stress, life transition, or risk group in question. For example, well-controlled epidemiological surveys (Berkman & Syme, 1979; Kraus & Lilienfeld, 1959) indicate that death, divorce, or separation from a spouse places individuals at risk for both physical and psychological disability. Furthermore, the evidence concerning death of a spouse indicates that young widowers are at greater risk than young widows. An intervention aimed at this risk group obviously could not prevent spouse death, but could be aimed at smoothing the readjustment needed in response to a tragic event of this sort.

The Program or Intervention

What specific procedures are employed to deal with the risk elements in the environment; or what specific procedures are used to increase coping capacity?

TABLE 15.2   Specification of Target Groups, Program Elements, and
Expected Outcomes of Prevention Programs

The prevention target: Specifying target groups and situations

Generic Questions	*Examples of available data*
What is the evidence for the suspected vulnerability of the specific target group?	Base rate and correlational data concerning negative outcomes associated with specific population characteristics (e.g. data on disability, developmental delay, disadvantage or subjective distress associated with possible risk markers such as age, sex, race, family history, economic status, geographic location, etc. Data can be obtained from epidemiological or community surveys, social indicators or formal research reports.
What is the evidence for the risk potential of the specific target situation?	Base rate and correlational data concerning negative outcomes associated with specific settings or events (e.g. data on disability, developmental delay, disadvantage or subjective distress associated with settings such as work or school environments or events such as separation, loss, hospitalization, or school or work transitions. Data can be obtained from epidemiological or community surveys, social indicators or formal research reports.

The prevention program: Specifying program elements

Generic Questions	*Examples of program components*
What specific procedures are to be employed to increase the coping capacity of the target population?	Educational programs, skill training curricula, stress management workshops, social problem solving training – described in manuals, written outlines, recordings of training sessions, case examples, etc.
What specific procedures are to be employed to reduce the risk producing features of the environment?	*Setting selection components*: Matching persons to setting such as schools, day care centers, support or interest groups – described by detailed outline of matching procedures utilized. *Setting change components*: Designing programs in existing social institutions such as schools, churches, hospitals or recreational or religious settings. Program consultation and organization development – described by program manuals, written outlines and summaries of progress notes.

TABLE 15.2   Specification of Target Groups, Program Elements, and
Expected Outcomes of Prevention Programs (Cont)

Setting creation components: Establishing new settings such as interest and support groups, alternative schools, residential units, churches, community organizations, etc. — described by written outlines and summaries of progress notes.

Expected outcomes: Monitoring objectives and goals

Generic Questions	*Types of evidence*
What is the evidence that the program elements were successfully implemented?	Attendance records, dropout rates, behavior observation samples, contact documentation, survey feedback and recipient service delivery interviews.
What is the evidence that the proximal program objectives were met?	*Coping capacity*: criterion tests of new skills, knowledge, abilities, attitudes or behaviors of the target population. *Setting selection, change or creation*: documentation of change in attitude, knowledge or behavior of setting participants.
What is the evidence for program popularity; cost; and impact on other systems?	Citizen surveys, interviews with program participants; service load data, cost per unit of service delivery; changes in service load of other human service agencies.
What is the evidence that the distal prevention goals have been met?	Longitudinal evidence, follow-up studies, or epidemiological surveys indicating a reduction in specific negative outcomes for which the interventions were originally designed.

Is there any prior evidence concerning the expected effectiveness of the procedures employed?

Preventive interventions seem to fall into two general types: those oriented toward competence-building (for example, family life education, parent effectiveness training, stress management, or problem-solving skill-building), or those which are systems-change-oriented programs (such as organization development and consultation, linking and network-building strategies, the development of alternative settings, and community organization).

Regardless of type, the intervention should be specified clearly. In many cases, specification of who does what to whom should be done early in the planning of the project and can be clarified in project manuals. Role specifications, job descriptions, and program procedures should be made clear at the outset.

Prior evidence concerning the expected effectiveness of the procedures employed can come from a variety of sources—clinical case descriptions, field trials, laboratory experimentation, or even research with animals. For example, data reported by Suomi (1979) on the importance of peer interactions for the development of social competence in rhesus monkeys might serve as a basis for developing interventions based on peer interactions in human infants. According to Suomi, depriving young rhesus monkeys of the opportunity to interact with peers results in incompetent play and uncontrolled aggression. While fostering peer interactions may not offset deficient or absent parenting, it does seem to provide the opportunity for infant monkeys to develop social skills needed in normal adult social functioning. Suomi's work suggests that infant peer groups providing opportunity for interactive play might be beneficial for the social development of human infants who have limited access to peers. His work also suggests that the composition of such groups should be heterogeneous with respect to the level of social skills of the members, since if all or most group members were deficient in social skills, continued social interactions among group members might not be beneficial. Although the applicability of animal research to human behavior remains an empirical question, the monkey data can provide the prevention worker with some ideas and a starting point for developing an intervention. Evaluation of the outcome of the intervention will be able to answer questions regarding efficacy.

Expected Outcomes:
Monitoring Proximal Programmatic Objectives
and Distal End-State Goals

What specific end state is to be prevented?

What specific programmatic objectives could be expected to contribute to the reduced incidence of the end state in question?

Was the intervention successfully implemented?

What changes occurred as a result of the intervention? Were changes in targeted groups different from changes in comparison groups; or were changes in targeted groups different from changes in these same groups during initial baseline periods of nonintervention?

Were there any changes in significant others or nearby "systems"?

What were the financial and social costs associated with the intervention?

We start the evaluation of outcome with the recognition that reduction in incidence in a distal end-state goal may be unattainable in a single study. While end-state goals should be specified so that the eventual direction of the project can be seen, programs should be more realistically focused on the specification and attainment of proximal objectives.

Measuring the attainment of program objectives obviously requires careful attention to assessment issues. Whether the measuring instrument is a psychological test, a neurological technique, observer ratings of overt behavior, or changes in demographic statistics, traditional concerns for reliability and validity still apply.

An important part of the evaluation involves monitoring the program itself for consistency over time. It will be impossible to properly evaluate a project that was not fully implemented or one in which participation was inconsistent. For example, a consultation program offered to school teachers in a particular district might find that only some of the teachers actually participated or that teacher participation declined steadily throughout the course of the project. Testing for the effectiveness of consultation under these conditions of haphazard program administration would be virtually meaningless.

Testing for the presence of change that legitimately can be attributed to the intervention is the heart of the evaluation. The literature on experimental and quasi-experimental program evaluation procedures is extensive, and there is little we can add except to remind the reader of a few basic caveats of community evaluation. We need to look for effects not only among target groups but in significant others or nearby "systems" likely to be affected by the intervention indirectly. For example, anticipated increases in welfare costs or cases brought before the criminal justice system are the often-cited indirect effects of deinstitutionalization programs. Of course, indirect effects can be positive as well as negative, such as when improved parenting skill increases self-esteem among program participants and establishes a "ripple" effect through other spheres of functioning.

A related question concerns the costs of the intervention both to participants and to society more generally. Included here are costs associated with community-wide interventions which provide program benefits to all, including those who do not need them, as well as costs to individuals singled out for intervention and possibly stigmatized for participation. In some cases, the costs may be relatively minor as, for example, in the standard procedure of placing drops of silver nitrate in the eyes of newborn infants in order to avoid blindness in the child as a result of undiagnosed maternal gonorrhea. In other cases the costs may be more substantial, as in removing children from the care of parental child abusers only to find that parental separation and alternative placement for the child may result in greater long-term psychological damage to all participants.

It should be clear that answers to the questions posed in this section will require the sustained effort of groups of investigators approaching prevention questions from a number of different vantage points—that is, using different experimental methodologies on the same prevention question. The kind of research we are advocating will take at least five to ten years of research collaboration between research centers, local communities, and funding groups in order to provide meaningful research data. Answering questions about prevention effectiveness is not an easy task, but it can be accomplished *if* we are willing to invest the resources in long-term research. To do so requires vision, planning, and a commitment to prevention research that transcends immediate political expediency.

Conclusion

We close this chapter with a sense of guarded optimism. Primary prevention as applied to psychological difficulties is a concept of untested promise. Despite conceptual ambiguities that have retarded the generation of crisply defined research variables and methodological impediments that make research perfection extremely unlikely, good research can be done. With sustained effort, we can contribute to our slowly growing knowledge of the possibilities and limitations of primary prevention.

Price (Note 2) suggests that we adopt a "bootstrapping" perspective to research in primary prevention, explicitly recognizing that the way to acquire new knowledge in this field is to do the research that moves us along in slow incremental steps—"pulling ourselves up by our bootstraps, using our current but imperfect knowledge as a beginning point in reaching the goals of effective, well documented prevention programs."

An implication of this view emphasizes the importance of public and professional patience. The public, through its elected representatives and government administrators, must understand that a long-term commitment to research without immediate pay-off is required if primary prevention is to be pursued as a societal goal. Professional patience, too, is required because prevention research initially will appear unrewarding, since distal prevention questions cannot be adequately addressed until proximal program effects are established. For example, in determining whether social problem-solving skills have preventive potential for elementary school children, it will first have to be established that children can learn the problem-solving curriculum; that they use it in school and elsewhere in daily life to solve stressful social problems; and that the skills learned are retained over time. Only then would we be prepared for a meaningful answer to the question of whether those provided the training, who use and retain its key elements, are subject to less psychological disability later in life than those who do not receive the training.

Although distal prevention goals require that effects be demonstrated over an extended time period, we must be prepared for the possibility that prevention effects are likely to be more circumscribed. Behavior change may occur in specific situations but may not generalize across settings or persist over time. This may occur not because the intervention produced only weak effects, but as a result of intervening real-life events that pull for different behaviors. For example, it is unreasonable to expect that children exposed to a one-year Head Start enrichment program will maintain intellectual progress if they are exposed to impoverished school environments for the next ten years. While maintenance and generalization elements should be built into interventions (Heller & Monahan, 1977: 240) specifically to increase the likelihood that effects will persist (for example, teaching children how to concentrate in noisy environments), we must recognize that even the best programs can be eroded by undesirable environmental conditions. In this regard, we hope that the current popularity of competency enhancement programs (basically person-centered interventions) does not divert us from the importance of concurrent research on environmental change.

The list of still unanswered questions about primary prevention is long and includes issues of both theoretical and practical import. One particularly current example with obvious practical implications concerns the repeated claims for social support as a buffer against the deleterious effects of stress. It is believed that support can provide individuals with a generalized invulnerability. However, our reading of the relevant literature leads us to expect that the positive effects of support probably are more modest and circumscribed; and we believe that it is unrealistic to expect that social networks provide automatic stress "immunity." Note that not very long ago clinicians believed that close ties to others, particularly family members, were a significant source of stress for their patients. The goal of therapy often was to disengage from family influence in order to achieve independence. Obviously, families can be either sources of stress or support. What is crucial to the proper understanding and utilization of social support as a prevention strategy is to understand the specific conditions under which close ties to others lead to either positive or negative outcomes (Heller, 1979).

The point is that most of the still unanswered questions about prevention are amenable to research investigation. If we can avoid the pressures that push us toward demanding immediate answers to complex questions, we can improve our knowledge of primary prevention. Furthermore, no matter how much we may personally believe that prevention is a "good idea," without the accumulation of some supporting evidence, it is unlikely that public interest and funding can be sustained. Unfortunately, at this point, little prevention research has been published (Novaco & Monahan, in press). The goal of this chapter has been to demonstrate that the conceptual and methodological tools exist which can help to overcome this deficiency.

Notes

1. Eisenberg, L. A research framework for evaluating health promotion and disease prevention. Presented at the First Annual Alcohol Drug Abuse and Mental Health Administration Conference on Prevention, Silver Spring, Maryland, September 12-14, 1979.

2. Price, R.H. Evaluation research in primary prevention: Lifting ourselves by our bootstraps. Presented at the Primary Prevention Conference sponsored by the Community Mental Health Institute, National Council of Community Mental Health Centers, Denver, Colorado, June 11, 1978.

References

Albee, G.W., & Joffe, J.M. (Eds.). *Primary Prevention of Psychopathology. Volume I. The Issues.* Hanover, NH: University Press of New England, 1977.

Allen, G.J., Chinsky, J.M., Larcen, S.W., Lochman, J.E., & Selinger, H.V. *Community Psychology and the Schools: A Behaviorally Oriented Multilevel Preventive Approach.* Hillsdale, NJ: Lawrence Erlbaum, 1976.

APA Monitor, 1979, *5.* (Special issue focus on prevention)

Attkisson, C.C., Hargreaves, W.A., Horowitz, M.J., & Sorensen, J.E. *Evaluation of Human Service Programs.* New York: Academic Press, 1978.

Bennett, C.A., & Lumsdaine, A.A. (Eds.). *Evaluation and Experiment: Some Critical Issues in Assessing Social Programs.* New York: Academic Press, 1975.

Berkman, L.F., & Syme, S.L. Social networks, host resistance and mortality: A nine year follow-up study of Alameda County residents. *American Journal of Epidemiology,* 1979, *109,* 186-204.

Bloom, B.L. The "medical model", miasma theory, and community mental health. *Community Mental Health Journal,* 1965, *1,* 333-338.

Bloom, B.L. The evaluation of primary prevention programs. In L.M. Roberts, N.S., Greenfield and M.H. Miller (Eds.), *Comprehensive Mental Health: The Challenge of Evaluation.* Madison: University of Wisconsin Press, 1968.

Bloom, B.L. Prevention of mental disorders: Recent advances in theory and practice. *Community Mental Health Journal,* 1979, *15,* 179-191.

Bolman, W.M. Toward realizing the prevention of mental illness. In L. Bellak and H.H. Barten (Eds.), *Progress in Community Mental Health, Volume I.* New York: Grune & Stratton, 1969.

Brunswik, E. *Systematic and Representative Design of Psychological Experiments.* Berkeley: University of California Press, 1947.

Campbell, D.T. Reforms as experiments. *American Psychologist,* 1969, *24,* 409-429.

Caplan, G. *Principles of Preventive Psychiatry.* New York: Basic Books, 1964.

Caplan, R.B. *Psychiatry and the Community in Nineteenth Century America: The Recurring Concern with the Environment in the Prevention and Treatment of Mental Illness.* New York: Basic Books, 1969.

Cook, T.D., & Campbell, D.T. *Quasi-Experimentation: Design and Analysis Issues for Field Settings.* Chicago: Rand McNally, 1979.

Cowen, E.L. Social and community interventions. *Annual Review of Psychology,* 1973, *24,* 423-472.

Cowen, E.L. Some problems in community program evaluation research. *Journal of Consulting and Clinical Psychology,* 1978, *46,* 792-805.

Dohrenwend, B.S. Social stress and community psychology. *American Journal of Community Psychology,* 1978, *6,* 1-14.

Edwards, W., Guttentag, M., & Snapper, K. A decision-theoretic approach to evaluation research. In E.L. Struening and M. Guttentag (Eds.), *Handbook of Evaluation Research. Volume I.* Beverly Hills, CA: Sage, 1975.

Farberow, N.L. *Suicide.* Morristown, NJ: General Learning Press, 1974.

Fisher, L., & Jones, F.H. Planning for the next generation of risk studies. *Schizophrenia Bulletin,* 1978, *4,* 223-235.

Gesten, E.L., Flores de Apodaca, R., Rains, M., Weissberg, R.P., & Cowen, E.L. Promoting peer-related social competence in schools. In M.W. Kent and J.E. Rolf (Eds.), *Primary Prevention of Psychopathology. Volume III: Social Competence in Children.* Hanover, NH: University Press of New England, 1979.

Goldstein, A.P., Heller, K., & Sechrest, L.B. *Psychotherapy and the Psychology of Behavior Change.* New York: John Wiley, 1966.

Hammond, K.R. Representative vs. systematic design in clinical psychology. *Psychological Bulletin,* 1954, *51,* 150-159.

Hammond, K.R., & Adelman, L. Science, values and human judgment. *Science,* 1976, *194,* 389-396.

Heller, K. The effects of social support: Prevention and treatment implications. In A.P. Goldstein .and F.H. Kanfer (Eds.), *Maximizing Treatment Gains: Transfer Enhancement in Psychotherapy.* New York: Academic Press, 1979.

Heller, K., & Monahan, J. *Psychology and Community Change.* Homewood, IL: Dorsey Press, 1977.

Herbert, W. The politics of prevention. *APA Monitor,* 1979, *10,* 5, 7-9.

Heston, L.L. The genetics of schizophrenic and schizoid disease. *Science,* 1970, *167,* 249-256.

Joint Commission on Mental Illness and Health. *Action for Mental Health*. New York: Basic Books, 1961.

Kent, M.W., & Rolf, J.E. *Primary Prevention of Psychopathology. Volume III. Social Competence in Children*. Hanover, NH: University Press of New England, 1979.

Kraus, A.S., & Lilienfeld, A.M. Some epidemiologic aspects of the high mortality rate in the young widowed group. *Journal of Chronic Disease, 1959, 10*, 207-217.

Lamb, H.R., & Zusman, J. Primary prevention in perspective. *American Journal of Psychiatry, 1979, 136*, 12-17.

Muñoz, R.F., Snowden, L.R., & Kelly, J.G. *Social and Psychological Research in Community Settings*. San Francisco: Jossey-Bass, 1979.

National Center for Health Statistics. Divorce and divorce rates: United States. *Vital and Health Statistics, 1978, 21* (29).

Nisbett, R.E. Interaction versus main effects as goals in personality research. In D. Magnusson and N.S. Endler (Eds.), *Personality at the crossroads: Current Issues in Interactional Psychology*. Hillsdale, NJ: Lawrence Erlbaum, 1977.

Novaco, R.W., & Monahan, J. Research in community psychology: An analysis of work published in the first six years of the *American Journal of Community Psychology*. *American Journal of Community Psychology*, in press.

Price, R.H. Etiology, the social environment, and the prevention of psychological dysfunction. In P. Insel and R.H. Moos (Eds.), *Health and the Social Environment*. Lexington, MA: D. C. Heath, 1974.

Price, R.H. The social ecology of treatment gain. In A.P. Goldstein and F.H. Kanfer (Eds.), *Maximizing Treatment Gains: Transfer Enhancement in Psychotherapy*. New York: Academic Press, 1979.

Price, R.H. Risky situations. In D. Magnusson (Ed.), *The situation: An Interactional Perspective*. Hillsdale, NJ: Lawrence Erlbaum, 1980.

Price, R.H., & Politser, P. (Eds.). *Evaluation and Action in the Social Environment* New York: Academic Pres, 1980.

Riecken, H.W., Boruch, R.F., Campbell, D.T., Caplan, N., Glennan, T.K., Pratt, J., Rees, A., & Williams, W. *Social Experimentation: A Method for Planning and Evaluating Social Intervention*. New York: Academic Press, 1974.

Shure, M.B. Training children to solve interpersonal problems: A preventive mental health program. In R.F. Muñoz, L.R. Snowden, and J.G. Kelly (Eds.), *Social and Psychological Research in Community Settings*. San Francisco: Jossey-Bass, 1979.

Shure, M.B., & Spivack, G. Interpersonal problem solving thinking and adjustment in the mother-child dyad. In M.W. Kent and J.E. Rolf (Eds.), *Primary Prevention of Psychopathology. Volume III. Social Competence in Children*. Hanover, NH: University Press of New England, 1979.

Suomi, S.J. Peers, play and primary prevention in primates. In M.W. Kent and J.E. Rolf (Eds.), *Primary Prevention of Psychopathology. Volume III. Social Competence in Children*. Hanover, NH: University Press of New England, 1979.

Task Panel Report on Prevention. Submitted to the President's Commission on Mental Health, Volume 4, 1978.

Zusman, J., & Lamb, H.R. In defense of community mental health. *American Journal of Psychiatry, 1977, 134*, 887-890.

ABOUT THE CONTRIBUTORS

Barbara C. Bader is Co-Director of the Center for Human Services Research in Ann Arbor, Michigan, and is affiliated with the Community Psychology Program at the University of Michigan. Ms. Bader received masters degrees in psychology and in social work from the University of Michigan and is completing a Ph.D. in community psychology and social work at the university. She has written extensively and conducted research in corrections, mental health, and the law, with recent research activities focusing on consultation, education, and prevention programs in community mental health. She has provided consultation and training to human service systems, focusing on such areas as organizational design, program evaluation, executive development, and patient rights. She serves on numerous boards and task forces in mental health and is currently participating in the writing of guidelines for consultation, education, and prevention in community mental health.

Bonnie E. Carlson, M.S.W., is currently on the faculty of the School of Social Welfare, State University of New York at Albany and is completing a Ph.D. in social work and psychology at the University of Michigan. She has done research on the father-child relationship, dual-career families, and battered women. In addition, she has been extensively involved at the community level in the development of services for families experiencing domestic violence.

Ralph Catalano is Associate Professor of Social Ecology at the University of California at Irvine. Professor Catalano, who holds a Ph.D. in social science from the Maxwell School of Syracuse University, is also Associate Director of the university's Public Policy Research Organization.

Saul Cooper was trained as a Clinical Psychologist at Boston University in the early 1950s. In addition to being the director of a comprehensive mental health center, he is Adjunct Professor of Psychology at the University of Michigan. During the past few years he has served as Chairman of the Region V Evaluation Steering Committee and Chairman of the Michigan Department of Mental Health Prevention Advisory Council. He continues to do consultation around the country with mental health boards and staff on issues related to prevention, consultation, and management.

Liane V. Davis, M.S.W., M.A. is currently on the faculty of the School of Social Welfare, State University of New York at Albany and is completing a Ph.D. in social psychology at the University of North Carolina-Chapel Hill. In addition to her interest in domestic violence, she is engaged in research on decision-making processes and community attitudes toward sex education.

David Dooley is Associate Professor in the Program in Social Ecology at the University of California, Irvine. He received his B.A. in economics from Harvard (1965) and his Ph.D. in psychology from UCLA (1973). His research interests include the relationship of economic change to behavioral disorder and the role and facilitation of nonprofessional mental health agents, including support from naturally occurring social networks. He is a research associate with the Public Policy Research Organization at UCI where he is currently co-principal investigator of an NIMH-sponsored longitudinal survey of economic change, stressful life events, social support, and behavioral symptoms in Los Angeles.

John C Erfurt has a long career in research on health and illness in working populations. His work includes research on the health consequences of rotating shift work, health and work performance of scientific work groups, the relationship of supervisory practices to worker health, and occupational differences in blood pressure. Since 1974 he has co-directed (with Andrea Foote) the Worker Helath Program at the University of Michigan's Institute of Labor & Industrial Relations. This program has concentrated on the development and testing of work-based systems for delivering health services to employed people. Mr. Erfurt, an associate research scientist at the University of Michigan, works closely with the Association of Labor-Management Administrators and Consultants on Alcoholism (ALMACA), and is a consultant to a number of different industries in the greater Detroit area on the establishment and evaluation of occupational programs.

Stephanie S. Farber is a doctoral candidate in clinical/community psychology at Union Graduate School. She received her B.A. from Barnard College and her M.A. in community psychology from the University of New Haven. Currently she is an associate in research and Co-Director of the Families in Transition Project at Yale University. Her research interests include life transitions and interdisciplinary collaborations for the development of social policy for children. She has co-authored several articles and papers in these areas.

Robert D. Felner is Assistant Professor of Psychology at Yale University. He received his B.A. from the University of Connecticut in Psychology and his M.A. and Ph.D. in clinical/community psychology at the University of Rochester. He has published a number of articles on life crisis and transitions and the development of preventive programs for individuals experiencing such events. He is Northeastern Regional Co-Coordinator for the Division of Community Psychology (Div. 27, APA) and Co-Director of the Families in Transition Project at Yale University. His other research activities involve the identification of factors leading to differential vulnerability in "at risk" children and adolescents, and an examination of the structure of transitional care facilities.

Andrea Foote is an associate research scientist at the University of Michigan. She has conducted research on work-related issues since earning her Ph.D. in sociology. She co-directs, with John C Erfurt, the Worker Health Program at the University of Michigan's Institute of Labor & Industrial Relations. This program pioneered the development of systems to improve the adequacy of hypertension control in working populations, and has subsequently expanded to include other types of health problems, including alcoholism and other behavioral/emotional problems. Dr. Foote does extensive consulting with industrial and health care organizations, and has taught courses in the area of the sociology of health care delivery systems.

James Garbarino is currently Associate Professor of Human Development at Pennsylvania State University, after having been a Fellow and Director of the Maltreatment of Youth Project at the Center for the Study of Youth Development at Boys Town. He received his Ph.D. in human development and family studies from Cornell University in 1973. Dr. Garbarino has pursued his study of the human ecology of child maltreatment in a program combining research and intervention, resulting in a series of articles and two books: *Protecting Children from Abuse and*

Neglect and *Understanding Abusive Families.* In 1975 he was named a Spencer Fellow by the National Academy of Education, and in 1979 won a Mitchell Prize from the Woodlands Conference on Growth Policy for his paper, "The Issue is Human Quality: In Praise of Children."

Benjamin H. Gottlieb is Associate Professor in the Department of Psychology at the University of Guelph, Ontario. He holds a joint Ph.D. in social work and psychology from the University of Michigan. His research interests center on the role of social support in moderating stress, the study of informal helping behaviors, and the organization of natural helping networks in neighborhoods. He is currently preparing a book which discusses methods of designing interventions which mobilize social support systems in the community.

Alan Hall is presently a research associate at the Dellcrest Children's Centre in Downsview, Ontario. He received his M.A. in community psychology from the University of Guelph. His major research interests are focused on examining the patterns of social service utilization by low-income populations. He is currently writing a review article which outlines a systems model for integrating the various psychological, sociological, organizational, and economical perspectives prominent in social service utilization research.

Kenneth Heller is Professor of Psychology at Indiana University. A Ph.D. of Pennsylvania State University, he has been Visiting Scholar at the University of Michigan Institute for Social Research, Visiting Professor at the University of California (Irvine), and Special Research Fellow and Visiting Lecturer at the Laboratory of Community Psychiatry at Harvard Medical School. He is an APA Fellow, and from 1974-1978 served on the Board of Consulting Editors of the *Journal of Consulting and Clinical Psychology.* He is a co-author with John Monahan of *Psychology and Community Change* and with A.P. Goldstein and L.B. Sechrest of *Psychotherapy and the Psychology of Behavior Change.* His current research interests are in prevention, social support, coping with stress, and the factors involved in individual, organizational, and community change.

Leonard A. Jason is currently Associate Professor of Psychology at DePaul University. He received his Ph.D. in clinical psychology in 1975 from the University of Rochester. Dr. Jason is on the editorial boards of *Professional Psychology* and the *American Journal of Community Psychology.*

In addition, he is the Co-Regional Coordinator of Division 27 (Community Psychology) of the American Psychological Association and the Co-Coordinator of the Community Research Special Interest Group of the Association for Advancement of Behavior Therapy.

Richard F. Ketterer is Co-Director of the Center for Human Services Research and has served as a lecturer in Social Work and Psychology at the University of Michigan. Dr. Ketterer holds M.S.W. and Ph.D. degrees from the University of Michigan's joint doctoral program in Social Work and Social Science. Dr. Ketterer has also written and consulted extensively in the area of consultation, education, and prevention services.

Marc Levy until recently had been the Director of Consultation, Education and Prevention at the Six Area Coalition Community Mental Health Center in Michigan. He is currently Agency Coordinator for United Neighborhood Centers of Dane County, Wisconsin. Previously he was State Prevention Coordinator for the Oregon Mental Health Division, and has consulted in the health and mental health promotion arena throughout the country. He has authored numerous prevention articles and presented them at national and state conferences.

Michael O. Miller is Court Psychologist with the Livingston County Juvenile Court in Howell, Michigan. He received his M.A. from Michigan State University in 1980. His doctoral dissertation, supervised by Martin Gold, addressed the behavioral and interpersonal effects of penetration into the juvenile justice system. He completed a clinical internship at the Howell-Area Community Mental Health Center, and has consulted and done workshops throughout Michigan on intervention programs with delinquent adolescents and young adult criminal offenders. His professional interests concern the interplay between psychodiagnostics, psychological intervention, and delinquent behavior.

John Monahan is a psychologist and Professor of Law at the University of Virginia. He was previously at the Program in Social Ecology at the University of California, Irvine. He has authored *Psychology and Community Change* (with K. Heller) and *The Clinical Prediction of Violent Behavior.* Monahan's primary interests are in the relationships between the mental health and legal systems. He has testified before Congress and several state legislatures on public policy in this area, and his work has been cited by the U.S. Supreme Court and other judicial bodies. He chaired the American Psychological Association's Task Force on the Role of Psychology in the Criminal Justice System, was a member of the Panel on Legal Issues of the President's Commission on Mental Health and of the Panel on Rehabilitation of the National Academy of Sciences, and is past-president of the American Psychology-Law Society.

Thomas F.A. Plaut received his Ph.D. from the Department of Social Relations and M.P.H., Harvard School of Public Health. He served on the staff of the Harvard School of Public Health Community Mental Health Program (1955-1962), and was Director of the Massachusetts Division of Alcoholism prior to moving to Stanford University (Institute for the Study of Human Problems) in the early 1960s. While at Stanford Dr. Plaut prepared *Alcohol Problems: Report to the Nation from the Cooperative Commission on the Study of Alcoholism.* He joined the National Institute of Mental Health in 1967 and has served there as Assistant Chief, National Center for the Prevention and Control of Alcoholism; Director, Division of Manpower and Training Programs; Associate Director for Program Coordination; Counsellor to the Director; and Deputy Director of the Institute. After five years as Deputy Director, he took his present position as Director, Office of Prevention. He is co-author of *Personality in a Communal Society: The Mental Health of the Hutterites* and author of over forty articles in professional and scientific journals.

Richard H. Price is Professor and Chairman of the Community Psychology Program at the University of Michigan. He received his Ph.D. from the University of Illinois in 1966. He served as Assistant and Associate Professor at Indiana University and Visiting Associate Professor at Stanford University. He is the author and editor of a number of books in the area of mental health and community mental health, including *Abnormal Behavior: Perspectives in Conflict* (1978), *Community Mental Health: Social Action and Reaction,* and *Evaluation and Action in the Social Environment.* He has served on the Editorial Review Board for the *Journal of Abnormal Psychology.* His research interests include primary prevention and coping and adaptation in the social environment. He is currently Director of the Prevention Evaluation Project at the University of Michigan, and is a Fellow of the American Psychological Association.

Judith Primavera is a doctoral candidate in clinical/community psychology at Yale University. She received her B.A. from Mount Holyoke College and her M.A. from Yale University. She is currently a clinical intern at the Yale

Child Study Center. Her research interests include the development of prevention programs in the schools for high-risk children and adolescents and the impact of family disruption on children and their families. Ms. Primavera has co-authored several articles in these areas.

Kenneth J. Sher is a doctoral candidate in clinical psychology at Indiana University. A graduate of Antioch College, he has been an NIMH predoctoral fellow in clinical psychology and currently is an NIAAA predoctoral alcoholism research trainee. His research interests include evaluation of clinical and community interventions, mental health epidemiology, factors in stress and coping, and etiological processes in alcoholism.

Carolyn F. Swift Ph.D., is Director of Prevention Services at the Southwest Community Health Center in Columbus, Ohio, and Research Associate with Warner-Amex Communications Corporation in Columbus. She is a member of the Council on Prevention of the National Council of Community Mental Health Centers, and has been its Chairperson from 1976 to 1980. As a member of the Staff College of the National Institute of Mental Health, she serves as faculty for a series of week-long workshops on the administration of consultation and education services in community mental health centers. At the Second National Conference on Consultation and Education, held in San Francisco in February 1980, she was presented an award for distinguished service to the field of consultation and education.

Betty Tableman, M.P.A., is a graduate of Vassar College and the University of Michigan. She has been with the Michigan Department of Mental Health in various capacities since 1970 and in other state health and planning agencies prior to that time.

Gary R. VandenBos, Ph.D., is Director of National Policy Studies for the American Psychological Association. Before joining APA, he directed the Howell-Area Community Mental Health Center in Michigan, served as consultant to several alternative service programs for adolescents—including the East Lansing Drug Education Center and the Family Effectiveness Training Project—and was senior research coordinator of the Michigan State University Research Project with Schizophrenics. He edited *Psychotherapy and National Health Insurance: A Sourcebook* with Charles Kiesler and Nicholas A. Cummings, and co-authored, with Bertram P. Karon, a text on clinical technique with schizophrenics (forthcoming).